The Art of Writing a Patholog[y]
What we Say ... and What we [Mean]
by Natasha Rekhtman, Diana Molavi, an[d]

What we Say:	What we M[ean:]
This is a difficult case	I have no idea what this is
This lesion is difficult to classify	I am not familiar with the new WHO classification
Dr. X concurs with the diagnosis	Sure am glad somebody else here knows what this thing is
Case was shown at the quality assurance conference	We're all going down together
Invasion cannot be excluded	Probably invasive but don't feel like searching too hard … and it's time for my coffee break!
Lesion is best seen on permanent sections	We missed it on frozen
Stains are suboptimal	Did not work at all
Stains are non-contributory	Stained the wrong block
Stains are non-evaluable	Forgot to order
Tissue with cautery artifact	PLEASE … turn down that bovie!
Tumor approaches the margin	Positive margin but am going to dinner with the surgeon, so gotta be nice…
Tumor approaches the margin (#2)	Positive margin but am afraid of the surgeon
Representative sections submitted	One
Innumerable (as in polyps or mitotic figures)	More than 10
Rare (as in mitoses)	I didn't see any, but if I say zero there will be three on the first field when I show this case
No specific pathologic changes/ Non-diagnostic findings/ Mild chronic cholecystitis (gallbladder) / Chronic inflammation and lymphoid hyperplasia (tonsil)/ Reactive epithelial changes (esophagus)	Completely normal
Specimen did not survive processing	Was dropped on the floor and stepped on
Specimen was entirely submitted	Can't send me back to the bucket!
Possible lymph nodes	Hunks of fat
Recommend clinical correlation	Not my problem anymore!

Chelsea R. Mehr, M.D.
2020 Walnut Street Apt. 17M
Philadelphia, PA 19103-5696
860-214-1143

Quick Reference Handbook
for Surgical Pathologists

Natasha Rekhtman · Justin A. Bishop

Quick Reference Handbook
for Surgical Pathologists

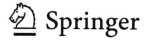 Springer

Natasha Rekhtman, MD, PhD
Assistant Attending
Memorial Sloan-Kettering Cancer Center
Department of Pathology
New York, NY
USA
rekhtman@mskcc.org

Justin A. Bishop, MD
Assistant Professor
The Johns Hopkins Medical Institutions
Department of Pathology
Baltimore, MD
USA
jbishop@jhmi.edu

ISBN 978-3-642-20085-4   e-ISBN 978-3-642-20086-1
DOI 10.1007/978-3-642-20086-1
Springer Heidelberg Dordrecht London New York

Library of Congress Control Number: 2011932990

Cover design: eStudioCalamar, Girona/Berlin

Printed on acid-free paper

Springer is part of Springer Science+Business Media (www.springer.com)

To Bob, Mark, Galina, and Katya.

Natasha Rekhtman

To Ashley, Riley, and Avery.

Justin Bishop

Preface

About this book

This book is a compilation of high-yield at-a-glance summaries for various topics frequently needed in a quick reference format at the microscope (or when cramming for the boards). As recently minted pathologists, we compiled this book from the perspective of pathologists-in-training and we gathered topics which we wanted to have in quick summary format during our recent residency and fellowships. Although written with the trainees in mind, the book may also be of interest to practicing pathologists as a practical quick reference by the microscope.

The book has a unique layout in that most of the information is presented in tables and diagrams accompanied by minimal explanatory text. Our motto for this book was to boil the information down to the essentials and key elements but with just enough commentary to be accessible to a newcomer to pathology. This book is not intended as a substitute for original resources or authoritative texts, but rather its purpose is to bring under one roof compact summaries for various types of information that trainees and practicing pathologists now search for in many different sources, and give the conceptual "lay of the land" with emphasis on "must know" facts. Certainly decisions about what constitutes "must know" and "high-yield" are highly subjective, and we apologize for any omissions which are inevitable by the nature of this book.

Our other main objective was to make the format of the book as user-friendly and easy to navigate as possible, such that one can quickly find the needed information. We thank our Springer editors for agreeing to publish this book in a non-standard format to help achieve this goal.

Contents

The focus is not organ-based morphologic criteria for which there are many excellent quick-summary resources, but rather the focus is everything else that helps a pathologist make a diagnosis (and pass the boards) with emphasis on the vast and fast-growing fields of immunohistochemistry (IHC) and molecular markers.

The book starts with unique introductory "primers" – at-a-glance 1-page summaries with diagrams on the main types of marker applications and high-yield facts (such as peculiar principles of cytokeratin designation). We highlighted the rules and biological principles behind various immunostains and special stains to help residents reason through a problem rather than having to resort to memorized panels. The other part of the IHC section contains a large compilation of general and organ-based applications of IHC with numerous immunopanels. This includes the classics (such as lung adenocarcinoma versus mesothelioma) and more recent applications (such as the work-up for mismatch repair proteins).

Other sections of the book contain various quick references that are often needed at the microscope but require frequent reminders. This includes a compilation of grading systems, common prognostic systems, and other criteria that are difficult to keep committed to memory (such as size cut-points for various micro-entities like thyroid papillary microcarcinoma). Also included are summaries for tumor syndromes with a particularly practical "slide-to-syndrome" summary where we highlighted which diagnoses or features should trigger consideration of a syndrome. In tumor genetics and cytogenetics we highlighted which tumors have unique molecular characteristics that can aid in the diagnosis or are used in prognostic/predictive testing.

Another high-yield section that is not usually covered in most pathology books is a compilation of quick clinical references geared for pathologists. This section contains resources that help pathologists interpret clinical information that may be highly informative in the differential diagnosis of tumors, including a primer on metastasis (what metastatic patterns are classic vs. exceptional for certain tumors) and serologic tumor markers. We also included a brief summary of targeted therapies for which pathologists may be asked to perform predictive marker testing.

Even though the focus of the book is not organ-based morphologic criteria, we included several sections with differentials that cut across all organs. For example, this section includes at-a-glance differentials for small round blue cell tumors, and classic differentials for certain morphologic features (such as which tumors are classically associated with granulomas or have staghorn vessels). We also included an illustrated guide to microorganisms. Finally, we compiled an illustrated glossary of histopathologic descriptors with illustrations of common objects these terms are said to resemble (such as storiform or palisaded, and what Orphan Annie's eyes actually look like!). Keep this by your side as you begin to tackle the large pathology books! We are also very excited to include a handy guide for pathology web resources by Terina Chen and a user-friendly CPT coding summary by Diana Molavi.

Sources

We used a variety of sources, including standard books and mountains of primary literature. However, most importantly our "world view" of pathology this early in our careers comes primarily from our outstanding teachers at The Johns Hopkins Hospital and Memorial Sloan-Kettering Cancer Center. From them we learned the approaches and principles that come only after years of experience but cannot be learned by reading books and papers. We were fortunate to learn pathology from these brilliant diagnosticians and generous educators, who shared their knowledge with us through sign outs, lectures and weekly unknowns during our residency at Johns Hopkins. We therefore can only take credit for organizing and presenting this stream of knowledge in a format easily accessible to a newcomer to pathology, and we give all credit for the many useful pearls and principles in this book to our teachers. On the other hand, we take full responsibility for any inaccuracies that may have inadvertently escaped our attention.

In conclusion

It is our hope that this book will be your best friend both at the microscope and in the late night hours of studying for the boards. Because the type of information covered in this book is rapidly evolving, please be sure to check the most current sources.

Natasha Rekhtman and Justin Bishop

How this book came about – part 1

I started working on this book in my second year of residency at The Johns Hopkins Hospital, although at that time I did not yet know that this was what I was doing. Like many pathologists, I am a very visual learner, and I firmly believe that a good table or diagram is worth many pages of text. Therefore I was desperately looking for resources that succinctly summarized the mountains of information I was trying to absorb, particularly in a format that was tabular or diagrammatic and was amenable to quick learning of the essentials. While there were many great resources for histologic criteria, what I felt was missing were quick references for the new and fast growing fields of immunostains and molecular markers, as well as other types of material frequently needed in pathologists' daily work but not available in a single source. I therefore started compiling these summaries and diagrams for my own use, and later started sharing them with my co-residents. After getting feedback that others were findings these summaries useful, and after I realized that creating them was an incredible motivator to learn and digest the information, I put together a small handbook which was generously printed by the Department of Pathology at Johns Hopkins as a Resident Manual in 2004 and 2007. Now in collaboration with Justin Bishop as my coeditor and main coauthor and with contributions from many former and current Hopkins residents and fellows and my current colleagues at Memorial Sloan-Kettering Cancer Center, this book has morphed into what it is today. Justin joined forces with me in the last two years, and I could not have dreamt of a more dedicated and talented collaborator, who made it possible to get this project completed.

Natasha Rekhtman

How this book came about – part 2

My first interaction with this book (universally known as the "Green Book" at Hopkins) was in 2006. The more senior residents had copies of a magical book that had all the answers I was seeking as a pathology intern. Desperate for something to boil down the massive amounts of information into one resource, my fellow first-year residents and I assembled crude bootleg copies of it. At the end of that year as she left Hopkins, Natasha distributed a new edition which remains a fixture at my microscope to this day. However, as the years passed and new waves of residents entered our program, original copies of the Green Book became increasingly scarce, and the quality of copies became increasingly poor as they became 2nd and 3rd generation. My chief resident year, I was frequently confronted with a question from the junior residents: "Where can I get a copy of that Green Book?" We had heard rumors about the possibility of it being published, but no one at Hopkins knew the status of the now-mythical Green Book. Intent on getting an answer, I contacted Natasha. As luck would have it, she needed a collaborator to push the project past the finish line, and that collaborator became me. Initially a great way to study for my boards, working on the book then became a means to stay on top of the newest information as I started signing out surgical pathology. Although perhaps it was a bigger commitment than I initially realized, it was well worth the effort, and I am extremely grateful to Natasha for allowing me to be a part of this very special project.

Justin Bishop

Acknowledgements

We were fortunate to learn pathology as residents and assistants in surgical pathology from the brilliant diagnosticians and dedicated educators of The Johns Hopkins surgical pathology team and other divisions. We are most grateful to all our teachers for sharing with us their knowledge and wisdom that serves as the foundation of this book.

We would like to sincerely thank all coauthors and reviewers for contributing their brainpower to this project with special thanks to Ashlie Burkart, Terina Chen, Amy Duffield, Diana Molavi and Janis Taube for lead-authoring various sections of this book. Very special thanks to Ashlie Burkart, Shien Michelli and Diana Molavi for reviewing various portions of this book, and penciling in multiple suggestions and question marks (as well as smiley faces...) and for being the constant source of encouragement over the years. We are most grateful to all Hopkins faculty and trainees for making suggestions/corrections and enthusiastic support over the years. This book would not be what it is today if it had not been vetted by several generations of keen Hopkins residents. We also want to thank our publishing team Gabriele Schroeder, Sandra Lesny, and Ellen Blasig at Springer and Patrick Waltemate at le-tex for all their efforts on behalf of this book.

Natasha also thanks her colleagues at Memorial Sloan-Kettering Cancer Center for their support and for generously sharing their knowledge and expertise.

Natasha Rekhtman and Justin Bishop

Editors and Main Authors:

Justin A. Bishop, MD
Assistant Professor
Department of Pathology
Surgical Pathology
The Johns Hopkins Medical Institutions
Baltimore, MD

Natasha Rekhtman, MD, PhD
Assistant Attending
Department of Pathology
Memorial Sloan-Kettering Cancer Center
New York, NY

Coauthors and Contributors:

Jennifer Broussard, MD
Franklin Square Hospital Center
Baltimore, MD

Ashlie L. Burkart, MD, CM
Assistant Professor
Department of Pathology, Anatomy and Cell Biology
Jefferson Medical College of Thomas Jefferson University
Philadelphia, PA

Terina S. Chen, MD
Good Samaritan Hospital of Maryland
Baltimore, MD

Amy S. Duffield, MD, PhD
Assistant Professor
Department of Pathology
Hematopathology Division
The Johns Hopkins Medical Institutions
Baltimore, MD

Tara Nikole Miller, MD
Pathology Resident and Clinical Instructor
Sanford School of Medicine of the University of South Dakota
Sioux Falls, SD

Ross Allen Miller, MD
Pathology Resident and Clinical Instructor
Sanford School of Medicine of the University of South Dakota
Sioux Falls, SD

Diana Weedman Molavi, MD, PhD
Sinai Hospital of Baltimore
Baltimore, MD

Janis M. Taube, MD
Assistant Professor
Departments of Dermatology and Pathology
The Johns Hopkins Medical Institutions
Baltimore, MD

Kathryn Villa, MD
Assistant Faculty in Surgical Pathology
Department of Pathology
The Johns Hopkins Medical Institutions
Baltimore, MD

Reviewers:

Meera Hameed, MD
Attending Pathologist
Memorial Sloan-Kettering Cancer Center, New York, NY
Professor of Pathology and Laboratory Medicine
Weil-Cornell Medical College
New York, NY

Jason T. Huse, MD, PhD
Assistant Attending
Department of Pathology
Memorial Sloan-Kettering Cancer Center
New York, NY

Peter B. Illei, MD
Assistant Professor
Director, Immunopathology laboratory
Department of Pathology
The Johns Hopkins Medical Institutions
Baltimore, MD

Anna Yemelyanova, MD
Assistant Professor
Department of Pathology
Gynecologic Surgical Pathology Division
The Johns Hopkins Medical Institutions
Baltimore, MD

Illustrator (for lymph node diagram in chapter 2 and non-microscopy objects in chapter 12)

Terry Helms
Medical Illustrator
Department of Media Services
Memorial Sloan-Kettering Cancer Center
New York, NY

Table of Contents – At a Glance

Detailed Table of Contents

Unless otherwise specified, subsection authors are Justin Bishop and Natasha Rekhtman.

Abbreviations, Acronyms, and Designations

**See IHC index for alternative designations of antibodies/antigens

AFIP – Armed Forces Institute of Pathology
AJCC – American Joint Committee on Cancer
ALL – acute lymphoblastic leukemia/lymphoma
AML – acute myeloid leukemia
BAC – bronchioloalveolar carcinoma
Bx – biopsy
CA – carcinoma
CD – cluster of differentiation (as in CD3, CD20, etc.)
CHR – chromogranin
CIS – carcinoma in situ
CK – cytokeratin(s)
CLL/SLL – chronic lymphocytic leukemia/small lymphocytic
    lymphoma
CMV – cytomegalovirus
CNS – central nervous system
CRC – colorectal carcinoma
CT – computed tomography
Derm – dermatopathology
DNA – deoxyribonucleic acid
DDx – differential diagnosis
DLBCL – diffuse large B cell lymphoma
Dx – diagnosis
EBV – Epstein-Barr virus
EM – electron microscopy
ER – estrogen receptor
FL – follicular lymphoma
GI – gastrointestinal
GIST – gastrointestinal stromal tumor
GU – genitourinary
GYN – gynecologic
HCC – hepatocellular carcinoma
H&E – hematoxylin and eosin
H&N – head and neck
Heme – hematopathology
HHV8 – Human Herpesvirus 8
HMWCK – high molecular weight cytokeratins
HPF – high-power field (40X)
HPC – hemangiopericytoma
HPV – human papillomavirus
HSV – herpes simplex virus

HTLV – Human T-lymphotropic virus
ID – identification or identify
IHC – immunohistochemistry
IPMN – intraductal papillary mucinous neoplasm
ISH – in situ hybridization
JHH – Johns Hopkins Hospital
LMWCK – low molecular weight cytokeratins
LN – lymph node
MCL – mantle cell lymphoma
MCN – mucinous cystic neoplasm
MD – moderately differentiated
ME – myoepithelial
MEC – myoepithelial cells
Met – metastasis
MPNST – malignant peripheral nerve sheath tumor
MSKCC – Memorial Sloan-Kettering Cancer Center
MZL – marginal zone lymphoma
NE – neuroendocrine
NK – natural killer
NLPHL – nodular lymphocyte predominant Hodgkin Lymphoma
NOS – not otherwise specified
PCR – polymerase chain reaction
PD – poorly differentiated
PEComa – perivascular epithelioid cell tumor
PET – positron emission tomography
PNET – primitive neuroectodermal tumor
PR – progesterone receptor
PTC – papillary thyroid carcinoma
RBC – red blood cell
RCC – renal cell carcinoma
R-S cell – Reed Sternberg cell
Rx – therapy, treatment
SmCC – small cell carcinoma
SqCC – squamous cell carcinoma
SRBCT – small round blue cell tumor
SYN – synaptophysin
TB – tuberculosis
vs. – versus
WD – well differentiated
WHO – World Health Organization

Immunohistochemistry reactivity code

+++	Overexpressed or consistently diffuse
+	Positive
+/–	Usually positive
–/+	Usually negative
–	Negative

Chapter 1 Immunostains: Introduction
by Natasha Rekhtman and Justin Bishop

Applications of Immunohistochemistry (IHC) in Anatomic Pathology
(select examples)

1. **DIAGNOSIS OF TUMORS:**
   a. **Classification of poorly differentiated neoplasms:**
      carcinoma (cytokeratin+) vs.
      lymphoma (CD45+) vs.
      melanoma (S100+, Melan-A+, HMB45+)
   b. **Diagnosis of carcinoma of unknown primary:**
      colon (CDX2+) vs.
      lung (TTF-1+) vs.
      prostate (PSA+)
   c. **Diagnosis of invasion:**
      loss of myoepithelial cells (breast cancer)
      loss of basal cells (prostate cancer)
      loss of basement membrane/collagen type IV (various carcinomas, rarely used)

2. **ASSESSMENT OF MARKERS REFLECTING PROGNOSIS ("PROGNOSTIC" MARKERS"):**
   Ki67/MIB1 (general proliferation marker)
   p53 (general marker of apoptosis)[1]
   HER2 (adverse prognosis in breast cancer)
   CD38 (adverse prognosis in chronic lymphocytic leukemia)

3. **ASSESSMENT OF MARKERS REFLECTING A THERAPEUTIC RESPONSE ("PREDICTIVE" OR "THERANOSTIC" MARKERS):**
   ER/PR (Tamoxifen for breast cancer)
   HER2 (Herceptin for breast cancer)
   c-kit (Gleevec for GIST, CML, other; mutations more predictive than IHC)

4. **DETECTION OF MICROMETASTASES:**
   melanoma (melanocytic markers)
   breast cancer (cytokeratins)

5. **IDENTIFICATION OF INFECTIOUS ORGANISMS[2]:**
   viruses (HSV, CMV)
   other organisms (Toxoplasma, Pneumocystis)

1. It may appear counterintuitive that p53, a well-known tumor-suppressor, is overexpressed in various tumors. This occurs because inactivating mutations in *p53* also disable protein degradation and lead to a robust p53 overexpression. In essence, robust overexpression of p53 is used as a surrogate marker for *p53* gene mutation.
2. Currently IHC is not widely used to identify bacteria and fungi (this is likely to change). These organisms are primarily evaluated by special stains (such as GMS), and some viruses may be identified by in situ hybridization (EBV, HPV).

N. Rekhtman, J.A. Bishop, *Quick Reference Handbook for Surgical Pathologists*,
DOI:10.1007/978-3-642-20086-1_1, © Springer-Verlag Berlin Heidelberg 2011

Markers of Differentiation at a Glance

Differentiation	Markers
Mesenchymal	Vimentin
Epithelial	Cytokeratins, EMA *[see "epithelial primer"]*
Smooth muscle	Desmin, muscle-specific actin, smooth muscle actin, Calponin, h-Caldesmon, smooth muscle myosin heavy chain *[see "muscle primer"]*
Skeletal muscle	Desmin, muscle-specific actin, myogenin, MyoD *[see "muscle primer"]*
Myofibroblastic	Partial smooth muscle phenotype: actins (MSA, SMA) in "tram-track" distribution, calponin, but not h-caldesmon *[see "muscle primer"]*
Myoepithelial	Polyphenotypic markers: smooth muscle (complete phenotype – smooth muscle actin, calponin, other), neural (S100), glial (GFAP), epithelial (CK), and basal/stem cell factor (p63) *[see "muscle primer"]*
Endothelial	CD34, CD31, Factor VIII, *Ulex europaeus I,* CD141, Fli-1, D2-40 *[see "vascular primer"]*
Lipomatous	S100 (immunos generally not used)
Melanocytic	S100, HMB45, Melan-A/MART-1, MITF, Tyrosinase *[see "melanocytic primer"]*
Neuroendocrine	SYN, CHR, NSE, CD56, CD57 *[see "neuroendocrine primer"]*
Glial	GFAP *[see "neuroglial primer"]*
Neuronal	Neurofilament, NeuN, SYN, CHR *[see "neuroglial primer"]*
Nerve Sheath (Schwannian)	S100 *[see "neuroglial primer"]*
Serous Acinar Cells	PAS (general), Trypsin, Chymotrypsin, and Lipase (pancreas)
Hematopoietic	CD45/LCA (pan-hematopoietic), CD3 (pan-T cell), CD20, CD79a, PAX5 (pan-B cell), CD138 & κ/λ light chains (plasma cell) *[see hemepath section]*
Histiocytic	CD68, CD163, HAM56, MAC 387, enzymes (Lysozyme/Muramidase, α1-antitrypsin) *[see hemepath section]*

Location, Location, Location!
Primer on Location of Antigens.

- In order to properly interpret immunoreactivity, it is important to know the expected location of the antigen of interest. Knowing the biological function of a molecule of interest can be very helpful in intuitively anticipating the site of reactivity.

- Transcription factors (TTF-1, CDX2, Myogenin, PAX2, WT1, p53, p63) and steroid hormone receptors (ER, PR) function in the nucleus, and therefore the expected IHC signal is **nuclear**. Ki67, a molecule with still unelucidated function, is also nuclear (except for peculiar membranous/cytoplasmic reactivity in hyalinizing trabecular adenoma of thyroid).

- In contrast, cytoskeletal, contractile, and other functional proteins are **cytoplasmic**. In fact, the majority of antigens in current use are cytoplasmic. This category includes all intermediate filaments (CK, Desmin, Vimentin, GFAP, Neurofilament), contractile proteins (Actin), melanosome-associated proteins (HMB45, Melan-A), secretory products (ACTH, Trypsin), and various other functional molecules.

- **Membranous** reactivity is expected for receptors (EGFR), adhesion molecules (E-Cadherin) and other surface molecules. This category includes virtually all CD (cluster of differentiation) antigens, such as CD3 (T cell marker) and CD20 (B cell marker). Occasionally, membranous reactivity may be difficult to distinguish from cytoplasmic signal; this distinction is important for several molecules where only membranous but not cytoplasmic reactivity counts as specific (HER2, EGFR).

- Although rare, several antigens have a characteristic **combined nuclear AND cytoplasmic** reactivity. This category most notably includes S100 and Calretinin. β-catenin is cytoplasmic in most cell types. However, it is a shift to nuclear reactivity that is a specific feature of several tumor types associated with mutations in adenomatosis polyposis coli /β-catenin pathway, such as deep fibromatosis and colon cancer.

- **Granular** reactivity usually indicates localization to cytoplasmic organelles (mitochondria, Golgi, secretory vesicles, etc). Distinctive granular cytoplasmic reactivity is typical of Racemase (mitochondrial/peroxisomal), Prostein/P501S (Golgi), and Napsin A (lysosomal). Dot-like CD30 in ALCL and classical HL, and CD15 in classical HL are attributed to Golgi staining, and are seen in conjunction with typical membranous staining generating the so-called "targetoid" or "ball and chain" appearance.

- Finally, **"punctate"** (aka peri-nuclear dot-like) reactivity is typical of some antigens that aggregate in the cytoplasm, most notably CK pattern in neuroendocrine carcinomas, including small cell carcinoma (pan-CK) and Merkel cell carcinoma (CK20). This occurs due to formation of CK tangles.

- Note that there are some instances in which the **lack of immunoreactivity** is what is significant. One example is the loss of DPC4, a protein deleted in 55% of pancreatic carcinomas, which supports the diagnosis of a pancreatic primary. Other examples are the loss of E-cadherin in lobular carcinoma of the breast and loss of INI1 in rhabdoid tumors and AT/RT.

- Beware of classic **false-positives** (tissue edge-effect, non-specific staining of hepatocytes due to high albumin content), and classic **false negative** as a result of failed IHC (always check controls, particularly normal structures serving as internal positive controls). Also beware of non-specific cytoplasmic reactivity for antigens with expected nuclear localization (such as TTF-1 or ER) – this should not be accepted as a specific signal!

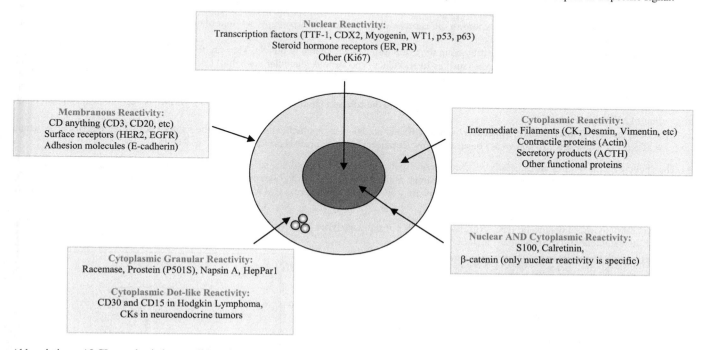

Abbreviations: ALCL anaplastic large cell lymphoma, HL Hodgkin lymphoma, CK cytokeratins

Primer on Cytokeratins

- Cytokeratins (CK) are cytoskeletal proteins that belong to a family of intermediate filaments (IFs). CKs are present in epithelial cells and are regarded as the most fundamental markers of epithelial differentiation. Other members of IF family are also used as markers of differentiation, including Vimentin (for mesenchyme), GFAP (for glia), Desmin (for muscle) and Neurofilament (for neurons).

- There are 20 distinct types of CKs (plus hair and nail-specific CKs).

- CKs were characterized by Moll et al. and the currently used CK designation system is known as the "Moll's catalogue." [1]

- CKs are designated in a somewhat non-intuitive fashion based their migration pattern in a two-dimensional (2D) gel electrophoresis, which separates proteins based on size and charge.

- Based on the 2D gel migration, CKs fall into two categories: basic (CK1 through 8) and acidic (CK9 through 20). Within each group, CKs are numbered in order of decreasing size, from high molecular weight (HMW) to low molecular weight (LMW), as diagramed below.

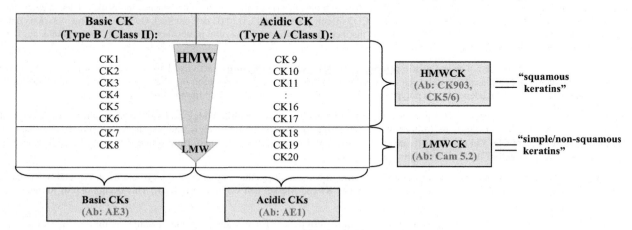

- In a cell, CKs exist as heterodimers, composed of acidic + basic subunits of a similar size. Therefore certain pairs of CKs (such as CK8/18, CK1/10) are expressed jointly.

- For diagnostic purposes, CKs are divided as LMWCK and HMWCK, as indicated on the diagram. This division corresponds to a distinctive distribution of these two groups of CKs in normal tissues:
  - **HMWCK**s are expressed predominantly in squamous epithelia (and in basal cells), and they are known as "**squamous keratins**". HMWCKs are large, and they are able to form a dense cytoplasmic network of filaments, accounting for resistance to mechanical stress of the surface epithelia. Large bundles of HMWCKs are known ultrastructurally (by electron microscopy) as "tonofilaments", and these structures are the hallmark of squamous epithelia and SqCC.
  - In contrast, **LMWCK**s are loosely distributed in the cytoplasm and are unable to bundle. They are therefore characteristic of visceral organs, which experience little mechanical stress (such as liver, kidney, and various glandular epithelia). LMWCK are known as "**non-squamous or simple keratins**". LMWCK are expressed in all epithelial tissues with the exception of keratinizing squamous epithelium. Note that some glandular epithelia (such as breast) do co-express HMWCK in addition to LMWCK, and HMWCK can be induced in non-squamous epithelia as a result of reactive conditions (such as inflammation). So the rule of thumb "squamous epithelium=HMWCK" vs. "non-squamous epithelium=LMWCK" is not 100%.
  - A designation of "**intermediate molecular weight CKs**" is occasionally applied, which refers to the lighter CKs within the HMWCK group (CK 5,6,17). These are also known as "**basal keratins**" because they are expressed preferentially in basal cells.

- The above patterns of CKs are generally retained in corresponding carcinomas, and can serve as useful diagnostic tools. As a word of caution – some carcinomas deviate from CK patterns of their parent epithelia. For example, high-grade SqCC frequently co-expression LMWCKs in addition to HMWCKs. In addition, some adenocarcinomas are well-known to co-express HMWCKs (such as carcinomas of pancreas, endometrium, and subset of breast).

- To increase the yield of diagnostic IHC, expression of CKs is usually analyzed by mixtures of various CK antibodies (Abs), known as "**Ab cocktails**". The commonly used Ab cocktails include:

Antibody Cocktail	What it detects
AE1	All **acidic** CKs except CK 9, 12, 17, 18
AE3	All **basic** CKs (CK1–8)
AE1/AE3 (pan-CK)	All types of CKs
OSCAR, PANK (MNF-116)	Broad-spectrum CK cocktail (similar to AE1/AE3)
Cam 5.2 (34βH11)	**LMWCK**s (CK 8, 18)
CK903 (K903; 34βE12)	**HMWCK**s (CK 1, 5, 10, 14)
CK5/6	**HMWCK**s (detects primarily CK5)

SUMMARY				
Epithelium Type	*Corresponding Carcinoma*	*CK profile*	*Antibody Reactivity*	
Squamous & basal cells	**Squamous cell carcinoma**	HMWCK[1]	**CK903** **CK5/6**	**Pan-CK** **(AE1/AE3)**
Glandular epithelia (bowel, prostate, etc) & **visceral parenchyma** (liver, kidney, etc)	Colon adenocarcinoma Prostate adenocarcinoma Hepatocellular carcinoma Renal cell carcinoma Etc	LMWCK[2]	**Cam5.2**	

1) HMWCKs (without LMWCKs) are expressed in keratinizing squamous epithelia, and in the majority of SqCC. However, some poorly differentiated non-keratinizing SqCC (particularly of mucosal surfaces and visceral organs, such as lung) do co-express LMWCKs.

2) Similarly, while majority of adenocarcinomas and carcinomas of visceral epithelia express LMWCKs only (e.g. prostate, HCC, RCC), some adenocarcinomas are well known to co-express HMWCK (e.g. pancreas, endometrium, breast). Urothelial carcinoma also co-express LMW and HMW CKs.

- **Practical applications:** The most common application of CKs is to identify a poorly differentiated malignancy as a carcinoma. In practical terms, expression of CKs (and to a lesser degree EMA) is what defines a poorly differentiated neoplasm as a carcinoma as opposed to sarcoma, lymphoma, melanoma, or glioma. For this "screening" purpose, CK antibodies are used as follows:
  - **AE1/AE3** (or another favorite pan-CK) is a good first-line marker: it recognizes both LMW and HMW CKs, and will identify virtually all types of carcinoma, squamous and non-squamous alike. The main caveat is that there are few carcinomas, most notably hepatocellular carcinoma (see table below for complete list), which are not recognized by AE1/AE3. This is because hepatocytes express CK18, which is omitted in AE1/AE3.
  - **Cam5.2** it a good complement to AE1/AE3. It does cover CK18 and will recognize those few carcinomas that are missed by AE1/AE3. The main drawback of Cam5.2 as a screening Ab is that it may not recognize SqCC (recall that squamous epithelium has HMW but not LMW CKs!). In this sense, AE1/AE3 and Cam5.2 are complimentary for screening purposes.
  - Note that **HMWCKs** have a more restricted expression profile than LMWCKs, particularly in the visceral organs where non-squamous carcinomas predominate. Therefore HMWCK antibodies (such as CK903) are generally not used for screening purposes, but are reserved for a number of specific differentials (see table below).
  - Examples of utilization of LMW vs. HMW CKs in DDx of carcinomas are:
    o DDx of prostate carcinoma (HMWCK−) vs. urothelial carcinoma (HMWCK+).
    o DDx of Paget's disease (Cam5.2+, CK903−) vs. SqCC in situ/Bowen's disease (Cam5.2−, CK903+).
  - Of particular diagnostic utility are CK7 and CK20, which have a striking organ-specific distribution. These are the workhorse Abs in the work-up of carcinomas of unknown primary (see table below).

- Other markers of epithelial differentiation include EMA, CEA, and p63 (although p63 may also be expressed by some non-epithelial neoplasms, such as lymphomas). One can broadly think of EMA and CEA as "LMWCK-equivalents" (markers of glandular epithelia) and p63 as "HMWCK"-equivalent (marker of squamous/urothelial epithelia and basal cells).

- Although expression of CKs (and EMA) is held as a defining feature of carcinomas, beware of epithelial marker reactivity in some **non-carcinomas**, including:
  1. tumors with **true epithelial differentiation** (intercellular junctions and keratin filaments by EM), yet not "classic carcinomas" (tumors of surface or glandular epithelia). This category includes several sarcomas (synovial sarcoma, epithelioid sarcoma, epithelioid angiosarcoma), non-seminoma germ cell tumors (yolk sac tumor, embryonal carcinoma), trophoblastic tumors, mesothelioma, chordoma, and thymoma. Reactivity for CK (and EMA) is usually strong.
  2. high-grade malignant neoplasms with **aberrant expression** of epithelial markers. This most notably includes leiomyosarcoma, melanoma, and MPNST. Reactivity is usually focal and seen mainly with Cam5.2.
  3. gliomas and reactive astrocytes. Beware of cross-reactivity with AE1/AE3 (Cam5.2 and EMA should be negative!).

Select References: [1–7]

Immunostains. Introduction

Epithelial Markers at a Glance		
Antibody	*Background*	*Applications*
AE1/AE3	AE1/AE3 is a **broad-spectrum CK** antibody (Ab) cocktail, which reacts with both LMWCK and HMWCK. It identifies virtually all types of epithelial neoplasms.	AE1/AE3 is the first-line epithelial marker in screening for carcinomas. Although AE1/AE3 reacts with virtually all epithelial neoplasms, there are few notable exceptions: • **Hepatocellular carcinoma** (HCC) is AE1/AE3– (Cam5.2+; CK903–, EMA–). • **Renal cell carcinoma** (RCC) is variably reactive with both AE1/AE3 and Cam5.2 (EMA is best). • **NE carcinomas**, including small cell carcinoma, show variable reactivity with both AE1/AE3 and Cam5.2 (Cam5.2 is best). • **Adrenocortical neoplasms** frequently do not react with AE1/AE3 or any other epithelial markers (Cam5.2, EMA).
Cam5.2 (34βH11)	Cam 5.2 is a **LMWCK** Ab cocktail. It reacts with virtually all non-squamous epithelia; squamous cells are usually (but not always) negative for LMWCK.	• Cam 5.2 is used in conjunction with AE1/AE3 to screen for carcinomas. In particular, Cam5.2 is useful for identification of carcinomas which may be missed by AE1/3 (see above).Cam 5.2 is also used for DDx of Paget's disease (Cam5.2+, CK903–) from Bowen's disease (Cam5.2–, CK903+)
CK903 (34βE12)	CK903 (aka K903) is a **HMWCK** Ab cocktail. It reacts with squamous, urothelial and few glandular epithelia. It also recognizes basal and myoepithelial cells.	Because of a more restricted distribution of HMWCKs, CK903 and CK5/6 are not generally used as screening Abs. Instead, they have several specific applications: • DDx of urothelial carcinoma (CK903+) vs. prostate cancer (CK903–) • DDx of mesothelioma (CK5/6+) vs. adenocarcinoma (CK5/6–) • ID of basal cells in prostatic lesions (CK903+): present in benign glands vs. absent in invasive cancer • ID of metaplastic breast cancer (CK903+) DDx of usual duct hyperplasia (CK903+ epithelial cells) vs. DCIS (CK903–)
CK5/6	CK5/6 is another **HMWCK** Ab. Reactivity is generally similar to CK903. Selection of CK903 versus CK5/6 for a particular application is usually empirically based.	
CK7 & CK20	CK7 and CK20 are LMWCKs, which show distinctive patterns of expression in various organs (see below).	CK7 and CK20 profiles are used to identify the origin of carcinoma of unknown primary: • **CK7+**: above-the-diaphragm organs (lung, breast, thyroid) and female Gyn tract (uterus, ovary) • **CK20+**: below-the-diaphragm organs (colorectum) and Merkel cell carcinoma • **CK7+, CK20+**: peri-diaphragmatic GI organs (pancreas, biliary tree, stomach) and urothelium • **CK7 & 20-negative**: simple visceral epithelia (except colon): liver, kidney, prostate and neuroendocrine cells
EMA (MUC1)	EMA is present in the majority of non-squamous carcinomas (see below for exceptions). Strongest expression is in carcinomas derived from secretory epithelia (eccrine, breast, pancreas). EMA is also present in several non-epithelial tissues and neoplasms (listed below). EMA is less sensitive and less specific for epithelial differentiation than CKs.	EMA is used in conjunction with CKs as a "CK-helper" to ID carcinomas. In particular, it is helpful in identifying renal cell carcinoma, which is EMA+ but is variably reactive for CKs. Other uses include: • DDx of renal cell carcinoma (EMA+) vs. adrenocortical neoplasms (EMA–) • ID of meningioma and few other EMA+ non-epithelial neoplasms (see table below)
CEA	CEA is expressed in some but not all carcinomas (see table below).	If positive, CEA confirms the diagnosis of carcinoma (as opposed to lymphoma, sarcoma, melanoma). However, negative CEA does not rule out a carcinoma since only a fraction of carcinomas are reactive.
Ber-EP4	Ber-EP4 reacts with majority of adenocarciomas of various sites.	Ber-EP4 is primarily used to differentiate lung adenocarcinoma (Ber-EP4+) from mesothelioma (Ber-EP4–). Favored marker in effusion cytology because it selectively labels adenocarcinoma, whereas background mesothelial cells are negative (CK would label both).

The main application of epithelial markers is to differentiate epithelial neoplasms (carcinomas) from non-epithelial neoplasms (lymphoma, melanoma, sarcoma, glioma). AE1/AE3, Cam5.2 and EMA are the first-line screening antibodies for this purpose. Note that in addition to carcinomas, epithelial marker reactivity may be seen in some non-epithelial neoplasms (e.g. synovial sarcoma); see above for details.

CK7 and CK20 Expression Profiles Diagram

CK7+ CK20–	CK7– CK20+
Above-the-diaphragm organs (lung, breast, thyroid, salivary gland) and **female GYN tract** (uterus, ovary) 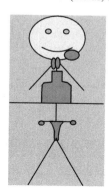	**Below-the-diaphragm** GI tract (colorectum) and Merkel cell carcinoma 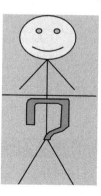
CK7+ CK20+	CK7– CK20–
Peri-diaphragmatic GI organs (pancreas, biliary tree, stomach) and **bladder** 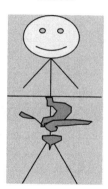	**Simple visceral** epithelia (except colon): liver, kidney, prostate 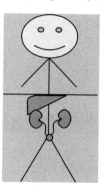

Abbreviations: CK cytokeratin, GI gastrointestinal, GYN gynecologic

CK7 and CK20 Expression Profiles

Predominant CK7/CK20 Profiles			
CK7+ **CK20+**	**CK7+** **CK20−**	**CK7−** **CK20+**	**CK7−** **CK20−**
Pancreaticobiliary Ovary (mucinous carcinoma) Stomach Bladder	Breast Ovary (non-mucinous) Endometrium Lung Mesothelioma Thyroid Salivary gland Kidney (papillary RCC)	Colorectum Merkel cell carcinoma	Liver (hepatocellular carcinoma) Kidney (clear cell RCC) Prostate Adrenal cortex

	CK7+ CK20+ (% positive)	CK7+ CK20− (% positive)	CK7− CK20+ (% positive)	CK7− CK20− (% positive)
Adenocarcinoma				
Breast, ductal	10	86	2	2
Breast, lobular	6	94	0	0
Cholangiocarcinoma	65	28	5	2
Colorectum[1]	8	0	82	10
Uterus	9	86	0	6
Lung	10	90	0	0
Ovary	2	98	0	0
Pancreas	64	28	5	3
Prostate	3	3	10	84
Salivary gland	0	100	0	0
Stomach	32	19	35	14
Thyroid	0	98	0	2
Squamous Cell Carcinoma				
Cervix	0	87	0	13
Esophagus	0	21	0	79
Head & neck	0	27	6	67
Lung	0	26	4	70
Neuroendocrine Neoplasms				
GI tract, carcinoid tumor	0	13	7	80
Lung, carcinoid tumor	0	22	0	78
Lung, liver and small bowel, neuroendocrine carcinoma	0	56	0	44
Lung, small cell carcinoma	0	24	0	76
Merkel cell carcinoma	0	0	78	12
Thyroid, medullary carcinoma	0	98	0	2
Other				
Adrenocortical tumor	0	0	0	100
Epithelioid sarcoma	0	0	0	100
Germ cell tumors	0	7	0	93
Hepatocellular carcinoma	5	15	2	78
Mesothelioma	0	67	0	33
Renal cell carcinoma	0	17	3	80
Thymoma	0	0	0	100
Urothelial (transitional cell) carcinoma	65	37	3	10

In contrast to the colon, rectal adenocarcinomas are frequently (~70%) CK7-positive. [8]

Reference: [3]

Expression of EMA, CEA and Vimentin in Carcinomas

1. EMA is present in conjunction with cytokeratins (CKs) in the majority of carcinomas and CK-positive non-epithelial tumors (e.g. epithelioid sarcoma, synovial sarcoma, desmoplastic small round cell tumor). The tumors that show a discordant expression of CKs and EMA are listed below:

CK+ / EMA–	CK– / EMA+
HCC (Cam5.2+, AE1/AE3–, CK903–)	Meningioma
Adrenocortical neoplasms (frequently negative for all CKs)	Perineurioma
Most neuroendocrine neoplasms	Plasma cell neoplasms
Embryonal carcinoma, yolk sac tumor	Anaplastic large cell lymphoma
Thyroid	Popcorn or lymphocyte predominant (LP) cells [formerly L&H cells] in Hodgkin lymphoma
	RCC (sometimes)

2. CEA is variably expressed in carcinomas as detailed below. However, CEA lacks specificity, and with the exception of canalicular staining in HCC, it is not routinely used to differentiate carcinomas.

CEA-positive carcinomas	CEA-variable carcinomas	CEA-negative carcinomas
HCC (canalicular pattern with pCEA*)	Urothelial carcinoma	Kidney
Colorectum	Breast	Adrenal
Stomach	Cervix	Prostate
Lung adenocarcinoma		Mesothelioma
Pancreaticobiliary		Ovary
		Endometrium

* Polyclonal but not monoclonal CEA cross-reacts with biliary epithelium in normal and neoplastic liver.

3. Vimentin is generally considered to be a mesenchymal marker, and it has been used in the past to differentiate sarcoma (vimentin-positive) from carcinoma (vimentin-negative). It is now known that vimentin is fairly non-specific and is variably expressed in many carcinomas. The table below is mainly of historic interest – vimentin is now rarely used to differentiate tumors. The main current application of vimentin is to confirm tissue immunoviability when all other markers are negative.

Vimentin-positive carcinomas	Vimentin-negative carcinomas
RCC, clear cell type	RCC, chromophobe type
Endometrium	Endocervix (adenocarcinoma)
Mesothelioma	Lung carcinoma
Salivary gland	Breast
Thyroid	Ovary
Sweat gland	Prostate
Spindle cell carcinoma of any site	Colorectum
	HCC

References: [5,6]

Primer on Markers of Muscle Differentiation

	Desmin	MSA (HHF-35)	SMA (α-actin)	Calponin	h-Caldesmon	SMMHC	MyoD*, Myogenin*, α-sarcomeric actin
Skeletal muscle	+	+	–	–	–	–	+
Smooth muscle and myoepithelial cells	+	+	+	+	+	+	–
Myofibroblast	+/–	+	+	+/–	–	–	–

* MyoD and Myogenin (both transcription factors) are nuclear; all other markers are cytoplasmic.

- **Desmin** is a universal marker of muscle cells. It is expressed both in smooth and striated muscle cells; expression is variable in myofibroblasts. Desmin is an intermediate filament (a counterpart to cytokeratins in epithelial cells).

- **Muscle specific actin (MSA)**, like desmin, is another pan-muscle marker. The antibody to MSA, HHF-35, recognizes the epitope common to α-skeletal, α-cardiac and γ-smooth muscle actins.

- **Smooth muscle actin (SMA)**, aka α-actin, is a smooth muscle specific isoform of actin; it is absent in striated muscle.

- **Calponin**, **h-Caldesmon**, and **Smooth Muscle Myosin Heavy Chain (SMMHC)** are contractile apparatus-associated proteins, which are unique to smooth muscle. Note that caldesmon and SMMHC are generally absent in myofibroblasts.

- **MyoD** and **Myogenin** are transcription factors (thus are nuclear), which are specific to striated muscle; they are absent in smooth muscle. **α-sarcomeric actin** is a cytoplasmic marker of striated muscle. These markers are used to differentiate rhabdomyosarcoma (positive) from leiomyosarcoma (negative). The pattern of reactivity can also be helpful, as embryonal rhabdomyosarcoma shows focal positivity while alveolar rhabdomyosarcoma is diffusely positive for MyoD/myogenin.

- **Myoepithelial cells** show differentiation as both smooth muscle and epithelial cells (they are therefore CK+). Myoepithelial cells express a COMPLETE smooth muscle phenotype in that they faithfully express all smooth muscle markers. In addition, these cells are curiously polyphenotypic and express markers of various other tissues: GFAP (glial), S100 (neural), and p63 (basal cell).

- **Myofibroblasts** show differentiation as both smooth muscle cell and fibroblast. Unlike myoepithelial cells, smooth muscle differentiation is INCOMPLETE, and only some muscle markers are expressed (actin-positive, desmin-variable, caldesmon- and SMMHC-negative). This feature may be used to differentiate myofibroblastic tumors (caldesmon –) from smooth muscle tumors (caldesmon +). Oddly, myofibroblasts are sometimes CK+ (as in inflammatory myofibroblastic tumor).

Applications:
- to ID smooth or skeletal muscle differentiation in poorly differentiated neoplasms. Reactivity may be variable, so actins and desmin are best used in conjunction.
- to diagnose myoepithelioma and myofibroblastic tumors (e.g. nodular fasciitis, fibromatosis)
- to diagnose invasive breast cancer: SMA, Calponin, and SMMHC (along with p63) may be used to identify myoepithelial cell layer which surrounds benign and in situ lesions, and is absent in invasive carcinoma
- some use desmin to differentiate reactive mesothelial cells (positive) from mesothelioma (negative)

Note: Several non-myogenic tumors/tissues are unexpectedly desmin+ (but actin–). This includes desmoplastic small round cell tumor, blastemal component of Wilms tumor, mesothelial cells (benign >> malignant), few other. Otherwise, desmin usually goes together with actins. On the other hand, actin is a bit more sensitive than desmin, and therefore actin+/desmin– reactivity is not unusual (such as in some leiomyosarcomas and myofibroblastic lesions).

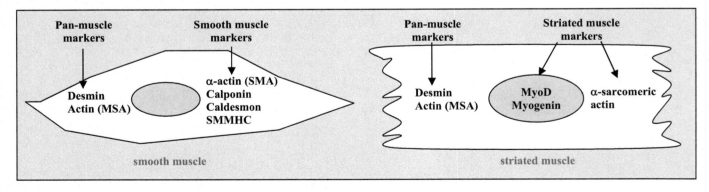

Abbreviations: MSA Muscle specific actin, SMA Smooth muscle actin, SMMHC Smooth Muscle Myosin Heavy Chain

Primer on Markers of Neuroendocrine (NE) Differentiation

- The classic list of "NE markers" includes **Synaptophysin (SYN)**, **Chromogranin A (CHR)**, **Neuron Specific Enolase (NSE)**, and **CD56** (NCAM or Neural Cell Adhesion Molecule). **CD57** (Leu-7) is sometimes used as a second-line NE marker. NE markers are usually strongly expressed in low-grade NE neoplasms (e.g. carcinoid), whereas expression may be weak/focal in high-grade NE neoplasms (e.g. small cell carcinoma).

- **SYN** and **CHR:**
  - These are the first-line markers of NE differentiation (along with CD56).
  - SYN and CHR mark neurosecretory granules and hence show granular cytoplasmic staining.
  - Overall, **SYN is more sensitive than CHR** but **CHR is more specific**. Some NE tumors will label for either CHR or SYN but not both, so **these are complementary and usually are ordered together**.
  - In addition to NE neoplasms, SYN and variably CHR are also present in neoplasms of neuronal origin (e.g. gangliocytoma) and primitive neuroectodermal neoplasms (neuroblastoma, medulloblastoma, PNET/Ewing).
  - There are few non-NE neoplasms which can be SYN + but are always CHR– (here staining is unrelated to NE granules). These include adrenocortical neoplasms and pancreatic solid-pseudopapillary tumor.

- Historically, **NSE** was considered to be a first-tier marker of NE neoplasms. It does have a high sensitivity, but also suffers from low specificity. In addition to NE lesions, it also reacts with astrocytomas, meningioma, schwannoma, and aderenocortical neoplasms, among others. NSE is therefore no longer considered a first-line marker (think of NSE as "neuron not-so-specific esterase").

- **CD56** is the most sensitive NE marker in every organ, but it is not entirely specific (also marks NK-cells, peripheral nerve sheath tumors, synovial sarcoma, etc.). Generally, SYN and CHR do a good enough job identifying low-grade NE neoplasms (e.g. carcinoid) and CD56 is not usually needed in this situation. However, CD56 can save the day when it comes to high-grade NE neoplasms, especially small cell carcinoma, which may be negative for all other NE markers, but are usually positive for CD56.

	SYN	CHR	CD56	NSE
Sensitivity	++	+	++	++
Specificity	+	++	+	–
++ best, + intermediate, – worst				

- **Peptide hormones** may occasionally be helpful in establishing the identity of a NE carcinoma. For example, calcitonin supports the diagnosis of medullary carcinoma (although it can also be positive in other NE neoplasms, especially atypical carcinoid of the larynx). In fact, most NE neoplasms are capable of producing ectopic hormones (e.g. pancreatic endocrine neoplasms may produce gastrin, ACTH, PTH, etc). In addition, some NE neoplasms are non-functional and will be negative for any hormones. Therefore, assigning the site of origin of an occult neuroendocrine tumor based on hormone expression is generally not recommended.

- **Cytokeratins (CK) in NE neoplasms:**
  - NE neoplasms fall into two categories: epithelial (e.g. carcinoid, pancreatic neuroendocrine tumor/islet cell tumor, small cell carcinoma) and non-epithelial/neural (e.g. pheochromocytoma, paraganglioma, PNET, neuroblastoma). Epithelial NE neoplasms are CK-positive, whereas non-epithelial NE neoplasms are CK-negative.
  - Although usually at least one of CK is positive, the reactivity is notoriously variable in NE neoplasms (particularly small cell carcinoma). Cam5.2 is considered to be a more reliable marker than AE1/AE3 in these lesions. To be safe, both Cam5.2 and AE1/3 should be performed if a NE tumor is in the differential. Be aware that expression can be focal and relatively unimpressive in small cell carcinoma because there is so little cytoplasm in the cells, requiring examination on high power.
  - In addition, distinctive feature of high-grade NE carcinomas (small cell and Merkel cell CAs) is that CK reactivity has a dot-like (punctate) perinuclear pattern. This pattern of reactivity applies to Cam5.2 and AE1:AE3 labeling of small call CA and Merkel Cell CA, and CK20 labeling of Merkel cell CA. Punctate reactivity is thought to be due to formation of CK tangles in these tumors. This is a helpful diagnostic feature because punctate reactivity for cytokeratins not only confirms that a tumor is epithelial, but also suggests that it is neuroendocrine.

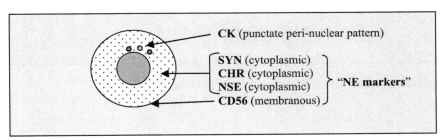

Abbreviations: CHR Chromogranin A, CK cytokeratin, SYN Synaptophysin, NE neuroendocrine, NSE Neuron Specific Enolase

Primer on Markers of Melanocytic Differentiation

- Key markers of melanocytic differentiation include **Melan-A/MART1, HMB45, S100** and **MITF**. Also available (but rarely used) are stains for **Tyrosinase** and special stains for melanin, such as Fontana Masson. **SOX10, PNL2,** and **MUM1** are more recent melanocytic markers, which identify epithelioid but not spindle cell melanoma.

- **Melan-A (A103)** and **MART-1** (<u>M</u>elanoma <u>A</u>ntigen <u>R</u>ecognized by <u>T</u> cells) are two distinct antibodies that recognize the same antigen.
  - 80–100% of epithelioid melanomas are positive.
  - Spindle cell and desmoplastic melanomas are generally negative or patchy.
  - Melan-A (A103) cross-reacts with steroid hormone-producing tumors (adrenocortical neoplasms and sex cord-stromal tumors of the gonads).

- **HMB45** (<u>H</u>uman <u>M</u>elanoma, <u>B</u>lack) recognizes the gp100 protein, which is present in premelanosomes.
  - 60–90% of epithelioid of melanomas are positive.
  - Spindle cell and desmoplastic melanomas are generally negative.
  - HMB45 is less sensitive than Melan-A and S100, but more specific (does not react with steroid hormone-producing tumors).
  - HMB45 is present specifically in immature melanocytes, whereas mature melanocytes are negative. This feature can be exploited to differentiate melanoma (+) from mature nevus cells (–) both at the *primary site* (melanoma shows no maturation toward the base → all cells HMB45+) vs. nevus (cell mature toward the base and become HMB45–) and in *lymph nodes* (metastatic melanoma is HMB45+ vs. intranodal nevus is HMB45–).

- **S100** protein, so named for its <u>s</u>olubility in <u>100</u>% ammonium sulfate, is a calcium binding protein.
  - > 90% of melanomas are positive, including spindle cell and desmoplastic type.
  - S100 is the most sensitive melanocytic marker. Negative staining for S100 makes melanoma highly unlikely.
  - S100 suffers from a low specificity because it reacts with many non-melanocytic neoplasms including nerve sheath tumors, myoepithelial neoplasms, granular cell tumor, Langerhans' cell histiocytosis, chordoma, gliomas, lipomatous tumors and some carcinomas, such as breast. Therefore S100 is usually used as part of a panel.

- **MITF** (<u>M</u>icrophthalmia <u>T</u>ranscription <u>F</u>actor) is a nuclear regulator. It is claimed to be as sensitive as Melan-A for epithelioid melanomas, but it is also sub-optimal (~40%+) for spindle cell and desmoplastic melanomas. It has the advantage of having nuclear reactivity, which can be easier to interpret.

- In addition to melanoma, all melanoma-associated antigens are also present in other melanosome-containing tumors, such as clear cell sarcoma/melanoma of soft parts, melanotic neurofibroma, melanotic schwannoma as well as PEComas (<u>p</u>erivascular <u>e</u>pithelioid <u>c</u>ell tumors) family, which include angiomyolipoma, lymphangioleiomyomatosis, pulmonary sugar tumor, and other rare clear cell tumors. PEComas are primarily positive for HMB45 and Melan-A; whereas S100 is positive in a subset (~30%).

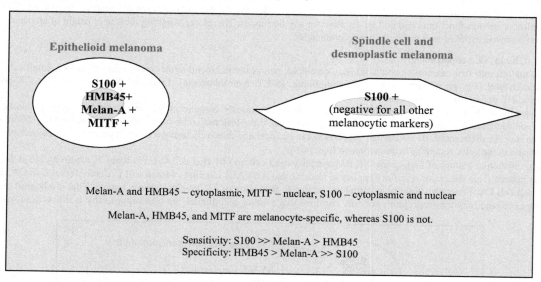

Abbreviations: HMB human melanoma black, MITF microphthalmia transcription factor

Primer on Markers of Neuroglial Differentiation

- **Neuronal Markers** include:
  - **Neurofilament (NF),** which includes Sm311 (pan-NF), Sm32 (cell body), Sm31 (axons)
  - **NeuN,** <u>Neu</u>ronal <u>N</u>uclei (nuclear marker)
  - **Synaptophysin (SYN)** and **Chromogranin (CHR):** react with synaptic vesicles in neurons and neurosecretory granules in neuroendocrine cells (more so SYN than CHR).
  - **Neuron Specific Enolase (NSE)** and **CD56** (Neural Cell Adhesion Molecule, NCAM): react with neurons and neuroendocrine cells. Despite the name, NSE is highly non-specific but it is sensitive.

- **Neuronal markers may be used to:**
  i. ID of tumors with neuronal/ganglion cell differentiation (e.g. gangliocytoma) or neuroblastic differentiation (e.g. neuroblastoma, medulloblastoma). SYN is best for this purpose.
  ii. ID of brain infiltration: Sm31 may be used to highlight normal axons to help identify the permeation of normal brain parenchyma by a glioma or meningioma.

- **Glia** (astrocytes, oligodendrocytes, and ependymal cells) and corresponding neoplasms (glioma, astrocytoma, and ependymoma) are identified by **GFAP** (<u>G</u>lial <u>F</u>ibrillary <u>A</u>strocytic <u>P</u>rotein). GFAP may be used to distinguish a glioma from non-glial neoplasms (lymphoma, carcinoma, melanoma) and inflammatory conditions (e.g. multiple sclerosis). GFAP also variably reacts with Schwann cells.

- **Schwann (nerve sheath) cells** are identified primarily by **S100**. S100 also reacts with gliomas as well as a number of other neoplasms, including melanoma. Note that S100 cannot be used to discriminate neuroglial neoplasms (e.g. MPNST) from melanoma. CD57 (Leu7) is a lymphoid marker that cross-reacts with myelin-associated protein. It has also been used as a second-tier marker for Schwann cells.

- **Neuroendocrine (NE) cells** react with SYN, CHR as well as NSE and CD56. Cytokeratin expression depends on the specific type of NE neoplasm: carcinoids are CK (+), whereas pheochromocytoma is CK (–). See section on NE markers for details. NE cells are S100-negative, but S100 marks supportive (sustentacular) cells in some NE neoplasms, most notably pheochromocytoma.

- **Cytokeratins:** All things glial/neuronal/nerve sheath are Cam 5.2 (–) and AE1/AE3 (–). However, beware of non-specific AE1/AE3 staining in normal and neoplastic brain, particularly in reactive astrocytes (Cam5.2 should be negative, though).

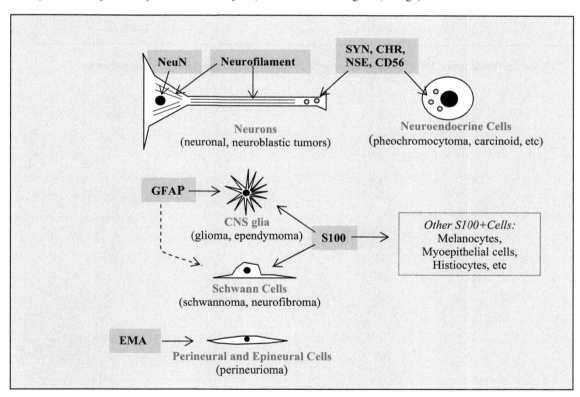

Abbreviations: CHR chromogranin, EMA epithelial membrane antigen, GFAP glial fibrillary astrocytic protein, NSE neuron specific enolase, SYN synaptophysin

Primer on Markers of Vascular Differentiation

- There are several markers of vascular differentiation in current use. They include **CD31**, **CD34**, **Factor VIII** (actual antigen is von Willebrand factor), ***Ulex europaeus I***, **CD141** (Thrombomodulin), and **Fli-1**. Stay tuned for ERG – a new promising vascular marker (which is also translocated in prostate cancer).

- These markers react with both blood vessels and lymphatics, although lymphatics are variably reactive for CD34.

- **D2-40** (Podoplanin) is a novel marker specific for the lymphatic endothelial cells.

- The most commonly used markers are CD31 and CD34. CD31 is more sensitive and more specific. CD34 also reacts with various soft tissue tumors and epithelioid sarcoma.

- Key applications of vascular markers are:
    1) to ID the vascular nature of a poorly differentiated or ambiguous neoplasm (such angiosarcoma, epithelioid hemangioendothelioma, Kaposi sarcoma, hemangiopericytoma);
    2) to highlight vessels to help identify lymphovascular invasion in tumors.

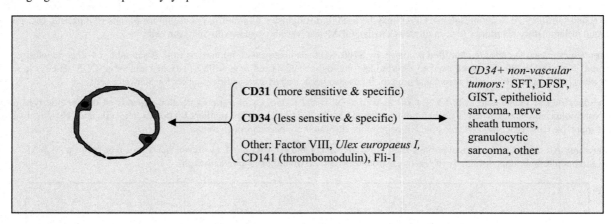

Abbreviations: SFT solitary fibrous tumor, DFSP dermatofibrosarcoma protuberans, GIST gastrointestinal stromal tumor

Primer on Assessment of Invasion

- Invasive carcinomas, by definition, extend beyond the surrounding basement membrane. Collagen type IV is a component of basement membrane. However, because of high background staining, this marker generally has a limited utility in the diagnosis of invasion.

- Alternative markers of invasion are basal cells and myoepithelial cells in the prostate and breast, respectively. These cells surround benign luminal cells and in situ lesions (such as PIN or DCIS), but are absent in the invasive carcinomas, as diagrammed below. Included in the diagram is Racemase, which is part of a standard "prostate cancer panel" (p63, CK903, Racemase). Racemase is highly expressed in malignant acinar cells (invasive and in situ), but is usually negative in benign cells.

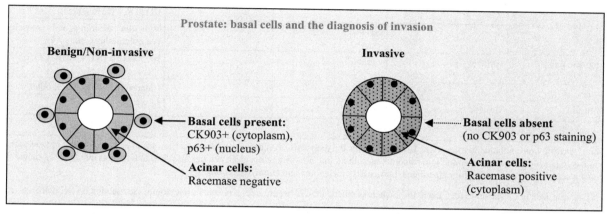

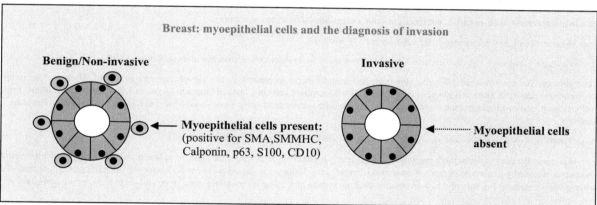

Abbreviations: SMA Smooth muscle actin, SMMHC Smooth Muscle Myosin Heavy Chain

Differential Diagnosis of Undifferentiated Malignant Neoplasm
(carcinoma vs. melanoma vs. lymphoma vs. sarcoma vs. other)

	Epithelial markers: CK, EMA	S100	CD45	Other
Carcinoma	+[1]	–[4]	–	see table below for site-specific markers
Melanoma	–	+	–	HMB45, Melan-A [8]
Lymphoma	–	–	+[7]	CD3 (T cell), CD20 & CD79a (B cell)
Sarcoma	–	variable[5]	–	Vimentin[9], desmin & actin (muscle), CD34 (vascular, other), etc
Neuroendocrine (NE) neoplasm	variable[2]	variable[6]	–	NE markers (SYN, CHR, CD56, NSE)
Mesothelioma	+	–	–	Calretinin, WT1, CK5/6, other
Germ cell tumor	variable[3]	–	–	PLAP, c-kit, other
Glioma	–	+	–	GFAP

1) In general, reactivity for epithelial markers (CK, EMA) confirms the diagnosis of a carcinoma. However, beware of epithelial marker expression in some non-carcinomas (e.g. synovial sarcoma, epithelioid sarcoma, mesothelioma, non-seminoma germ cell tumors). In addition, aberrant labeling mainly with Cam5.2 may be seen focally in some high-grade tumors, particularly melanoma and leiomyosarcoma.

2) Some NE neoplasms are CK-positive (e.g. carcinoid), whereas others are CK-negative (e.g. pheochromocytoma). See section on NE markers.

3) Non-seminoma germ cell tumors (embryonal carcinoma, yolk sac tumor) are CK-positive, whereas seminoma is CK-negative.

4) Carcinomas are generally S100-negative, but there are some exceptions (30% of breast cancer).

5) Sarcomas of nerve sheath and adipocytic differentiation are S100-positive.

6) Pheochromocytoma/paraganglioma and olfactory neuroblastoma show S100 reactivity in sustentacular (supportive) cells.

7) CD45 is highly specific for hematopoietic cells. However, few hematopoietic neoplasms are notoriously negative for CD45. These include lymphoblastic lymphoma (variable), anaplastic large cell lymphoma (variable), Reed-Sternberg cells in Classical Hodgkin lymphoma, plasma cell neoplasms, follicular dendritic cell sarcoma, and myeloid sarcoma (variable). Other markers are needed to identify these lesions, such as CD79a for plasmacytoma and CD43 for myeloid sarcoma.

8) Spindle cell and desmoplastic melanoma are (+) for S100 only (HMB45 and Melan-A are absent or focal).

9) Vimentin is historically used to distinguish carcinoma and glioma (vimentin-negative) from sarcoma, lymphoma and melanoma (vimentin-positive). However, vimentin is actually expressed in many carcinomas (thyroid, lung, kidney, uterus, other) and is no longer considered a particularly useful discriminating marker. Positive staining for vimentin is occasionally used to confirm that tissue is "immunoviable" when all other markers are non-reactive.

Primary panel usually includes cytokeratins (AE1/AE3 and Cam5.2), S100 and CD45.

Carcinoma of Unknown Primary (CUP): Site-Specific Markers[1]
Summary of Key Organ-specific Markers

Site	Marker
Breast	ER/PR (60%+), GCDFP-15 (50%+), Mammaglobin (50%+), HER2 (10–25%+, not specific for breast)
Prostate	PSA, PSAP, Prostein (P501S), PSMA
Lung	TTF-1 (75% non-mucinous adenocarcinoma; 90% small cell carcinoma[2]), Napsin A, Surfactant (PE10)
Thyroid: papillary and follicular CA	TTF-1, Thyroglobulin, PAX8
Thyroid: medullary CA	TTF-1, Calcitonin
Liver	HepPar-1, canalicular CD10, other
Pancreas	Loss of DPC4 expression (in 55% of adenocarcinomas)
Kidney	PAX2, PAX8, CAIX, RCC and CD10 (last 2 markers have low specificity)
Adrenal	Inhibin, Melan-A (not specific for adrenal)
GYN tract	PAX8, ER/PR (endometrioid ~100%+, serous 50%+, cervical – negative), WT1 (serous carcinoma)
Neuroendocrine organs: – Pituitary – Parathyroid – Pancreatic islet cells	Prolactin, GH, ACTH, TSH, LH/FSH PTH Insulin, Glucagon, Somatostatin, other[3]
Bladder	p63, Thrombomodulin (not specific), Uroplakin, GATA3
Intestine	CDX2, Villin
Gallbladder, stomach	no specific markers available
Squamous cell cancer of cervix, anus, and tonsil[2]	HPV (by ISH), p16

Marker	Site
TTF-1	lung (non-squamous) and thyroid (papillary/follicular/medullary). Beware of expression in subset of GYN tumors. Small cell carcinoma of lung (90%) and extra-pulmonary origin (40%)
Napsin A	lung, RCC (especially papillary), rarely thyroid (weak)
ER/PR	breast, uterus/ovary (endometrioid>>serous). Can label subset of other carcinomas (~5% of lung carcinomas).
GCDFP	breast and salivary gland – low sensitivity and specificity
Mammaglobin	breast. Reportedly more sensitive than GCDFP, but also reacts with GYN tumors.
CDX2, Villin	intestinal differentiation: carcinomas of large and small bowel. Carcinomas with GI phenotype (e.g. adenoCA of urinary bladder, mucinous BAC) are also variably reactive.
PAX8	pan-renal (broader than PAX2), pan-Mullerian (uterus, ovary), thyroid (papillary/follicular>>medullary)
PAX2	pan-renal
DPC4	loss of expression fairly specific to pancreaticobiliary carcinoma, though present in only 55% of cases (loss of expression confirms pancreaticobiliary primary, but positive labeling is non-contributory). Few colon cancers (11%) also show the loss of expression.
Prostate markers (PSA, PSAP, Prostein, PSMA)	highly specific for prostate, though few non-prostate tumors are reactive (e.g. PSAP-reactivity in rectal carcinoids, PSA in salivary tumors)
HepPar1	hepatocellular differentiation – specific for HCC (also positive in rare hepatoid variants of carcinomas at other sites)

1) These markers are used to determine the site of origin of metastatic CUP. None of the markers are 100% site-specific; therefore they must be interpreted in context of morphology, clinical findings, and in conjunction with CK7/CK20 and other less specific markers (see sections on specific organs).

2) Note that the above site-specific markers apply only to ADENOCARCINOMAS. Squamous cell cancers of various organs generally cannot be distinguished based on their immunoprofile. Exceptions are squamous cancers of cervix, oropharynx (tonsil and base of tongue), and anus, subsets of which are HPV-related and can be distinguished by in situ hybridization for HPV DNA or by expression of p16 (a sensitive but nonspecific marker of high-risk HPV infection).

3) Note that hormone expression is not considered sufficiently specific to assign the origin of a metastasis.

For details on each marker please refer to the alphabetical index and the organ systems sections.

Differential Diagnosis of Small Round Blue Cell Tumors (SRBCT)

	CK & EMA	CD45	CD99/O13	NE Markers[2]	TTF-1	WT1	Desmin	Other
SRBCT of childhood								
Lymphoblastic Lymphoma[1]	–	+ (few –)	+	–	–	–	–	TdT+, CD34+ 80% are T cell: CD3+
Rhabdomyosarcoma, solid alveolar type	– (few + focally)	–	– (few +)	– (SYN+)	–	–[3]	+	Actin+, Desmin+, Myogenin+, MyoD+
Wilms tumor, blastema-predominant	+	–	–	–	–	+	+ blastema	
PNET/Ewing sarcoma	– (20% + focally)	–	+	+ NSE, SYN	–	–	–	PAS+
Neuroblastoma	–	–	– always	+ mainly SYN	–	–	–	
Medulloblastoma	–	–	–	+ mainly SYN	–	–	–	Variable GFAP
Small cell osteosarcoma	–	–	+/–	–	–	–	–	Osteocalcin+
SRBCT of adulthood								
Lymphoma	–	+	–	–	–	–	–	B cell: CD20+, CD79a+ T cell: CD3+
Small cell carcinoma	+[5]	–	–	+	+/–[4]	–	–	
Merkel cell carcinoma	+[5]	–	–	+	– always	–	–	CK20+[4], Neurofilament+, Merkel cell polyomavirus+
Desmoplastic small round cell tumor	+	–	– (few +)	– (+ NSE only)	–	+	+[4]	actin–
Mesenchymal chondrosarcoma	–	–	+	–/+[6]	–	–	–	Sox-9+, S100+ focally in small blue cell component

1) Beware of lymphoblastic lymphoma: it may be CD45– & CD99/O13+, thereby masquerading as Ewing sarcoma. However, unlike Ewing sarcoma, lymphoblastic lymphoma is reactive for blast markers (TdT, CD34) and either T-cell markers (CD3) or B-cell markers (CD20, CD79a).

2) NE markers include SYN, CHR, CD56 and NSE.

3) Rhabdomyosarcoma often shows cytoplasmic, but not nuclear, WT1 expression. [9]

4) TTF-1 is expressed in small cell cancers of lung (90%) and non-lung origin (>40%). In contrast, Merkel cell carcinoma is ALWAYS TTF-1-negative.

5) "Dot-like" peri-nuclear reactivity. This is typical pattern of cytokeratin reactivity in neuroendocrine carcinomas (small cell CA, Merkel cell CA).

6) The small cell component of mesenchymal chondrosarcoma can be positive for the nonspecific NSE and CD57, but not SYN, CHR, or CD56.

Differential Diagnosis of Spindle Cell Tumors

Differentiation	Neoplasm	CK & EMA	S100	SMA	Desmin	CD34	other
Muscle	LM	–	–	+	+	–	
	LMS	rare +	–	+	+	–	variable CD99/O13
	RMS	–	–	–	+	–	Myogenin+, MyoD+
Nerve Sheath	Neurofibroma	–	+ focal	–	–	+	
	Schwannoma	–	+ diffuse	–	–	+	
	MPNST	+ focal	+ focal	–	–	+	
Vascular	e.g. Angiosarcoma, Kaposi, etc	–	–	–	–	+	Factor VIII+, CD31+
Myofibroblastic[1]	Fibromatosis	–	–	+	–/+	–	nuclear β-catenin+ [2]
	Nodular Fasciitis	–	–	+	–	–	CD68+
	IMT	–/+ variable	–	+/–	+/–	–	ALK+ (subset)
Fibrohistiocytic[5]	DF	–	–	–	–	–	Factor XIIIa+
	DFSP	–	–	–	–	+	Factor XIIIa –
Adipose	Dedifferentiated liposarcoma	–	+	–	–	–/+	CDK4+, MDM2+[6]
Other	GIST	–	–	+30%	–	+ 70%	c-kit+ 95%, DOG1+ 85%, Bcl-2+
	SFT & HPC [3]	–	–	–	–	+	Bcl-2+
	Synovial sarcoma	+ focal	+30%	–	–	– always	calponin+, Bcl-2+, CD56+, variable CD99/O13, TLE1
Non-sarcomas	Spindle cell CA	+	–	–	–	–	For SqCC: CK903+, p63+; various site-specific markers
	Spindle cell melanoma	–	+ diffuse [4]	–	–	–	

1) Caldesmon helps to differentiate smooth muscle tumors (caldesmon +) from myofibroblastic tumors (caldesmon –). In addition, "tram-track" pattern of actins (due to peripheral cytoplasmic accentuation) is characteristic of myofibroblastic lesions (such as nodular fasciitis) but not smooth muscle tumors (such as leiomyosarcoma), which have diffuse expression.

2) Nuclear β-catenin (reflecting mutations of either β-catenin or APC genes) is found in deep fibromatoses (desmoid tumors) but not superficial fibromatoses. [10]

3) HPC is now generally accepted as a cellular variant of SFT, except in the brain and sinonasal tract where HPC and SFT are still regarded as distinct entities. In the brain, stains may be used to differentiate SFT (diffusely CD34+, reticulin-negative) versus HPC (focally CD34+, reticulin-positive in pericellular pattern). Sinonasal HPC (also known as glomangiopericytoma) is SMA+, Factor XIIIa+, and negative for CD34 and Bcl-2.

4) Spindle cell melanoma is usually reactive for S100 only; other melanocytic markers (HMB45, Melan-A) are generally negative or focal.

5) Fibrohistiocytic tumors, including MFH, are described to be variably reactive for histiocytic markers, such as CD68.

6) CDK4 and MDM2 are not specific for liposarcoma, but positivity in the context of a spindle cell tumor in the retroperitoneum supports dedifferentiated liposarcoma. They are most useful in the differential of a well-differentiated liposarcoma/atypical lipomatous tumor (CDK4 and MDM2+) and a benign lipoma (CDK4 and MDM2 –). [11]

Abbreviations: DF dermatofibroma, DFSP dermatofibrosarcoma protuberans, GIST gastrointestinal stromal tumor, HPC hemangiopericytoma, IMT inflammatory myofibroblastic tumor, LM leiomyoma, LMS leiomyosarcoma, MFH malignant fibrous histiocytoma, MPNST malignant peripheral nerve sheath tumor, RMS rhabdomyosarcoma, SMA smooth muscle actin (α-actin), SFT solitary fibrous tumor

Differential Diagnosis of Neuroendocrine (NE) and Neuroectodermal Neoplasms

	NE markers (SYN, CHR, CD56, NSE)[1]	Epithelial markers (Cam5.2, AE1/3)[2]	S100	Other
Carcinoid	+	+	–[3] (most)	TTF-1+ (lung)[4] or CDX2+ (intestinal)[4] hormones (variable)
Pancreatic endocrine neoplasm (formerly islet cell tumor)	+	+	–	hormones (variable): insulin, glucagon, somatostatin, etc[5]
Medullary carcinoma of the thyroid	+	+	–[3] (most)	TTF-1+, Calcitonin+, CEA+ (Thyroglobulin negative)
Pheochromocytoma & Paraganglioma	+	–	+ (sustentacular/ supportive cells)	
Small cell NE carcinoma	+/–	+/–	–	TTF-1+[4]
Merkel cell carcinoma	+	+	–	CK20+, Neurofilament (both punctate perinuclear)+, Merkel cell polyomavirus+, always TTF-1–
Pituitary neoplasms	+	+	–	PRL, GH, ACTH, TSH, LH/FSH
Parathyroid neoplasms	+	+	–	PTH+
Neuroblastoma	+	–	+[6]	
PNET/Ewing sarcoma	+ (mainly NSE)	–/+ (20%+)	variable	CD99/O13+, PAS+

1) See section on NE markers for background.

2) Cytokeratin (CK) expression is variable in NE carcinomas: Cam5.2 reactivity is more consistent than AE1/AE3. Note that CK's (Cam5.2 & AE1/3) show punctate (dot-like) perinuclear reactivity in NE neoplasms. Same applies to CK20 staining in Merkel cell carcinoma. This is a helpful diagnostic clue.

3) Some medullary thyroid carcinomas and carcinoid tumors show a sustentacular staining pattern with S100.

4) TTF-1 is expressed in >90% of small cell NE carcinomas of lung and several non-lung sites (see above). TTF-1 is positive in pulmonary (50%) but usually not intestinal carcinoids. On the other hand, CDX2 is positive in up to two-thirds of intestinal but not pulmonary carcinoids.

5) Insulin and glucagon may be expressed not only by pancreatic endocrine neoplasms but also by NE neoplasms of other sites (although pancreas is more common). Because of the lack of specificity, these and other hormones are not generally used to assign the source of a metastatic NE neoplasm.

6) S100 reacts with schwannian stromal cells.

Semiquantitative Assessment of Predictive Markers

Estrogen and Progesterone Receptor Expression Interpretation in Breast Cancer (only nuclear staining is scored)

Criteria	Interpretation
≥1% staining of any intensity	POSITIVE
<1% staining with appropriately staining internal control tissue	NEGATIVE
Internal control tissue not staining or specimen handling did not conform to guideline requirements (e.g., fixation <6 hr or >72 hr, fixation solution other than 10% buffered formalin)	UNINTERPRETABLE

- Also report % of tumor cells staining, staining intensity (strong, medium, or weak), internal and external controls (positive, negative, or not present), and whether standard assay conditions were met/not met.
- Hormone receptor-positive cancers are treated with Tamoxifen. Studies suggest that as few as 1% positive tumor cells may be associated with significant clinical responses.

Reference: [12]

HER2 (c-erbB-2) Dako HercepTest Interpretation (only membranous staining is scored)

Criteria	Score and Interpretation
<30%	0 = NEGATIVE
>30%, partial membrane staining	1+ = NEGATIVE
>30%, complete membrane staining, weak to moderate	2+ = WEAKLY POSITIVE (EQUIVOCAL)
>30%, complete membrane staining, moderate to strong	3+ = STRONGLY POSITIVE

- Cases that are negative by IHC (0 & 1+) are reported out as "negative", and strongly positive cases (3+) are reported out as "positive". Weakly positive (2+) or equivocal IHC should be further analyzed for HER2 gene amplification by FISH (or CISH).
- FISH criteria are:
  - HER2 amplified: >6 HER2 gene copies/nucleus or FISH ratio (HER2 gene signals to chromosome 17 signals) > 2.2
  - HER2 non-amplified: <4.0 HER2 gene copies/nucleus or FISH ratio < 1.8
- HER2-positive cancers are treated with Trastuzumab (Herceptin), a monoclonal antibody directed against HER2.
- According to the recent ASCO/CAP guidelines, the recommended cut-off for "positives" is changed from previous 10% to 30%.

References: [13,14]

EGFR PharmDx Assay Interpretation (only membranous staining is scored)

Criteria	Score and Interpretation
no staining	0 = NEGATIVE
≥1%, weak (partial or complete membrane staining)	1+ = POSITIVE (weak)
≥1%, moderate (partial or complete membrane staining)	2+ = POSITVE (moderate)
≥1%, strong (partial or complete membrane staining)	3+ = POSITIVE (strong)

- EGFR (Epidermal Growth Factor Receptor) staining is currently validated only for metastatic colorectal carcinomas.
- Erbitux (cetuximab) and Vectibix (panitumumab) are monoclonal antibodies directed against EGFR, which is currently approved for the treatment of patients with metastatic colorectal cancer. Clinical response does not appear to correlate with the level of EGFR expression, but are best predicted by the absence of KRAS mutations.
- Note that EGFR mutations and NOT IHC is not used to predict response to EGFR-targeted therapies in the lung.

Reference: [15]

Chapter 2 Immunostains: Organ Systems

by Natasha Rekhtman, Ashlie Burkhart, Amy Duffield, Janis Taube, Justin Bishop

Breast

Breast: Key Markers at a Glance	
Marker [location]	Applications
E-cadherin (CAD-E) [membranous]	E-cadherin is an adhesion molecule expressed in normal ductal and lobular cells. Loss of staining is a hallmark of lobular carcinoma (in situ and invasive) – remember that lobular lesions are discohesive! The main application of E-cadherin is to differentiate DCIS/ADH (+) from LCIS/ALH (–). p120 catenin is an E-cadherin-binding protein, which is advocated by some experts for E-cadherin-equivocal cases [membranous p120 = DCIS, cytoplasmic p120 = LCIS].
ER and PR [nuclear]	ER and PR are present in normal and neoplastic breast epithelium. ER controls the synthesis of PR. Therefore ER+/PR– tumors are not uncommon, but the opposite should raise a suspicion of a false result. ER and PR are weakly favorable prognostic factors (expression correlates with better differentiation). Most importantly, expression of ER and PR is a strongly favorable predictive factor because these patients can be treated with Tamoxifen (see above for quantitative scoring of ER and PR). In addition, ER and PR are used to identify metastatic breast cancer (~60%+), but note that ovarian, endometrial and few other non-mammary carcinomas are also positive (see antibody index for complete list).
GCDFP (GCDFP-15, BRST2) [cytoplasmic]	GCDFP is a marker of apocrine cells, which are present in breast and sweat glands. Main application is to identify breast metastases. Note that in general staining is patchy at best and overall only ~50% of tumors are positive. In addition, it is highly non-specific and many other tumors, such as lung carcinoma, can express GCDFP. Therefore GCDFP is always used in conjunction with ER and PR. Lobular carcinomas have more of an apocrine differentiation and stain reliably with GCDFP. Because it is a marker of apocrine differentiation, note that GCDFP is also positive in salivary duct carcinoma and some skin adnexal tumors.
Mammaglobin [cytoplasmic]	Mammaglobin is a newcomer to the breast-marker scene. It is present in ~50% of breast cancer and is not as focal as GCDFP. Like GCDFP, it recognizes apocrine differentiation (breast, sweat glands). In addition, mammaglobin is also expressed in tumors of female genital tract (ovary, endometrium, cervix). Therefore it is less specific but more sensitive than GCDFP.
HER2 [membranous]	HER2 is a growth factor receptor, which is absent or rare in normal breast cells. Overexpression (as a result of gene amplification) is present in 10–30% of tumors. HER2 is a poor prognostic factor, though a weak one. Most importantly, HER2 is a strongly favorable predictive factor in that it predicts a response to Herceptin, the anti-HER2 antibody. See above for quantitative scoring of HER2. Note that better differentiated tumors are ER+, PR+ and HER2–, whereas opposite is true for tumors with poor differentiation. Exceptions are medullary CA (triple negative), basal-like CA (triple negative), and micropapillary CA (triple positive). HER2 is overexpressed in several non-mammary carcinomas, including lung and GYN tract. Considering that <30% of breast tumors are positive, HER2 is not generally used as a marker of metastatic breast cancer.
Myoepithelial (ME) markers [variable]	**SMA, Calponin, SMMHC, p63** are the usual ME markers of choice (see below). ME layer is intact in benign and in situ lesions, and is absent in invasive carcinomas. In addition, ME markers may be used to distinguish papilloma (intralesional ME cells present) from papillary carcinoma (intralesional ME cells absent). • False negatives: microglandular adenosis lacks myoepithelial cells • False positives: rare invasive ductal carcinomas focally retain myoepithelial cells

Abbreviations: ADH atypical ductal hyperplasia, ALH atypical lobular hyperplasia, DCIS ductal carcinoma in situ, LCIS lobular carcinoma in situ, SMA smooth muscle actin, SMMHC smooth muscle myosin heavy chain

Markers for Myoepithelial Cells (and what else they stain)				
	SMA (α-actin) [cytoplasmic]	Calponin [cytoplasmic]	SMMHC [cytoplasmic]	p63 [nuclear]
Myoepithelial cells	+	+	+	+
Myofibroblasts	+	–/+	–	–
Vessels, pericytes (smooth muscle)	+	+	+	–

p63 and SMMHC are superior to SMA and Calponin in specificity because they do not react with myofibroblasts (less background). Other myoepithelial markers in use include S100, HMWCK, and CD10.

Abbreviations: SMA smooth muscle actin, SMMHC smooth muscle myosin heavy chain

Reference: [1]

Breast: Immunoprofiles at a Glance	
Diagnosis	Immunoprofile
Breast carcinoma, general	CK7+, CK20–, ER/PR (~60–75%+), GCDFP (~50%+), Mammaglobin (~50%+), HER2 (10–30%+)
Lobular carcinoma (in situ and infiltrating)	loss of E-cadherin, GCDFP (~100%+)
Metaplastic breast carcinoma	CK903+, p63+, variable AE1/AE3, Cam 5.2 and CK7 (most reliable epithelial marker is HMWCK, such as CK903)

N. Rekhtman, J.A. Bishop, *Quick Reference Handbook for Surgical Pathologists*, DOI:10.1007/978-3-642-20086-1_2, © Springer-Verlag Berlin Heidelberg 2011

Breast Differentials

DDx of In Situ Proliferations

	ALH/LCIS	ADH/DCIS	UDH
E-Cadherin	–	+	+
HMWCK (CK903, CK5/6)	+	–	+
ER	+	+ (diffuse)	+/– (patchy)
p120 catenin	cytoplasmic	membranous	

HMWCK represents a marker of "differentiation": expression is present in normal breast epithelium as well as UDH, whereas DCIS shows the loss of differentiation and concurrent loss of HMWCK expression. This may aid in the distinction of UDH from ADH/DCIS, but the gold standard is morphology in H&E. Loss of E-cadherin and presence of mucin vacuoles (rarely used) supports LCIS.
Abbreviations: ADH atypical ductal hyperplasia, ALH atypical lobular hyperplasia, DCIS ductal carcinoma in situ, UDH usual ductal hyperplasia
References: [2,3]

DDx of Papillary Lesions

	Papilloma[1]	Papillary DCIS	Encapsulated papillary carcinoma[2]	Solid papillary carcinoma[3]	Invasion associated with papillary DCIS
Intralesional myoepithelial cells[4]	+	–	–	–	–
Peripheral myoepithelial cells	+	+	–	+/–	– (at the site of invasion)
NE markers and mucicarmine	–	–	–	+/–	–

The above are the "idealized" criteria. In general, IHC is notoriously unreliable in the Dx of papillary lesions, and the distinction mainly relies on morphology.
1) Intralesional myoepithelial cells (MEC) may be focally present in carcinoma and absent in sclerosing papilloma.
2) The entity known as "encapsulated papillary carcinoma" or "intracystic papillary carcinoma" (papillary DCIS-like lesion forming a single mass) is usually negative for peripheral MECs, but whether this represents invasion is controversial.
3) Instead of discrete papillae, fibrovascular cores cut in cross section are seen among a solid cellular proliferation in solid papillary carcinoma. It may or may not have MECs at its periphery. Like encapsulated papillary carcinoma, it is controversial whether it is a form of DCIS or an invasive carcinoma with a pushing border.
4) MEC markers include p63, SMMHC, actin, and calponin.
References: [4,5]

DDx of Low Grade Spindle Cell Proliferations in the Breast

	CK903, p63	SMA	Desmin	ER	Nuclear β-catenin	CD34
Metaplastic carcinoma[1,2]	+	–	–	+/–	–/+	–
Phyllodes tumor (stromal component)	–	–	–	+/–	+/–	+
Fibromatosis	–	+	–/+	–	+	–
Nodular Fasciitis	–	+	–	–	–	–
Myofibroblastoma/pseudoangiomatous stromal hyperplasia/myoid hamartoma	–	+	+	+		+

1) Metaplastic carcinoma is frequently AE1/AE3 and Cam5.2-negative, therefore CK903 and p63 should always be used to rule it out.
2) There is even a "fibromatosis-like" variant of metaplastic carcinoma (!) that is very bland and can stain with myofibroblastic markers, emphasizing that any spindle cell lesion of the breast should be worked up with epithelial markers.
DDx also includes various primary sarcomas (which are uncommon relative to phyllodes tumor and metaplastic CA), most notably angiosarcoma (CD31+, CD34+).
References: [6,7]

DDx of Pagetoid Proliferations in the Nipple

	LMWCK (Cam5.2), EMA	HER2	Mucicarmine	GCDFP	Melanocytic markers[1]	HMWCK (CK903)
Paget's disease of the nipple[2]	+	+ 70–100%	+ 40–70%	+ ~50%	–	–
Melanoma in situ	–	–	–	–	+	–
Bowen's disease (SqCC in situ)	–	–	–	–	–	+

1) Melanoma markers include S100, Melan-A, and HMB45 (S100 is positive in some Paget's cells but HMB45 is always negative).
2) Paget's disease of the nipple ALWAYS has an underlying high grade DCIS; invasive carcinoma is present in ~50% of cases. Paget's cells are CK7+/CK20–. Toker cells are the clear cells in the normal nipple epidermis, which may mimic Paget's; these cells are Cam5.2 (+) but HER2(–) and mucin (–).
Reference: [8]

Prostate and Bladder

Prostate: Key Markers at a Glance	
Marker [compartment]	Applications
PSA & PSAP [cytoplasmic]	In general, PSA (prostate-specific antigen) is more specific and PSAP (Prostate-specific acid phosphatase) more sensitive*. These markers may be used to identify metastatic prostate cancer. They are highly specific for prostate, but are known to cross-react with a few non-prostatic tumors. Most notably, PSAP shows reactivity with rectal carcinoid, which should not be misinterpreted as prostate cancer! In addition, PSA is positive in some salivary gland tumors (especially salivary duct carcinoma). See antibody index for details. * The specificity/sensitivity profile of PSA versus PSAP is related to the type of antibodies commonly used to detect these antigens: PSA antibody (Immunotech) is monoclonal (=more specific), whereas PSAP antibody (Dako) is poly-clonal (=more sensitive).
Prostein (P501S) [cytoplasmic, dot-like], **PSMA** [membranous]	Prostein and PSMA (Prostate Specific Membrane Antigen) are the two newer prostate-specific markers. Prostein is particularly promising for both sensitivity and specificity. Reference: [9]
Basal cell markers: • **p63** [nuclear] • **CK903** [cytoplasmic]	These markers are used to distinguish invasive prostate cancer (basal cells absent) from PIN or adenosis (basal cells present). Note that basal cells are occasionally patchy or even absent in some cases of PIN and adenosis. Therefore stains must be interpreted in the context of morphology. Reference: [10]
Racemase (P504S, AMACR) [cytoplasmic]	**Racemase** is a marker that is overexpressed in prostate cancer cells, both in situ (PIN) and invasive, but is absent in benign cells. There are few exceptions: **Racemase (+) benign lesions:** 10% adenosis, 60% nephrogenic adenoma **Racemase (–) carcinomas:** 20% conventional, 65% foamy, 65% atrophic, 75% pseudohyperplastic Reference: [10]

Prostate: Immunoprofiles at a Glance	
Diagnosis	Immunoprofile
Prostate adenocarcinoma	Prostate-specific markers: PSA, PSAP, Prostein, PSMA Epithelial markers: CK7–/CK20–; Cam5.2+; CK903–
Prostate, Stromal Tumor of Uncertain Malignant Potential (STUMP)	CD34+, PR+, ER usually–, actin –/+, desmin+/– (vs. muscle neoplasms are CD34–)
Prostate, Stromal Sarcoma	same as STUMP, but usually negative for actin and desmin
Prostate and bladder, Inflammatory Myofibroblastic Tumor (IMT)	vimentin+, actin+/–, desmin+/–, CK variable, ALK+ in a subset (2/3)

Prostate and Bladder: Differentials

Reactive Urothelial Atypia vs. Carcinoma in Situ		
	Normal urothelium or reactive urothelial atypia	**Urothelial carcinoma in situ**
p53	–	+ (80%)
CK20	+ in umbrella cells only	+ in all layers
E-cadherin	+ in all layers	– or reduced expression
CD44	+ in basal layer	– or reduced expression
		References: [11,12]

Dx of the Depth of Invasion by Urothelial Carcinoma		
	Muscularis propria (detrusor muscle)	**Muscularis mucosa or Desmoplastic myofibroblasts**
Smoothelin	+ (strong)	– or focal
Vimentin	–	+
Urothelial carcinoma invading the muscularis propria is an indication for cystectomy, while cancers that do not invade detrusor muscle can be managed conservatively.		
		References: [13,14]

DDx of Adenocarcinoma Involving the Bladder		
	Primary Vesical Adenocarcinoma	**Colorectal Adenocarcinoma (metastatic or direct extension)**
β-catenin (nuclear)	– (~100%)	variable (~50% +)
CDX2, CK20	variable	+ (~100%)
Thrombomodulin, CK7	variable	–
Most informative markers are positive β-catenin (= colon primary) or negative CDX2 (= bladder primary). Otherwise, the immunoprofiles are not sufficiently specific and colon primary needs to be ruled out clinically.		
		References: [15,16]

Adenocarcinoma of Bladder and Prostate vs. Mimics			
	Nephrogenic Adenoma	**Primary Vesical Adenocarcinoma[1]**	**Prostate adenocarcinoma**
Racemase	+	–	+
PAX2 or PAX8	+	–	–
PSA, PSMA, Prostein	– (or weak)	–	+
1) The exception is clear cell adenocarcinoma of the bladder, which has the same immunoprofile as nephrogenic adenoma.			
			References: [17–19]

Urothelial Carcinoma vs. High-Grade Prostate Carcinoma		
	Urothelial carcinoma	**Prostate adenocarcinoma**
HMWCK (CK903), p63[1]	+	–
Thrombomodulin, Uroplakin, GATA3[2]	+	–
PSA, PSAP, Prostein, PSMA	–	+
CK7, CK20[3]	usually 7+,20+	usually 7–,20–
1) p63 is more specific (but less sensitive) for urothelial carcinoma than CK903. [20]		
2) Uroplakin is not widely used. It is reported as having a high specificity but low sensitivity.		
3) Strongly CK7+/CK20+ profile favors bladder, whereas CK7 (–) profile is highly unusual for bladder. Any other CK7/CK20 pattern is not informative.		
		References: [10,21]

Kidney and Adrenal

Kidney: Key Markers at a Glance	
Marker [compartment]	Applications
PAX2 and **PAX8**	New pan-RCC markers. PAX8 is broader than PAX2: both label clear cell and papillary RCC; PAX8 also detects chromophobe, medullary, collecting duct carcinomas while PAX2 does not.
CAIX (Carbonic Anhydrase)	When membranous and diffuse is the most sensitive and specific marker of clear cell RCC. CAIX is expressed as a result of VHL mutations in CC-RCC (100% inherited, 75% sporadic). VHL normally regulates the degradation of HIF (hypoxia inducible factor). VHL mutation → ↑HIF → ↑expression of HIF-regulated genes (CAIX, VEGF). Targeted therapies for CC-RCC (Sunitinib) inhibit this pathway, therefore distinction of CC subtype of RCC is important. Focal expression of CAIX may be seen focally in various tumors in areas of necrosis/ischemia (such as in papillary RCC).
RCC, CD10	Older markers of RCC (prior to PAXes and CAIX) – poor sensitivity and specificity.
Epithelial markers	Cam5.2 & AE1/3 are usually positive, but may be variably reactive. Most reliable epithelial marker for RCC is EMA. RCC is CK7–, CK20–.

Kidney: Immunoprofiles at a Glance	
Diagnosis	Immunoprofile
RCC, conventional (clear cell) type	CAIX+ (strong, diffuse)
RCC, papillary type	CAIX-negative (except in areas of necrosis), usually CK7+ and Racemase+
RCC, chromophobe type	Hale's colloidal iron (HCI): chromophobe RCC (blue cytoplasmic staining) vs. oncocytoma (no cytoplasmic staining, though apical blush may be present). EpCam (+) – new marker for chromophobe RCC. c-kit: chromophobe (c-kit +) versus conventional RCC (c-kit –). Usually CK7+. Reference: [22]
Angiomyolipoma (and other PEComas)	**Melanoma markers** (HMB45+ and Melan-A+; S100+ in 30%) and **muscle markers** (actin+, desmin +). Coexpression of melanoma and muscle markers is essentially **pathognomonic** for angiomyolipoma. c-kit+, epithelial markers –. Recently reported that subset is TFE3+, cathepsin-k+ [23]
Mixed epithelial stromal tumor (MEST)	Stromal component ER/PR+, desmin+, SMA+, CD10+
Translocation carcinomas of the kidney	TFE3 [Xp11 translocation], TFEB [t(6;11) translocation], cathepsin-K (both translocations) References: [24,25]
Wilms tumor	Epithelial component: WT1+, CK+, EMA+; Blastemal component: desmin +
Clear cell sarcoma of kidney	Hallmark is absence of any differentiation markers (only vimentin +).

Adrenal: Immunoprofiles at a Glance	
Diagnosis	Immunoprofile
Adrenocortical neoplasms	Melan-A+ (other melanocytic markers, S100 and HMB45, are negative), Inhibin+ CK (AE1/3 and Cam5.2) usually – but may be focally +, EMA– variable SYN and NSE, CHR–
Pheochromocytoma	Neuroendocrine markers (CHR, SYN, NSE, CD56) +, S100+ (sustentacular), CK–
Neuroblastoma/ Ganglioneuroblastoma	Neuroendocrine markers (CHR, SYN, NSE, CD56) + especially in ganglion cells, S100+ in septae, always CD99–

Kidney and Adrenal: Differentials

DDx of Main Types of Renal Cortical Neoplasms				
	Clear Cell RCC	Papillary RCC	Chromophobe RCC	Oncocytoma
PAX2	+	+	–	+
PAX8	+	+	+	+
CAIX (membranous)	+ (strong diffuse)	– (+ in perinecrotic areas)	–	–
CK7	–/+	+ (diffuse)	+ (cytoplasmic, peripheral)	–/+
Racemase	+/–	+ (100%)	–/+	–/+
c-kit	–	–	+	+/–
CD10, RCC	+ (diffuse)	+/–	+/–	–
Vimentin, GST-α	+	+	–	–
EpCam	–/+ (focal)		+ (diffuse)	+/–
Hale's Colloidal Iron	–	–	+	– (+ apical blush)
				References: [26–28]

DDx of Cytologically Bland Renal Tumors with Tubulo-papillary Architecture			
	Papillary RCC (type 1, solid variant)	Metanephric adenoma	Wilms tumor (epithelial-predominant with tubular architecture)
CK7	+ diffuse	–	–/+ (weak/focal)
WT1	–	+	+
Racemase	+	–/+ (weak/focal)	–
CD57	–	+	–
			Reference: [29]

DDx of Renal Tumors with Clear Cells						
	Clear cell RCC	Papillary RCC with clear cells	Chromophobe RCC	Clear cell papillary RCC[1]	Xp11 transloca-tion RCC	Angiomyolipoma
CAIX	++	–	–	+	–/+	–
CD10	+	+/–	–/+	–	+	–
CK7	–	+	+	+	–/+	–
Racemase	–	+	–	–	+	–
c-kit, Hale's Colloidal Iron	–	–	+	–	–	–
TFE3, Cathepsin-K	–	–	–	–	+	–/+
HMB-45, Melan A, Actin	–	–	–	–	–/+	+
Vimentin	+	–	–	–	–	+

1. Clear cell papillary RCC is a recently recognized entity that frequently occurs in the context of end-stage renal disease. It does not have the genetic changes of clear cell RCC (chromosome 3p loss), papillary RCC (trisomy 7 and 17), or Xp11 translocation RCC. It has low grade nuclei that typically show reverse polarization similar to secretory endometrium. [30]

References: [23–25,30–32]

Renal Cell Carcinoma vs. Adrenocortical Neoplasm		
	Renal Cell Carcinoma	Adrenocortical Neoplasms
PAX2, PAX8, CD10, RCC	+	–
EMA	+	–
CK AE1/AE3, Cam 5.2	+ / –	–/+ (generally –)
Melan A (A103), Inhibin	–	+
SYN	–	+
D2-40	–	+
		Reference: [33]

Testis

Testicular Neoplasms: Key Multipurpose Markers at a Glance	
Marker [compartment]	Applications
OCT4 (POU5F1) [nuclear]	Relatively recent stem cell marker, very sensitive and specific for seminoma and embroynal carcinoma. [34]
SOX2 [nuclear]	Relatively recent stem cell marker, expressed in embryonal carcinoma.
SALL4 [nuclear]	Most recent stem cell marker, and a pan-germ cell tumor marker. Primary utility is to identify Yolk Sac Tumors, which are negative for OCT4. Fairly specific to germ cell tumors (also labels leukemic cells, but only rarely expressed in other tumor types). [35]
D2-40 (Podoplanin) [membranous]	Mesothelial and lymphatic marker, which also identifies seminoma (100%+) and embryonal carcinoma (30%+). [36]
Epithelial markers (cytokeratins and EMA)	All non-seminoma germ cell tumors are cytokeratin-positive (though EMA-negative), whereas seminoma (conventional and spermatocytic) are negative for all epithelial markers.

Testicular Neoplasms: Immunoprofiles at a Glance							
	Cam5.2 & AE1/3	EMA	OCT4	SALL4	PLAP	D2-40	Other
Seminoma and ITGCN	–	–	+	+	+	+	PAS+, c-kit+ [1]
Spermatocytic seminoma	–	–	–	+	–	–	PAS–
Embryonal carcinoma	+	–	+	+	+	–/+	CD30+, SOX2+
Yolk sac tumor	+	–	–	+	+	–	α-fetoprotein+ (not specific), Glypican-3 +(focal)
Choriocarcinoma	+	+ (50%)	–	+/–	+/–	–	βHCG+, Inhibin+, hPL+, HLA-G+, Glypican-3+
Teratoma	+	+	–	+/–	–	–	
Sex cord-stromal tumors (Sertoli, Leydig)	– (rare +)[2]	–	–	–	–		Inhibin+, Melan-A+, CD10+, CD99+, Calretinin+

1) c-kit shows membranous staining in seminoma vs. cytoplasmic staining in other germ cell tumors.
2) Although cytokeratins may mark some Sertoli cell tumors and granulosa cell tumors, EMA is always negative.

Abbreviation: ITGCN Intratubular germ cell neoplasia

References: [21,37,38]

Thyroid, Parathyroid, and Sinonasal Tract

Thyroid and Parathyroid Neoplasms: Immunoprofiles at a Glance					
	TTF-1	Thyroglobulin	PAX8[5]	CKs (Cam5.2, AE1/AE3)	Other
Thyroid: Papillary and Follicular CA [1]	+	+	+	+	
Thyroid: Anaplastic CA	–	–	+/–	+ (25% negative[2])	
Thyroid: Medullary CA	+	–	–/+	+	Calcitonin+, mCEA[4]+, NE markers[3]+, amyloid deposits (Congo red +)
Parathyroid neoplasms	–	–	–	+	PTH+, NE markers[3]+ Parafibromin loss in CA[6]

1) CK903, CK19, HBME-1, and Galectin-3 have been reported to favor papillary CA over benign follicular lesions but none of these markers are sensitive or specific enough for routine use.
2) Essentially any malignant spindle cell neoplasm centered in the thyroid should be presumed to be anaplastic CA, regardless of CK positivity. [39]
3) Standard NE markers include SYN, CHR, CD56.
4) Proportion of Calcitonin-negative versus mCEA-positive cells is reported to have an inverse relationship in medullary CA. Expression of CEA (and therefore decreased expression of calcitonin) is postulated to reflect a more aggressive disease. [40]
5) PAX8 is a relatively new thyroid marker (also positive in carcinomas of renal and Mullerian origin) that is positive in about 75% of anaplastic thyroid carcinomas (compared with only rare positivity with TTF-1 and thyroglobulin). [41,42]
6) Parafibromin is a new nuclear marker that is diffusely expressed in sporadic parathyroid adenomas but lost or only weakly/focally expressed in most parathyroid CAs (as well as adenomas of the hyperparathyroidism-jaw tumor syndrome). [43]

DDx of Poorly Differentiated Neoplasms in the Sinonasal Tract				
	Epithelial markers (CK, EMA)	NE Markers (SYN, CHR, CD56)	EBV[1]	Other
Olfactory neuroblastoma/ Esthesioneuroblastoma	–/+ (at most focal)[2]	+ (SYN 100%)	–	S100+ (stromal/sustentacular) cells
Sinonasal undifferentiated carcinoma (SNUC)	+ (LMWCK)[3]	–/+ (SYN in 25%)	–	p63+/–, usually patchy
NUT Midline Transloca- tion Carcinoma	+	–	–	CD34+/–, p63+, NUT+. NUT translocation confirms the diagnosis.
Nasopharyngeal carci- noma (NPC)[4]	+ (HMWCK)[2]	–	+ (especially in lymphoepithelial-type)[5]	p63+
Nasal NK/T-cell lym- phoma (lethal midline granuloma)	–	– (CD56+[6])	+	CD45+, CD2+, cytoplasmic CD3ε+ (pan-T cell markers such as CD3 usually absent), cytotoxic proteins (e.g. perforin)+

1) EBV can be detected by in-situ hybridization (EBER) or IHC for EBV-LMP.
2) Olfactory neuroblastoma can be focally CK+, but EMA should be negative. [44]
3) SNUC shows no squamous differentiation by H&E and is typically HMWCK (CK903, CK5/6)–negative.
4) NPC arises, of course, in nasopharynx but may secondarily involve sinonasal tract. It is a type of squamous cell cancer (HMWCK+).
5) It has been reported that a subset of nasopharyngeal carcinomas are EBV negative but HPV positive [45,46], but these often represent carcinomas extending from the oropharynx [47], where HPV is a well-recognized causative agent. [48]
6) NK/T-cell lymphoma is CD56+ (CD56 is a marker of both NE cells and NK cells).
DDx also includes neoplasms not unique to these sites, including basaloid squamous cell carcinoma (p63, HMWCK), melanoma (S100, HMB45, Melan-A), small cell carcinoma (NE markers, TTF-1), rhabdomyosarcoma (actin, desmin, myogenin), and PNET/Ewing sarcoma (CD99).

References: [49,50]

DDx of Basaloid Carcinomas of the Head and Neck						
	HMWCK	CK7	p63	ME markers other than p63	NE markers	Other
Basaloid squamous cell carcinoma	+	–	+ (diffuse)	–	–	
Adenoid cystic carcinoma (particularly solid pattern)	+	+	+ (peripheral)	+	–	c-kit+
HPV-related squamous cell carcinoma	+	–	+ (diffuse)	–	–	p16+[2], high risk-HPV+[1]
Small cell carcinoma	–	–	+/–[3]	–	+	TTF-1+/–
Basal cell adenocarcinoma (of salivary gland origin)	+/–	+	+ (patchy)	+ (patchy)	–	c-kit +/–

1) Some HPV-related SqCCs are morphologically identical to basaloid SqCC. The distinction is critical, however, because while basaloid SqCC carries a poor prognosis, HPV-related SqCCs respond very well to therapy. HPV-related SqCC almost always arises in the oropharynx. HPV testing is the only way to definitively distinguish the two entities. [51]
2) p16 is sensitive, but not specific, for the diagnosis of HPV-related SqCC.
3) Unlike the situation in the lung, p63 is not consistently negative in small cell carcinoma of the head and neck, and therefore cannot reliably differentiate SmCC from basaloid SqCC. [52]

References: [51–54]

Salivary Gland

Salivary Gland Neoplasms: Immunoprofiles (and Special Stains) at a Glance	
Tumors with epithelial (glandular) and myoepithelial components: adenoid cystic carcinoma, epithelial-myoepithelial carcinoma, pleomorphic adenoma	Epithelial component: CK, EMA, CEA (Lumen: c-kit+) Myoepithelial component: CK, p63, calponin, SMA, S100, GFAP
Mucoepidermoid carcinoma	Mucicarmine+ (goblet cells), p63+ (intermediate cells)
Acinic cell carcinoma	PAS+, PASD+
Oncocytoma, Oncocytic carcinoma	PTAH+
Salivary duct carcinoma	Androgen receptor+ (90%), GCDFP+, HER2 Amplification –/+
Low grade cribriform cystadenocarcinoma	Characteristically S100+
IHC has a limited role (except to confirm myoepithelial differentiation); diagnosis is primarily based on H&E histology.	

References: [55,56]

DDx of Salivary Gland Tumors with Clear Cells	
Epithelial-Myoepithelial Carcinoma	Epithelial component: CK, EMA, CEA (Lumen: c-kit+) Myoepithelial component: CK, p63, Calponin, SMA, S100, GFAP
Mucoepidermoid carcinoma	Mucicarmine+ (goblet cells), p63+ (intermediate cells); negative for ME markers
Acinic cell carcinoma	Clear cells are PAS negative, mucin negative. ME markers negative
Tumors with oncocytic cells (oncocytoma, oncocytic carcinoma, Warthin's tumor)	Clear cells are PAS+/diastase-sensitive, ME markers negative; oncocytic cells are PTAH+ and often c-kit+
Myoepithelioma or Myoepithelial carcinoma	Myopeithelial markers
Clear cell adenocarcinoma	Clear cells PAS+/diastase-sensitive, mucin negative, ME markers negative
Metastatic carcinoma (especially RCC)	Organ specific markers (e.g. PAX8, RCC, CD10 for RCC)
For the most part, appropriate sampling will reveal a component of the tumor that shows classic features for that tumor (i.e., not dominated by clear cells).	

References: [55,56]

Pancreas

Pancreas: Immunoprofiles at a Glance	
Adenocarcinoma	Gene mutation and loss of expression of **DPC4** is found in 55% of pancreatic ca (loss of expression supports the diagnosis of metastases from pancreatic primary, but positive staining does not rule it out). Negative nuclear AND cytoplasmic staining counts as negative. Few other neoplasms show a loss of DPC4, although much less frequently: gallbladder 19%, colon 11%, and 0% ovary, appendix, small bowel, stomach, endocervix [57,58]
	CK7+, CD20+ (usually), CA19.9+, CEA+
Pancreatoblastoma	acinar markers (trypsin, lipase, chymotrypsin), neuroendocrine markers (CHR, NSE, SYN), and ductal markers (CK, CEA)
Mucinous cystic neoplasm	ER+/PR+/ Inhibin+ (ovarian stroma)
Intraductal Papillary Mucinous Neoplasm (IPMN)	MUC1–, MUC2+, CDX2+ (intestinal immunophenotype) vs. **PanIN** (MUC1+, MUC2–, CDX2–). MUC4 present in both. Note that IPMN and IPMN-associated carcinomas have intact DPC4. References: [59,60]
Serous Cystadenoma	CK+, EMA+ (1/3), inhibin+ , MUC-6+, calponin+, CD31 and Factor VIII– (vs. **Lymphangioma**: CK–, EMA–, CD31 and Factor VIII+) References: [61,62]
Lymphoplasmacytic sclerosing (autoimmune) pancreatitis	Infiltration by IgG4+ plasma cells (usually >20/HPF), except in "type 2" which is instead characterized by granulocytic epithelial lesions (GELs). [63] Recent criteria require >50 IgG4+ plasma cell per high-power field for diagnosis. [64]

DDx of Pancreatic Neoplasms with Cellular (no desmoplastic stroma) Acinar/Solid Growth Pattern			
	Pancreatic Neuroendocrine Tumor (formerly Islet cell tumor)	**Acinar Cell Carcinoma (and pancreatoblastoma**)**	**Solid-Pseudopapillary Neoplasm**
Cytokeratins (AE1/AE3, Cam5.2)	+	+	– (30% focally +)
Vimentin	–	–	+ (100%)
NE Markers **(SYN, CHR)**	+	–/+*	–/+ (CHR always negative)
Acinar Markers (trypsin, chymotrypsin, lipase, PAS/D)	–	+ (trypsin/chymotrypsin most sensitive)	–
CD10	– (25% focally +)	–	+
Nuclear β-catenin	–	–/+ (25% +)	+
Hormones (glucacon, insulin, etc)	+ (variable)	–	–
ER/PR	ER – / PR +		ER – / PR +

*   Focal neuroendocrine component is present in up to 40% of acinar cell carcinomas.
** Acinar cell carcinoma and pancreatoblastoma have similar immunoprofile of acinar component (entities distinguished by presence of squamoid nests and younger age of the latter).

Reference: [65]

Tubular Gastrointestinal Tract

DDx for the Site of Origin of Intestinal Metaplasia at the GE junction			
	CK7	CK20	Other
Esophagus (Barrett's mucosa)	+ (surface and deep)	+ (surface only)	Das–1+, MUC1+, MUC2+
Cardia (Intestinal metaplasia of the gastric cardia)	–	+ (variable pattern)	Das–1–, MUC1–, MUC2–

Note that stains are not entirely reliable in this differential; diagnosis mainly relies on clinical information. Some studies show that the risk of malignancy is substantially higher for Barrett's esophagus than for the cardiac intestinal metaplasia.

References: [66–68]

Evaluation of Dysplasia in IBD		
	Nuclear β-catenin	p53
DALM (dysplasia associated lesion or mass)	–	+
Sporadic tubular adenoma	+	– (+ late in disease progression)

The diagnosis of DALM carries a worse prognosis than a tubular adenoma and is treated by resection.

Reference: [69]

Diagnosis of Autoimmune Metaplastic Atrophic Gastritis (AMAG)/ "Pernicious Anemia"

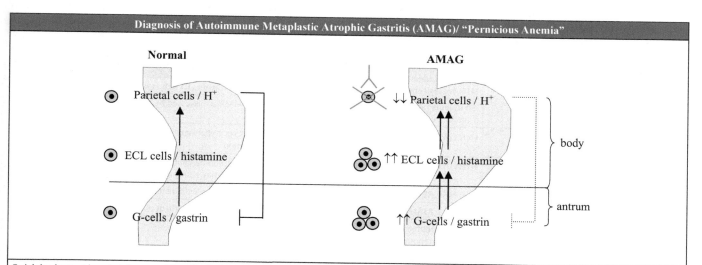

Quick background on Autoimmune Metaplastic Atrophic Gastritis (AMAG):
- Acid is produced by parietal cell, which are located in the gastric body. Acid release is stimulated by gastrin (product of G cells, located in the antrum) through an intermediary action on histamine (product of ECL cells, located in the body).
- AMAG is caused by autoantibodies to parietal cells, which secrete intrinsic factor (IF) in addition to acid. As a result, parietal cells are wiped out and the body begins to look histologically like the antrum (gets "antralized"), except there are no G cells.
- Hypochlorhydria ($\downarrow$H$^+$) causes compensatory increase in antral G cells and hypergastrinemia. High gastrin stimulates ECL cell to grow, which manifests as nodular and linear ECL cell hyperplasia in the body.

Immunostains aid in the diagnosis of AMAG as follows:
- **Chromogranin** (CHR) is a marker of NE cells; it marks both ECL cells in the body and G cells in the antrum. Normally only rare ECL and G cells are present. In contrast, these cells are abundant in the setting of AMAG, which are highlighted by CHR.
- **Gastrin** identifies gastrin-secreting G cells, which are located exclusively the antrum and not in the body (even when the body is "antralized" as a result of AMAG). IHC for gastrin serves two purposes in the diagnosis of AMAG:
  1) Gastrin highlights G cell hyperplasia in the antrum (same as CHR).
  2) Gastrin should be negative in the body: "antralized" body looks identical to the antrum minus the G cells. Negative gastrin stain confirms that the biopsy is indeed taken from the body rather than inadvertently from the antrum.

Immunohistochemical Testing of DNA Mismatch Repair (MMR) Proteins

by Ashlie L Burkart

- Loss of expression of DNA mismatch repair (MMR) proteins can occur by two mechanisms: one is promoter hypermethylation, which silences gene expression and occurs in sporadic colorectal carcinoma (CRC) (10–15% of CRC) [70] and second is germline mutation, which occurs in hereditary cases (aka Lynch Syndrome/HNPCC) (~3% of CRC). [71] Testing for the loss of protein expression is done by IHC as summarized below.

- The consequence of defective MMR is instability of microsatellites (small repetitive sequences of DNA). Testing for microsatellite instability (MSI) is done by PCR. In tumors with defective MMR there is instability in ≥2 out of 5 microsatellite markers (called "MSI-high"). PCR testing is not discussed further here.

- The advantage of IHC is that it tells which MMR protein is defective. There are four main DNA MMR proteins – **MLH1, PMS2, MSH2, MSH6**. If all 4 proteins are utilized, IHC identifies ~95% of tumors with defective MMR. The specificity of IHC is virtually 100%. [71]

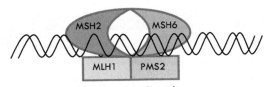

MMR Protein Complex

- There are five possible patterns of NUCLEAR IHC staining for the 4 DNA MMR proteins. Understanding these patterns requires a basic understanding of how these proteins work in pairs.
  - MLH1 and PMS2 are partners, and if MLH1 (the dominant partner) is lost, PMS2 also disappears. On the other hand, if PMS2 is lost, MLH1 persists.
  - Similarly, MSH2 and MSH6 are partners, and if MSH2 (the dominant partner) is lost, MSH6 disappears. On the other hand, if MSH6 is lost, MSH2 persists.

MLH1	PMS2	MSH2	MSH6	IHC Interpretation	Implication for germline mutation (Lynch syndrome) vs. sporadic loss
				Interpretation of IHC for DNA MMR proteins	
+	+	+	+	**No defects** (all DNA MMR proteins expressed)	No evidence of defective MMR as assessed by IHC
–	–	+	+	**Defective MLH1**	~90% sporadic loss (promoter hypermethylation) ~10% germline gene mutation
+	–	+	+	**Defective PMS2**	Germline mutation most common mechanism of gene inactivation (reportedly, rare cases of MLH1 mutations may result in this staining pattern)
+	+	–	–	**Defective MSH2**	Germline mutation most common mechanism of gene inactivation*
+	+	+	–	**Defective MSH6**	Germline mutation most common mechanism of gene inactivation

+ Retained nuclear expression by the invasive adenocarcinoma (expression can be patchy or faint)
– Complete loss of nuclear staining by invasive adenocarcinoma (patchy loss does not count)
* Recent data shows that the loss of MSH2 can be caused either by inherited mutation in MSH2 gene OR inherited deletion of 3' end of *EPCAM gene* leading to inactivation of adjacent MSH2 gene through methylation induction of its promoter.

Note: It is very important to have a positive internal control on the slide to make sure the stain worked properly (such as normal colon epithelial cells, stromal cells or lymphocytes).

Reference: [72]

- Applications:
  - The primary application of IHC for MMR proteins is to screen for Lynch syndrome (to identify patients at higher risk for additional colonic and extracolonic tumors and with at-risk family members).
  - Other applications include evaluation of prognosis and chemosensitivity in sporadic CRC. MMR deficient/MSI-high CRC 1) have a better prognosis per stage, 2) may not have the same response to 5-FU chemotherapy, and 3) may have improved outcome with irinotecan. [71,73,74]
  - Testing of adenomas is controversial. IHC may be performed on adenomas of patients with a clinical concern for Lynch syndrome but normal staining does not exclude Lynch syndrome as the test is less sensitive in adenomas compared to CRC. [75–78]
  - Classically, IHC has been used to test CRC; however other tumors, such as endometrial carcinomas, are now beginning to be included in screening for Lynch syndrome.
  - MMR deficient/MSI-high colorectal (and endometrial) carcinomas have distinct pathologic features (see page 117).

Abbreviations: HNPCC Hereditary nonpolyposis colorectal cancer, CRC colorectal carcinoma, MMR mismatch repair, MSI microsatellite instability

Liver

Hepatocellular carcinoma vs. Cholangiocarcinoma vs. Metastatic Adenocarcinoma			
	Hepatocellular carcinoma	**Cholangiocarcinoma**	**Metastatic adenocarcinoma**
HepPar-1	+ 95% (fairly specific)	–	–
α-FP	+ 30–60% (not specific)	– (rare +)	variable
mCEA	–	+	+
pCEA	+ 80% (canalicular, highly specific)	+ (cytoplasmic)	+ (cytoplasmic)
CD10 and villin	+ (canalicular)	–	site-dependent
CK7	–	+	site-dependent
CK20	– (but up to 20%+)	+ (usually)	site-dependent
CK AE1/AE3 (pan-CK)	– (but 5–20%+)	+	+
Cam 5.2 (LMWCK)	+	+	+
CK903 (HMWCK)	–	+	site-dependent
Glypican-3 and Arginase-1 (new markers of hepatocellular differentiation)	+	–	–
Markers of glandular epithelium: **EMA, MOC-31, Mucicarmine**	–	+	+
other	~50% α1-Antityrpsin+ Cytoplasmic TTF-1+ Fibrolamellar carcinoma is CK7+ and α-FP–	CK19+ (70–100%) There are no good markers which are specific for cholangiocarcinoma (cannot differentiate metastasis by immunostains)	

References: [21,79–81]

Hepatocellular carcinoma vs. Benign Hepatocellular Nodule		
	Hepatocellular carcinoma	**Benign hepatocellular nodules** (adenoma, focal nodule hyperplasia, regenerative nodule in cirrhosis)
Reticulin	thickened hepatocyte plates (> 3-cell thick)	normal thickness of hepatocyte plates (1–2 cell thick)
CD34, Factor VIII	+ ("sinusoidal capillarization")	–
Glypican-3	+	–
p53 (not routine)	–/+	–

References: [82–85]

Lung and Mediastinum

Lung: Immunoprofiles at a Glance								
	TTF-1	Napsin A	CK7	CK20	p63	CK5/6, CK903	NE markers[1]	Other
Non-mucinous adenocarcinoma	85%+	+	+	–	–/+	–/+	–	
Mucinous adenocarcinoma[2]	–/+ (10–20%+)	–/+	+/–	+/–	–/+	–/+	–	May have focal CDX2
Squamous cell carcinoma	–	–	–/+	–	+	+	–	
Small cell carcinoma	90%+[3]	–	–/+	–	–	–	+	Punctate Cam5.2 and AE1/3 Diffuse CK903 or CK5/6 exclude SmCC
Carcinoid	50%+[3]	–	–	–	–	–	+	
Mesothelioma	–	–	+	–	–	+	–	WT1, Calretinin, D2–40

All above entities are AE1/3+ and Cam5.2+, although reactivity is variable in NE tumors (e.g. carcinoid, small cell carcinoma).

1) Standard NE markers include SYN, CHR, NSE and CD56. These may be variably expressed in small cell carcinoma, but morphology trumps the immunophenotype in this diagnosis.
2) Metastatic pancreatic and upper GI adenocarcinoma may be difficult to distinguish from primary lung mucinous adenocarcinoma by either morphology or immunoprofile (both may be CK7+/CK20+ and TTF-1 –). DPC4 may be helpful: it is deleted in 55% of carcinomas of the pancreatic but not lung origin.
3) TTF-1 is not specific for small cell carcinoma of the lung because >40% of extra-pulmonary small cell carcinomas are also TTF-1-positive. In contrast, TTF-1 is positive in pulmonary but usually not intestinal carcinoids.

Common differentials for lung primary carcinoma include:
  – adenocarcinoma (TTF1+/–, p63 variable) vs. squamous cell carcinoma (consistently TTF1-, p63+) [86,87]
  – small cell carcinoma (TTF1+/–, NE marker+/–, p63–, HMWCK–) vs. basaloid SqCC (consistently TTF1–, NE marker–, p63+, HMWCK+)[88]

DDx of Neuroendocrine Neoplasms of the Lung				
	Typical Carcinoid	Atypical Carcinoid	Large Cell Neuroendocrine Carcinoma	Small Cell Carcinoma
TTF-1	+/– (~30%+, weak)		50%+	90%+
Cytokeratins	+/– (~80%+)		+	+ (dot-like)
CHR, SYN, CD56	+ strong diffuse		+ diffuse to focal	+ usually weak focal
Ki67[1]	<2% (mean 1%)	<20% (mean 10%)	>>20% (mean 50%)	>>20% (mean 70%)

1) Ki67 rate is very helpful in evaluating small specimens, particularly if crushed. Carcinoids can have a crush artifact, and can be over interpreted as small cell carcinoma in the absence of Ki67.

Reference: [88]

Carcinoid Tumorlet vs. Minute Meningothelial-like Nodule		
	Carcinoid tumorlet	Minute meningothelial-like nodule ("chemodectoma-like body")
CHR, SYN	+	–
CK	+	–
EMA	+	+
PR	–	+

Reference: [89]

DDx of Thymic Epithelial Neoplasms					
	TdT, CD99, CD1a (markers of immature/thymic T lymphocytes)	CD5 (dual marker of T cells and malignant thymic epithelium)	c-kit	GLUT1	Cytokeratins
Thymoma	+ (lymphocytes)	+ (lymphocytes only)	–	–	+ (epithelium)
Thymic carcinoma*	–	+ (epithelium & lymphocytes)	+ (epithelium)	+	+ (epithelium)
Non-thymic carcinoma	–	–	–/+	–/+	+

* Epithelial cells in thymic carcinoma are also positive for CD70 [90]

References: [91–93]

Mesothelioma

Mesothelioma vs. Adenocarcinoma			
		Mesothelioma [1]	Adenocarcinoma
Immunohistochemistry	Mesothelial markers		
		Calretinin +	–
		WT1 +	–
		CK5/6 +	–
		Thrombomodulin (CD141) +	–
		HBME-1[#], N-Cadherin[#], D2-40[#], Mesothelin[#] +/–	–/+
	Adenocarcinoma markers		
		TTF-1, Napsin A – (always)	+/–
		BerEP4 –	+/–
		mCEA –/+	+/–
		CD15 (Leu-M1) –	+
		B72.3[#], BG8[#], MOC-31[#] –/+	+/–
	Epithelial markers		
		EMA –/+ (membranous)	+/– (cytoplasmic)
		Cytokeratins (AE1/3, Cam5.2) [2] + perinuclear accentuation	+ peripheral (membrane) accentuation
Special stains [3]			
		Mucicarmine –	+/–
		PAS → PAS/Diastase + → –	+ → +
		AB →AB/hyaluronidase + → –	+ → +
EM		Length of microvilli	
		long (length to width ratio >10:1)	short

A standard panel includes mesothelial markers (Calretinin, WT1, CK5/6) versus adenocarcinoma markers (TTF-1, Napsin A, BerEP4 +/– mucicarmine).

[#] indicates markers which are reported as variably useful, and not as widely used.

1) This immunoprofile applies primarily to epithelioid mesothelioma. In contrast, sarcomatoid mesothelioma is usually less reactive or negative for mesothelial markers (cytokeratin positivity is consistently retained).

2) Both mesothelioma and adenocarcinoma are CK7+/CK20–.

3) Special stains distinguish mucin (mucicarcmine+, PAS+) produced by some adenocarcinoma from hyaluronic acid (AB+/hyaluronidase sensitive) and glycogen (PAS+/diastase sensitive) produced by mesothelioma.

References: [21,94,95]

DDx Malignant vs. Reactive Mesothelial Proliferations		
	Mesothelioma	Reactive mesothelial proliferations
p53, EMA, CD146	+	–
Desmin	–	+
GLUT1*	+	–

There markers are reported as variably useful. In practice, the distinction of malignant from reactive mesothelial proliferations is based on morphologic criteria.

*   GLUT1 also positive in lung carcinoma.

References: [96–98]

Immunostains: Organ Systems

Soft Tissue

Select Mesenchymal Tumors: Immunoprofile at a Glance		
Diagnosis	*Immunophenotype*	*Genetic markers*
Adenomatoid tumor	calretinin+, epithelial markers (CK, EMA) +	
Alveolar soft part sarcoma	nuclear TFE3+; desmin (focal in 50%), actin (10%), S100 (25%); PAS+/Diastase Resistant rhomboid cytoplasmic crystals (pathognomonic by EM)	
Angiomatoid fibrous histiocytoma	Desmin+ (50%), CD68+/–	FUS/TLS-ATF1 EWS-ATF1
Clear Cell Sarcoma of Tendon Sheath/ Melanoma of Soft Parts	S100+, HMB45+, Melan-A+ (generally, HMB45 and Melan-A are not as high as in melanoma)	EWS-ATF1
Dermatofibroma	Factor XIIIa+/D2-40+/CD34– (vs. **DFSP**: Factor XIIIa–/D240–/CD34+)	
Epithelioid sarcoma	CK+ (strong), EMA+, CD34+ (50%), CEA+ (focal), vimentin+ (CK and CD34 co-expression is **unique** to epithelioid sarcoma and epithelioid angiosarcoma) Loss of INI1 (hSNF5/BAF47) expression [99]	
Ewing sarcoma/PNET	CD99+, focal CK+ in 20% (SYN/NSE+ favors PNET)	EWS-FLI1 EWS-ERG
Fibromatosis (myofibroblastic differentiation)	nuclear β-catenin+ (only deep but not in superficial fibromatoses are positive), actin+, CD34– (vs. solitary fibrous tumor: actin–, CD34+), c-kit variable; abdominal fibromatosis ER/PR +	
Gastrointestinal stromal tumor (GIST)	c-kit+ (>95%, diffuse staining), DOG1, CD34+ (70%), bcl2+, actin+ (30%)	c-kit, PDGFRA mutations
Glomus tumor	SMA+, calponin+, caldesmon+, desmin–, pericellular type IV collagen	
Granular cell tumor	S100+, CD68+, Inhibin+, PAS+	
Hemangiopericytoma	CD34+(often weak/focal), bcl2+, EMA–	
Inflammatory myofibroblastic tumor (IMT)	ALK+ (35%), actin* (80%) , desmin (40%), vimentin, CK+/– *actins have distinctive "tram track" pattern (peripheral cytoplasmic accentuation) in IMT, whereas actins in smooth muscle tumors have diffuse cytoplasmic distribution	
Desmoplastic small round cell tumor	Polyphenotypic marker expression: WT1+, CK+, EMA+, desmin+ (dot-like), actin–, NSE+, SYN–, CHR–, CD99 variable	EWS-WT1
Leiomyoma/ Leiomyosarcoma	desmin, actin, caldesmon, variable Cam5.2+ (aberrant reactivity in LMS)	
Nodular Fasciitis (myofibroblastic differentiation)	SMA+, calponin+; desmin–, caldesmon– (vs. LMS: caldesmon +)	
PEComas	Smooth muscle (SMA+, desmin+/–) and melanocytic differentiation (HMB45+, Melan-A+, MITF+, S100 –/+), c-kit+, cathepsin-K+, TFE3+ (subset)	TFE3 rearrangements or amplification in a subset [23]
Rhabdomyosarcoma	Desmin+, MSA+, myogenin+ (alveolar >> embryonal), MyoD, PAX5+ in translocation+ alveolar RMS, CD99+ in a subset; p53+ in anaplastic RMS; muscle marker expression is typically focal	Alveolar – PAX3-FKHR PAX7-FKHR
Solitary Fibrous Tumor	CD34+, bcl2+, muscle markers (SMA/desmin)–, c-kit–, EMA–	
Synovial Sarcoma (SS)	TLE1 – new excellent marker for SS (focal reactivity in schwannoma, GIST, other) [100,101] always CD34–, bcl2+, focal CK+, focal EMA+, calponin+, S100+ in 30%; always desmin–; poorly differentiated SS is usually CD99+	SYT-SSX1 SYT-SSX2
Abbreviations: MSA muscle specific actin, PNET peripheral neuroectodermal tumor		

Central Nervous System

Reviewer: Jason Huse
Please see "Primer on Markers of Neuroglial Differentiation" for marker overview.

Tumors/Lesions of Central Nervous System (CNS) at a Glance	
Gliomas (astrocytoma, oligodendroglioma, ependymoma)	GFAP + and reticulin – except pleomorphic xanthoastrocytoma (PXA), which is reticulin +. See below for DDx of astrocytoma vs. oligodendroglioma
Meningioma	EMA+ (but CK–), Progesterone Receptor + (>50%), S100 variable • **Fibrous meningioma**: S100+ (80%) • **Secretory meningioma**: CK+ (>50%), cytoplasmic inclusions are CEA+ and PAS+
Neuronal/glioneuronal/ neurocytic neoplasms	Generally neuronal cells are SYN+, Neurofilament/Sm32+ (NeuN works best for normal neurons, but it is not as reliable for tumors) • **Gangliocytoma**: SYN/Sm32/NeuN+ • **Ganglioglioma**: neurons (SYN/Sm32+/NeuN+) & glia (GFAP+) • **Central neurocytoma**: SYN+, usually NeuN+, may be GFAP+
Primitive neuroectodermal neoplasms	All SYN+ • **Medulloblastoma**: may show divergent differentiation – neuronal (SYN+) and/or glial (GFAP+) • **PNET** (primitive neuroectodermal tumor): SYN+ & GFAP+ (unlike PNET of soft tissues, CD99 is negative in the brain!)
Atypical teratoid/rhabdoid tumor (AT/RT)	INI1 (hSNF5/BAF47) – loss of expression (due to 22q11 deletion); EMA+, GFAP+, CK+, vimentin+, SMA+, variable SYN & CHR
Dysembryoplastic neuroepithelial tumor (DNT)	S100+, NeuN focally+, SYN–
Pituitary neoplasms	SYN+, CHR+, hormones (ACTH, GH, PRL, etc)
Pineal neoplasms	SYN+
Choroid plexus tumors	CK+, EMA–, S100+ (may be focal in carcinoma), patchy GFAP in minority, usually transthyretin +
Demyelinating disorders	Luxol fast blue (myelin stain) – rarely used, NF staining should reveal relative axonal preservation
Reticulin in CNS at a glance	**Negative:** all gliomas (except PXA), meningioma, SFT. **Pericellular:** HPC, fibrosarcoma, schwannoma, PXA, lymphoma, sarcomatous areas of gliosarcoma. **Nested:** hemangioblastoma, pituitary (enlarged irregular lobules in adenoma vs. small nests in normal).

CNS: Differentials

Astrocytoma vs. Oligodendroglioma		
	Astrocytoma	**Oligodendroglioma**
GFAP	+	variable
p53[1]	+ (in 30% of cases)	–
1p/19q deletion[2]	– (vast majority of cases)	+ (most cases)

1) p53 may be used to distinguish astrocytoma (p53+ in ~30% of cases) from oligodendroglioma (p53–).
2) 1p/19q deletion is specific for oligodendroglioma: molecular detection of this deletion is used to confirm the diagnosis.

References: [102,103]

DDx of Clear Cell Nested Tumors in CNS		
	Hemangioblastoma	**Metastatic Renal Cell Carcinoma**
Inhibin	+	–
EMA, Cytokeratin	–	+ (CK is variable)
PAX2/8, CAIX, RCC, CD10	–	+
Reticulin (nested and pericellular)	+	–
Other	Oil red O+ (requires unfixed tissue), Aquaporin-1+, NSE (variable)	

References: [104–108]

DDx of Dural-Based Spindle Cell Tumors			
	Meningioma (fibrous)	**Solitary Fibrous Tumor**	**Melanocytoma**
EMA, Progesterone Receptor	+	–	–
CD34, bcl-2	–	+	–
Melanocytic markers	–	–	+

DDx of Myxoid and Chondromyxoid Lesions of the CNS/Coverings				
	Chordoma	**Myxoid Chondrosarcoma**	**Myxopapillary ependymoma**	**Chondroid meningioma**
Cytokeratin	+	–	–	–
EMA	+	–	–	+
GFAP	–	–	+	–
S100	+	+/–	+/–	–
D2-40	–	+	+/–	+/–
Brachyury	+	–	–	–
Typical location	Sacrum, Clivus (extra-dural)	Bone and soft tissue	Filum terminale (intra-dural)	Dural
Also exclude metastatic mucinous adenocarcinoma!				References: [109–111]

Gynecologic Tract

Reviewer: Anna Ymelyanova

Gynecologic Tract: Key Markers at a Glance	
Marker [localization]	Applications
ER/PR [nuclear]	ER/PR are used to identify metastasis from the GYN tract. ER/PR expression is highest in endometrioid carcinoma (>90% of cases) and is lower in serous carcinoma (50% of cases). HPV-related cervical adenocarcinomas are negative, which may be used to differentiate cervical from endometrial primary.
WT1 [nuclear]	WT1 (Wilms Tumor 1 protein) is expressed in serous carcinoma of the ovary and serves as a good marker for ovary as a source of a carcinoma of unknown primary. Note that nuclear WT1 is also present in benign and neoplastic mesothelium. If needed, calretinin, PAX8, and ER/PR may be used to distinguish a serous carcinoma (calretinin–/PAX8+/ER+/PR+) from a mesothelioma (calretinin+ /PAX8–/ER–/PR–).
PAX8 [nuclear]	Novel pan-Mullerian (endometrial and ovarian) marker. Also expressed in renal and thyroid carcinomas. Useful in the differential of ER/PR positive tumors, e.g. breast vs. gynecologic (breast is PAX8 negative)
p53 [nuclear]	p53 is a tumor suppressor protein. Overexpression of p53 is seen in many malignant tumors. It seems counterintuitive that a tumor suppressor would be overexpressed in a malignancy. It turns out that p53 protein is mutated in those tumors, and overexpression is a reflection of defective degradation of a mutant p53. Although not specific for a particular tumor, robust overexpression of p53 is used as a marker of serous carcinoma and its putative precursor tubal intraepithelial carcinoma (TIC).
p16 [nuclear and cytoplasmic]	In GYN tract p16 it is used in two different settings: One use of p16 is as a surrogate marker of high-risk HPV infection. As such, p16 is used to distinguish SIL (p16+) from atypical squamous metaplasia (p16–), as well as cervical adenocarcinoma (p16+) from endometrioid carcinoma (p16– or focal). Because the majority of LSIL are associated with high-risk HPV, p16 is NOT used to determine the grade of SIL. Second use of p16 is unrelated to HPV. Analogously to p53, diffuse overexpression of p16 is a feature of serous carcinoma and may be used to distinguish serous carcinoma (p16 strong, diffuse) from endometrioid carcinoma (p16 negative or focal).
ProExC [nuclear]	ProExC is a new marker of cellular proliferation that is composed of 2 monoclonal antibodies specific for topoisomerase II alpha and minichromosome maintenance protein 2. It is used by some institutions in a manner similar to, or in combination with, Ki67 and/or p16 in distinguishing HPV-related vs. unrelated lesions. [112–114]

Gynecologic Tract: Immunoprofiles at a Glance (All carcinomas of GYN tract are CK7+ and CK20–)	
Diagnosis	Immunoprofile
Uterus, endometrioid carcinoma	PAX8+, ER+/PR+(>90%), p16 (negative or patchy), CA125+
Uterus, serous carcinoma	PAX8+, ER/PR (50%+), p53 and p16 (diffuse; p53 in nearly every cell), ↑↑ Ki67 Unlike ovarian serous carcinoma, WT1 usually (–) in serous carcinoma of endometrial origin.
Ovary, serous carcinoma	PAX8+, WT1+, ER/PR (50%+) [vs. breast ca: also ER/PR+ but PAX8–, WT1–, GCDFP (2/3+)] and [vs. mesothelioma: also WT1+ but PAX8–, calretinin+] <div align="right">References: [115–117]</div>
Ovary, mucinous neoplasms	CK7+, CK20– (or focal), CDX2– (or focal) [vs. metastasis from lower GI adenocarcinoma: CK7–, CK20+, CDX2+]
Ovary, clear cell carcinoma	HNF-1beta+ (can be seen in endometrial clear cell carcinoma and small proportion of non-clear cell endometrial carcinomas)
Ovary, sex cord-stromal tumors (Granulosa Cell tumor, Sertoli/ Leydig cell tumors, Thecoma, Fibroma)	Classic markers: Inhibin+, Melan-A+, CD10+, CD99+, Calretinin+ New markers: SF1+ [118] and FOXL2 Epithelial markers: CK (–) or patchy, EMA– <div align="right">References: [119,120]</div>
Cervix, adenocarcinoma	HPV in situ and p16+ (diffuse), p53 (completely negative or focal, not all cells like serous CA), ↑↑ Ki67, ER/PR-negative or weak
Endometriosis (any site)	ER/PR+ (both glands and stroma), CD10+ (stroma)

Ovarian Germ Cell Tumors at a Glance								
	PLAP	c-kit	OCT-4	SALL4	D2-40	Cam 5.2 & AE1/3	EMA	Other
Dysgerminoma (counterpart to testicular seminoma)	+	+	+	+	+	–	–	PAS+, OCT4 (POU5F1)+
Embryonal carcinoma	+	–	+	+	–/+	+	–	CD30+
Yolk sac tumor	+	–	–	+	–	+	–	α-FP+ (not specific)
Choriocarcinoma	+/–	–	–	+/–	–	+	+ (50%)	βHCG+, Inhibin+, hPL+, CD146+ (in intermediate trophoblast cells)

Gynecologic Tract: Differentials

DDx of Dysplastic vs. Reactive Squamous Intraepithelial Lesions (SIL) of the Cervix

	High grade squamous intraepithelial lesion (HSIL)	Atypical Immature Metaplasia (& normal squamous mucosa)
p16 and HPV (in situ hybridization)	+	–
Ki67	+++ (extending up to the surface)	rare + (parabasal cells only or only rare cells above the parabasal area)

p16 (nuclear and cytoplasmic stain) indicates that high risk HPV is present. p16 does NOT distinguish most low-grade squamous intraepithelial lesions (LSIL) from HSIL because ~80% of LSIL and all HSIL harbor high risk HPV.
Same panel may be used to distinguish adenocarcinoma in situ (p16+, ↑↑ Ki67) from benign mimics, such as microglandular hyperplasia and tubal metaplasia (p16–, ↓Ki67).

DDx of Uterine Carcinomas

	Endometrioid carcinoma	Serous carcinoma	Clear Cell Carcinoma
ER/PR	+ (>90%)	+/– (50%)	–/+
Ki67	low	high	intermediate (variable, can be low)
p53	–/+ (patchy/rare weakly + cells)	+++ (diffuse)	–
p16	–/+ (patchy)	+++ (diffuse)	+/–
HNF-1beta	–	–	+
WT1	–	+ in the ovary, but –/+ in endometrium	–

Note that in serous carcinoma, expression of p16 is unrelated to HPV. Here overexpression of p16 is used analogously to p53, in that it is an indicator of a highly proliferative malignancy. PAX8 is positive if all of the above carcinomas.

References: [121–124]

Endometrial vs. Endocervical Adenocarcinoma

	Endometrioid carcinoma	Endocervical adenocarcinoma
p16 and HPV in situ hybridization	– (patchy p16)	+++ (diffuse)
ER/PR	+	– (or low)
CEA (low specificity)	–	+
Vimentin (low specificity)	+	–

DDx of Uterine Spindle Cell Neoplasms

	Smooth muscle tumors of the uterus (leiomyoma and leiomyosarcoma)	Endometrial stromal tumors of the uterus (endometrial stromal nodule and endometrial stromal sarcoma)	Uterine tumors resembling ovarian sex cord tumors (UTROSCT)
SMA and Desmin	+	–/+	+/–
h-Caldesmon[1]	+	–	–
CD10	–/+	+	+/– (focal)
ER/PR	+	+	+
Sex-cord stromal markers (CD99, Inhibin, Calretinin, Melan-A)	–	–	+/– (calretinin is most sensitive)
Cytokeratins	–/+	–	+/–
JAZF1-JJAZ1 gene fusion	–	+/– (50%)	–

1) h-Caldesmon is the most sensitive and specific marker for the above DDx.

References: [125–127]

DDx of Serous Tubal Intraepithelial Carcinoma (TIC)

	Tubal Intraepithelial Carcinoma (TIC)	Stratified benign tubal epithelium
p53	+	– (rare weakly positive cells)
Ki67	high	low

Reference: [128]

DDx of Ovarian Tumors with Tubular/Trabecular Pattern

	Sertoli Cell Tumor/ Granulosa cell tumor	Endometrioid Carcinoma	Carcinoid tumor	Struma Ovarii
Sex cord-stromal markers (CD99, Inhibin, Calretinin, Melan-A)	+ (variable)	–	–	–
EMA	–	+	variable	+
Neuroendocrine markers (SYN, CHR)	– (variable)	–	+	–
TTF-1, Thyroglobulin	–	–	–	+

Reference: [129]

Gynecologic Tract: Differentials – continued

	DDx of Trophoblastic Tumors[1]				
	Tumors of Implantation Site Intermediate Trophoblast		Tumors of Chorionic-type Intermediate Trophoblast		Tumor of Mixed-type Intermediate Trophoblast
	Exaggerated Placental Site	Placental Site Trophoblastic Tumor	Placental Site Nodule	Epithelioid Trophoblastic Tumor	Choriocarcinoma
hPL, Mel-CAM (CD146)	+++		–/+		+ (in IT and CT)
p63	–		+++		+ (in CT)
Ki67	<1%	>8%	<8%	>10%	>50%
Other			Cyclin E–	Cyclin E++	hCG+ (in ST)

1) All types of trophoblastic cells (ST, CT, IT) are + for CKs, CK18, Inhibin, and HLA-G.
2) HSD3B1 is a new marker that is positive in IT and ST in all trophoblastic tumors

Abbreviations: IT intermediate trophoblast, ST syncytiotrophoblast , CT cytotrophoblast

Reference: [130]

	DDx of Hydatidiform Moles[1]		
	Complete mole	Partial mole	Hydropic abortus
Cytogenetics	XX or XY (both paternal)	XXY or XXX (2:1 paternal:maternal)	Normal or variable
p57(KIP2)[2] – paternally imprinted gene, transcribed entirely from a maternal allele	Loss of expression	Intact expression	Intact expression

1) Hydatidiform moles are lesions of trophoblastic tissue (CK+, Inhibin+, HLA–G+).
2) p57 is a paternally imprinted gene, which is normally transcribed entirely from a maternal allele. Complete moles contain paternal DNA only and therefore show the loss of expression of p57 (in villous stroma and villous cytotrophoblast), whereas maternal tissue (decidua) and intermediate trophoblast (IT) islands retain expression and serve as internal positive controls (retained expression in IT is surprising because these are fetal cells, but this is proposed to be due to incomplete imprinting in this cell type). In contrast, p57 expression is intact in partial moles and in a hydropic abortus.

References: [131,132]

Skin

by Janis Taube, Natasha Rekhtman, Justin Bishop

Key Melanocytic Markers at a Glance	
S100	• Most sensitive marker of melanocyte differentiation (>95% of all melanomas, including desmoplastic melanoma). • Normal melanocytes are positive. • Not specific—seen in dendritic cells, cartilage tumors, nerve sheath tumors, myoepithelial tumors, etc.
HMB45	• Antibody to gp100. • Normal melanocytes are negative. • In conventional nevocellular nevi, junctional nests, papillary dermal nests, and nests around adnexal structures are positive. Lost with increasing dermal depth, consistent with maturation. • Blue nevi show more diffuse positivity. • Melanomas tend to show relatively patchy superficial and deep staining. • Non-specific—PEComa family, pheochromocytomas, gliosarcomas (generally not in DDx of melanocytic lesions)
Melan-A (A103)	• Antibody to MART-1. • Normal melanocytes are positive. • Stains more nevi and more cells per nevi than HMB45. • Expression does not vary by maturation status throughout a lesion. • Non-specific—PEComa family, steroid hormone producing cells (adrenal, ovarian, Leydig, Sertoli).
MITF	• Since transcription factor, is a nuclear stain. • Normal intraepidermal melanocytes are positive. • Non-specific staining of macrophages limits its use in lymph node. MITF is most reliable when assessing intraepidermal melanocytic proliferations. Reference: [133]
SOX10	• Newly described transcription factor (nuclear stain) target • Early results suggest increased specificity over MITF, in that it lacks non-specific macrophage staining • Particular useful for the evaluation of desmoplastic melanoma (+) vs. scar (−) • May have sensitivity of S100 with improved specificity, additional studies needed. References: [134,135]

General reference: [136]

Select Skin Lesions: Immunoprofiles at a Glance	
Melanoma (epithelioid)	S100+, HMB45+, Melan-A+, MITF+, AE1/3− – Melan-A is more sensitive than HMB45 for epithelioid melanoma – Beware of pitfalls in sentinel node evaluation: S100 reacts with dendritic cells, and HMB45 may react with melanophages and rarely nodal nevi. Melan-A is most specific. [137]
Melanoma (desmoplastic)	S100+, HMB45−, Melan-A−
Mycosis Fungoides (MF)	T cells (CD45+, CD3+, CD20−) often with aberrant loss of T-cell markers (CD2, CD5, and CD7). Vast majority are of T-helper cell origin (CD4+), and rare cases are of a cytotoxic T-cell origin (CD8+). Normally CD4:CD8 ratio is ~2:1, but this ratio is abnormally elevated in MF. Clonal T cell receptor (TCR) gene rearrangement may be of assistance. In early stage disease, the differential diagnosis includes reactive inflammatory infiltrates, which are also often CD4-predominant, demonstrate loss of CD7, and can show clonal gene rearrangements. Clinical-pathologic correlation is of great utility in securing a definitive diagnosis. Additionally, matching T-cell clones from two separate biopsy sites can increase specificity for the diagnosis of MF. Reference: [138]
Granuloma annulare and lupus erythematosus	PAS-AB or colloidal iron highlight interstitial mucin
Urticaria pigmentosum (and other mast cell diseases)	immunostain (c-kit) and special stains (Giemsa, Tryptase, Toluidine blue, Leder's)

Skin: Differentials

DDx of Melanocytic Lesions		
	Melanoma	Intradermal nevus
HMB45*	Superficial and deep cells	Superficial cells only (deep/mature nevocytes are negative)
Ki67	+++	− (rare cells +)

* HMB45 is a marker of immature melanocytes. In benign nevus, there is diminution of HMB45 from the surface (immature, HMB45-positive cells) toward the base (mature, HMB45-negative cells). In contrast, no maturation is seen in melanoma (both superficial and deep cells are HMB45+).

S100 and Melan-A react with both immature and mature melanocytes. Therefore these markers are uniformly positive in both nevus and melanoma and cannot be used to differentiate the two lesions.

Reference: [136]

Skin: Differentials – continued

DDx of Cutaneous Storiform Spindle Cell Lesions		
	Dermatofibroma (DF)	Dermatofibrosarcoma protuberans (DFSP)
Factor XIIIa	+	–
CD34	–	+
D2-40	+	–

Reference: [139]

DDx of Cutaneous High-Grade Neuroendocrine Carcinomas		
	Merkel cell carcinoma	Metastatic small cell carcinoma
CK20	+ (dot-like peri-nuclear pattern)	–
TTF-1	–	+
Neurofilament	+ (100%)	–
NE markers (SYN, CHR, NSE)	+	+
Cytokeratins (AE1/3, Cam5.2)	+	+
Merkel cell polyomavirus*	+	–

* Viral antigen can be detected by IHC (recent data). [140]

DDx of Ugly-Looking Spindle Cell Neoplasms of the Skin				
	Atypical Fibroxanthoma (AFX) *	True sarcoma (e.g. MFH, leiomyosarcoma)	Spindle cell variant of SqCC (sarcomatoid carcinoma)	Melanoma
Cytokeratins, p63	–	–	+	–
Melanoma markers (especially S100)	–	–	–	+
CD10	+	–	–	–
Actin, Desmin	–	–/+	–/+	–

* AFX is especially likely in sun-exposed areas, especially of the head and neck.

References: [141–143]

DDx of Pagetoid Proliferations in the Skin			
Squamous cell carcinoma in situ (Bowen's disease)	Melanoma in Situ	Sebaceous carcinoma	Paget's disease (see table below for subtypes)
HMWCK (CK903) +	S100+, Melan A+, HMB 45+, MITF+	BerEP4+, EMA+, CK7+	LMWCK (Cam 5.2) +, Mucin+, PAS-AB+ EMA+, CEA+/– Nipple: GCDFP+, HER2+, ER+

DDx of Mammary vs. Extra-mammary Paget's Disease				
	GCDFP[1]	ER, HER2	CK7	CK20, CDX2
Mammary Paget's disease (always secondary)	+/– (~50%+)	+/–	+	–
Extra-mammary (anal or vulvar) Paget's disease – PRIMARY (aka "apocrine intraepidermal adenocarcinoma")	+/– (~30%+)	–	+	–
Extra-mammary (anal or vulvar) Paget's disease – SECONDARY (= Paget's with an underlying anorectal, urothelial or cervical carcinoma)	–	–	variable[2]	variable[2]

Note: Primary Paget's disease = apocrine intraepidermal adenocarcinoma vs secondary Paget's = epidermis colonized by an underlying malignancy (breast, anorectal, bladder, cervix). Mammary Paget's disease always has an underlying DCIS; invasive carcinoma is present in ~50% of cases. Similarly, anal Paget's is usually secondary, whereas Paget's disease of the vulva is usually primary.

1) GCDFP is a marker of breast epithelium as well as apocrine cells in general; hence both mammary and extra-mammary Paget's are (+).

2) CK7/CK20 pattern of Paget's cells reflects an underlying neoplasm: urothelial CA (CK7+/CK20+) vs. anorectal CA (CK7variable/CK20+ plus CDX2+) vs. cervical CA (CK7+/CK20–). In general, positive CK20 and negative GCDFP suggest that Paget's disease is secondary rather than primary.

References: [8,144]

Cutaneous Lymphomas

by Janis Taube

	CD3	CD4	CD8	Cyto-toxic mark-ers[1]	CD56	βF1	EBV	T cell receptor gene rearrangements	other
Classification of Cutaneous T Cell Lymphomas (CTCLs) other than MF/Sezary Syndrome and Primary Cutaneous CD30+ Lymphoproliferative Disorders*									
Subcutaneous panniculitis-like T-cell lymphoma (SPTL)[4]	+	–	+	+	–	+	–	+	
Extranodal NK/T-cell lymphoma, nasal type	+ (cytoplasmic, not surface)	–	–	+	+	–	+	–	Latent membrane protein (LMP)+/– CD2+, CD5–
CD4+CD56+ hematodermic neoplasm/ Plasmacytoid dendritic cell tumor[5]	–	+	–	–	+	–	–	–	CD123+,TCL1+, MPO–[2] CD43+, CD7+/–, CD2+/–, CD45RA+, TdT+/–, CD68+/–,
Adult T-cell Leukemia/ Lymphoma	+	+ (rare–)	(rare+)	–	–/+	+	–/+	+	CD25+, serologies for HTLV-1+ CD2+, CD5+, CD7–
Aggressive epidermotrophic CD8+ CTCL[6]	+	–	+	+	–	+	–	+	CD45 RA+/– CD45 RO– CD2–/+, CD5–, CD7+/–
Cutaneous γ/δ T-cell lymphoma	+	–	– (rare+)	+	+	–	–	+ (of γ chain)[3]	CD2+, CD5–, CD7 +/–
Primary cutaneous CD4+ small/medium-sized T-cell lymphoma[6]	+	+	–	–	– (rare+)	+	–	+	May have loss of pan-T-cell markers
Primary cutaneous peripheral T-cell lymphoma, NOS[7]	+	+	–	– (rare+)	+/–	+	–	+	Variable loss of pan-T-cell markers

* In many of these entities, a diagnosis of mycosis fungoides should be excluded by history and clinical exam.
1) Cytotoxic markers include TIA-1, granzyme, perforin.
2) Need MPO– to exclude myeloblastic entities which have significant overlap.
3) TCR-β is not expressed secondary to rearrangement or deletion.
4) Must be restricted to the subcutaneous tissue (no dermal and/or epidermal involvement), and only cases with an α–β T-cell phenotype (cases expressing γ phenotype are classified as primary cutaneous γ/δ T cell lymphoma).
5) Derived from precursors of plasmacytoid dendritic cells, thus related to myeloid neoplasms, but listed here due to CD4+.
6) Provisional entities by WHO classification
7) Primary cutaneous peripheral T-cell lymphoma NOS is reserved for those entities which do not fall into any of the above categories.

Reference: [145]

	CD20 or CD79a	Bcl-2	Bcl-6	CD10	MUM1	Monotypic κ or λ[1]	Other
Classification of Primary Cutaneous B-cell Lymphomas							
Primary cutaneous MZL[2]	+	+	–	–	–	+	IgM+/–, CD5–, CD23–, CD43+/–
Primary cutaneous FCL[3]	+	– (staining is weak if present)	+	+/– (diffuse lesions more often CD10–)	–	–	CD5–, CD43– IgM– (cytoplasmic)
Primary cutaneous DLBCL, Leg-type	+	+	+/–	–	+	+	IgM+ (cytoplasmic)

1) If monotypia cannot be demonstrated by stains for kappa or lambda, consider IgH gene rearrangement studies.
2) May be associated with reactive germinal centers, which are Bcl6+, CD10+, and Bcl2–.
3) Strong expression of Bcl2 and CD10 should raise suspicion for secondary cutaneous involvement by nodal follicular lymphoma

In a B-cell lymphoma, the demonstration of a B-cell clone by PCR is helpful, although two different biopsies may show two different clones. T-cell clones are less helpful singularly, but if matched are more meaningful.

Abbreviations: MZL marginal zone lymphoma, FCL follicle center lymphoma, DLBCL diffuse large B cell lymphoma

Reference: [145]

Hematopoietic System

by Amy Duffield, Justin Bishop, Tara Miller, Ross Miller, Natasha Rekhtman

Hematopoietic Markers at a Glance	
Pan-hematopoietic	CD45/LCA (Leukocyte Common Antigen)*
B cell markers:	(also see diagram on B-cell development)
Pan-B cell	CD19, CD20, CD22, CD79a, PAX5. CD79a is the widest pan-B cell marker (see diagram on B-cell development). Note: B-cells in patients who have been recently treated with Rituximab (anti-CD20 antibody) will not stain with CD20
Naïve B cell	CD5+, CD23+ (origin of a subset of CLL) CD19, CD20, CD22, CD79a, PAX5. Note: CD5+ B-cells can be increased in children and patients with rheumatologic disorders
Mantle cell	CD5+, CD23– (origin of MCL) CD19, CD20, CD22, CD79a, PAX5, Bcl-2
Germinal center cell	CD10+, Bcl6+, Bcl-2– (germinal center cells are the origin of FL, many DLBCLs, and Burkitt lymphoma) CD19, CD20, CD22, CD79a, PAX5 Note: Bcl-2 is not expressed by the B-cells in germinal centers, although it is positive on scattered T-cells in the germinal centers. The expression of Bcl-2 on germinal center B-cells in follicular lymphoma is due to the BCL2-IGH translocation [t(14;18)].
Plasma cell	CD138, Ig κ or λ light chain, CD38 (bright), MUM1, CD79a. Normal κ:λ ratio is 2–3:1 Negative for CD45. Abnormal plasma cells may aberrantly express CD19, CD20 (dim), CD56, c-kit and CD10.
Follicular dendritic cell	CD21, CD23, CD35, Clusterin, Fascin
Pan-T cell	CD2, CD3, CD5, CD7, CD43 Mature T-cells express either CD4 or CD8 (see diagram on T-cell development)
NK cell	CD56+, cytotoxic proteins (perforin, granzyme B, TIA-1)+; negative for pan-T cell markers (CD3, CD5); cytoplasmic CD3ε+ (origin of nasal type NK/T cell lymphoma)
Activated B or T cell	CD30, CD25 Note: large CD30-positive cells may be immunoblasts (i.e. activated B-cells) and are not necessarily Reed-Sternberg cells
Myeloid cells	Myeloperoxidase (MPO), CD43, *CD11b, CD13, CD15, CD33* CD34 and/or c-kit are positive in myeloid progenitor cells (myeloid blasts)
Monocyte (histiocyte)	CD4, CD68, CD163, Lysozyme, HAM56, MAC 387, *CD11b, CD14, CD15, CD64* Note: the expression of CD4 on histiocytes tends to be somewhat dimmer than the expression of CD4 on CD4+ T-cells
Megakaryocyte	Factor VIII, *CD41 (GPIIb), CD42b (GP1b alpha), CD61 (GPIIIa)*
Erythrocyte	Hemoglobin A, spectrin, *Glycophorin (CD235a), Transferrin (CD71)*
Mast cell	c-kit, mast cell tryptase, Giemsa (special stain). Neoplastic mast cells are CD2+ and CD25+.

* Several hematopoietic entities are CD45 negative: R-S cells in Classical Hodgkin, B- & T-lymphoblastic lymphoma (variable), ALCL (variable), plasma cell neoplasms, follicular dendritic cell sarcoma, granulocytic sarcoma (variable). If a hematopoietic neoplasm is suspected but CD45 is negative, CD43 is a useful marker as it is also positive in many hematologic neoplasms.
The *italicized markers* may only be available by flow cytometry.

Markers for Identification of Blasts							
	CD34	**TdT**	**CD10**	**c-kit**	**HLA-DR**	**Lineage-specific markers**	**sIG**
Myeloblast[1]	+/–	– (rarely + in M0)	– (rarely +)	+/–	+/–	CD13, CD33, CD15, CD11b, c-kit	–
B-lymphoblast[2]	+ (may be –)	+	+ (occasionally –)	–	+ (rarely –)	CD19, CD79a, CD20 (+/–)	– (or dim +)
T-lymphoblast	+/–	+	+/–	– (very rarely +)	– (rarely +)	CD3 (often cytoplasmic only)	–

1) CD34 and/or c-kit are typically present in AML, although some forms of AML may be entirely negative for CD34 and c-kit, notably AML with monocytic differentiation. Most AMLs express HLA-DR, but some myeloid leukemias [i.e. acute promyelocytic (M3) and AML with NPM1 mutations and cup-like nuclear invaginations] are HLA-DR negative.
Myeloid sarcoma (chloroma) can be identified by immunostains for blast markers (CD34, c-kit), myeloid/monocytic markers (MPO, Lysozyme), and CD43.
2) DDx: Burkitt lymphoma has a mature B cell phenotype (sIG+ i.e. kappa or lambda+, CD20+, CD10+, Bcl-2–) and is negative for blast markers (CD34, TdT).
3) Mast cells are intensely c-kit+ and often have small processes extending from the cells; blasts are less intensely c-kit+

Cytochemistry for Identification of Blasts*		
Type of Blast	**Stain**	**Comment**
Myeloblast (neutrophil precursor)	Myeloperoxidase (MPO) Sudan Black B (SBB) Chloracetate esterase (Leder stain)	Flow cytometry is more sensitive than cytochemistry in the detection of MPO
Monoblast	Nonspecific esterase (α Naphthyl Acetate and Butyrate)	Reactivity is inhibited by sodium fluoride (NaF).
Lymphoblast, Erythroblast, Megakaryoblast	PAS	Erythroblasts show chunky globular staining. Burkitt lymphoma is PAS-negative.
Burkitt lymphoma (mature B cell phenotype)	Oil Red O	Oil Red O highlights lipid vacuoles.

* These methods have been largely supplanted by flow cytometry and immunohistochemistry.

Reference: [145]

Stages of Lymphocyte Differentiation and Corresponding Lymphomas

Normal stages of B cell development and corresponding lymphomas

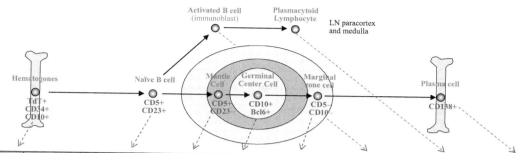

Cell of origin	Progenitor B-cell	Precursor B-cell	Naïve B cell	Mantle cell	Germinal center (centroblast → centrocyte)	Marginal zone cell (memory B cell)	Activated B cell (immunoblast)	Plasmacy-toid Lym-phocyte	Plasma cell
Corresponding Lymphoma/ Leukemia	B-ALL	B-ALL	CLL/SLL (some) [5+10–23+]	MCL [5+10–23–]	FL, Burkitt, many DLBCL (GC-type) [5–10+Bcl6+]	MZL [5–10–]	some DLBCL (non-GC type)	LPL	Myeloma
CD45	–/dim	–/dim	+	+	+	+	+	+	–
TdT	+	+	–	–	–	–	–	–	–
CD34	+	+/–	–	–	–	–	–	–	–
CD19, PAX5	+	+	+	+	+	+	+	+/–	–
CD20	–	–/dim	+	+	+	+	+	+/–	–
CD79a	+	+	+	+	+	+	+	+	+
CD5	–	–*	+	+	–	–	–	–	–
CD23	–	–	+	–	–	–	–	–	–
CD10	–/+	+	–	–	+	–	–	–	–
Bcl-6	–	–	–	–	+	–	–	–	–
CD138	–	–	–	–	–	–	–	+	+
cIg	–	µ chains	–/weak +					+ (IgM)	+ (IgG, A)
sIg	–	–*	+ (IgD, M)		+ (Ig M, G, A)			+/– (IgM)	–

* A subset of hematogones can express dim CD5 or surface light chain; however, this is typically only appreciated by flow cytometry

Normal stages of T cell development and corresponding lymphomas

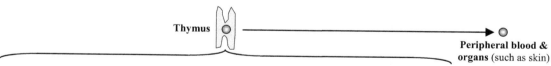

Cell of origin	Pro-T cell	Pre-T cell	Cortical Thymocyte	Medullary T-cell	Mature T-cell
Corresponding Lymphoma	T Lymphoblastic Lymphoma				Peripheral T cell lymphoma
CD45	dim/+	dim/+	dim/+	dim/+	+
TdT*	+	+	+/–	–/+	–
CD34	–/+	+/–	–	–	–
CD1a	–	–	+	–	–
CD2	–	+	+	+	+
CD7	+	+	+	+	+
Cytoplasmic CD3	+	+	+	+	+
Surface CD3	–	–	–	+	+
CD4, CD8	Double negative	Double negative	Double positive	Single positive	Single positive

* CD99 expression is often seen in TdT positive neoplasms; an immunostain for CD99 may aid in the identification of T-lymphoblasts

Reference: [145]

Normal Stages of B Cell Development, Immunostains and Corresponding Lymphomas

Diagram created by Tara Miller, Ross Miller, Amy Duffield, Natasha Rekhtman.
Illustrator Terry Helms.

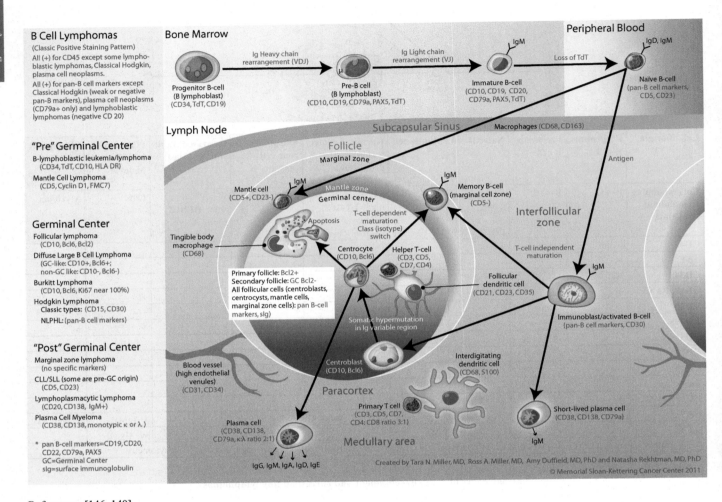

References: [146–149]

B cell Lymphomas

Reactive Hyperplasia versus Follicular Lymphoma		
	Reactive Follicular Hyperplasia	**Follicular lymphoma (FL)**
BCL2 in germinal center cells[1]	–	+ (90%)[3]
Germinal center markers (CD10, BCL6)	Restricted to germinal centers	Germinal centers and interfollicular zones
Ki67 staining (proliferation index)	Very high; polarized	Lower (except in high grade tumors)
Monoclonal κ or λ light chain restriction (best determined by flow)	–[2]	+
Morphology	Polarized follicles of varying sizes with distinct mantle zones. The germinal centers contain mitotic figures and tingible body macrophages.	Atypical follicles are uniform and tightly packed with attenuated poorly-defined mantle zones. Follicles may extend into the perinodal fat. In low grade FL (WHO 1–2) the atypical follicles lack tingible body macrophages and mitotic figures are rare.

1) Do not mistake primary (resting) follicles for FL based on Bcl-2 expression: primary follicles are composed entirely of mantle cells (Bcl-2+), but these follicles do not have germinal center cells and are negative for CD10 and Bcl-6. In addition, primary follicles are IgD-positive, whereas FL is IgD-negative.

2) Occasionally florid follicular hyperplasia may show light chain restriction, particularly in children or adolescents.

3) Bcl-2 can be negative in high grade FL, pediatric FL or cutaneous FL.

Low-grade B cell lymphomas (LGBCL) All LGBCLs are positive for CD45, pan-B markers CD19/20/22/79a and sIg							
	CD10 Bcl6	**Bcl-2**	**CD5**	**CD23**	**CD43**	**Other markers and molecular**	**Morphology**
CLL/SLL[1]	–	+	+	+	+/–	CD38+ and ZAP-70+: adverse prognosis *Flow: small FMC7– B-cells, light chain dim, CD20 dim*	Involves lymph nodes. Proliferation centers or scattered larger prolympho-cytes.
MCL	–	+	+	–	+/–	Bcl-1 (CyclinD1)[2] +; blastoid variant is also CyclinD1+ *Flow:small FMC7+ B-cells, light chain bright, CD20 bright* t(11;14)(CCND1-IgH)	Monotonous – no large neoplastic lymphocytes.
FL	+[3]	+[4] (90%)	–	–	– (rare +)	*Flow: small-medium size light chain restricted CD10+ B-cells* t(14;18)(IgH-BCL2)	Mixture of small (centrocytes) and large (centroblasts) cells.
MZL	–	+/–	–	–	–/+ (30%)[5]	There is no specific marker for MZL. *Flow:often mixture of neoplastic& non-neoplastic B-cells; may be CD23+*	Variable numbers of large cells. Mono-cytoid cells can be prominent.
LPL	–	+/–	–	–	–/+ (20%)	CD20, CD138+ (plasmacytic cells), IgM+, sIG (κ or λ) *Flow: light chain restricted small B-cells + plasma cells*	
HCL	–		–	–		CD20+, CD22+, CD25+, TRAP+ (cytochemical stain) *Flow: CD20 bright, CD22 bright, CD103+, CD11c+, CD25+; very few monocytes in PB or BM*	Rarely involves lymph nodes. Uniform cells with abundant clear cytoplasm.

1) Two prognostic subgroups of CLL/SLL are recognized:
   a. *Pre-GC (naïve) B-cell type* – unmutated IgV_H, CD38+, ZAP-70+, associated with 17p (10%) or 11q (25%) deletions, poor prognosis.
   b. *Post-GC center type* – mutated IgV_H, CD38–, ZAP-70–, associated with isolated 13q deletion, good prognosis.
2) Cyclin D1 is not specific for MCL; it is also expressed in other LGBCL, including HCL (50%) and LPL. It is also expressed in the blastoid variant of MCL (100%).
3) Interfollicular neoplastic lymphocytes may lose CD10 and Bcl-6 expression and some high grade FLs are CD10-negative.
4) Bcl-2 differentiates FL (Bcl-2+) from reactive follicles (Bcl-2–). Bcl-2 may be negative in a subset of FL, particularly in high grade FL, pediatric FL and cutaneous FL.
5) CD43 is positive in approximately 50% of nodal MZL and gastric & salivary gland MALT MZL. CD43 is less frequently + in MZL in other soft tissue sites and skin. CD43 is typically – in splenic MZL. CD43 expression can be seen in non-neoplastic B-cells in the terminal ileum.

Quick marker overview:
- CD10 and Bcl-6 are markers of germinal center B cells (origin of FL, Burkitt lymphoma and some DLBCL).
- CD5 and CD23 are markers of naïve B cells (origin of CLL/SLL). CD23 (along with CD21) also marks follicular dendritic cell network. CD5 is present in normal T cells.
- CD43 is a T cell marker, but may be aberrantly expressed in all LGBCLs (very rare in FL).
- Assessment of light chain expression by immunohistochemistry is often not possible in LGBCL (except LPL and MZL or other LGBCL with plasmacytic differentiation); flow cytometry is a preferred method.

Typical panel (CLL, MCL): CD20, CD3, CD5, CD23, Cyclin D1, Ki67
Typical panel (FL): CD20, CD3, CD10, Bcl-6, Bcl-2, Ki67
Typical panel (MZL): CD20, CD3, CD43, Ki67; if there is plasmacytic differentiation then add kappa and lambda light chain
Typical panel(LPL): CD20, CD3, CD43,kappa,lambda, Ki67, IgM, IgG, IgA
Typical panel (HCL): CD20, CD3, CD10, CD5,CD23, CD22, CD25, Ki67. HCL is difficult to Dx using immunohistochemistry alone; flow cytometric analysis of the peripheral blood is recommended since even if there is not clinically evident leukemia it is usually possible to identify a small population of hairy cells.

Reference: [145]

Hodgkin Lymphoma and DDx of Plasma Cell-Rich Neoplasms

Hodgkin Lymphoma (HL)		
	Classical HL (Nodular Sclerosis, Mixed Cellularity, Lymphocyte Rich, Lymphocyte Depleted)	**Nodular lymphocyte predominant HL (NLPHL)**
Neoplastic cells — **Designation**	Reed-Sternberg/ Hodgkin cells and variants	Lymphocyte predominant (LP) cells or "popcorn cells" [formerly called L&H cells]
Pan B-cell markers (CD45, CD20, PAX5, OCT2/Bob.1)	CD45–, weak PAX5+ & OCT2+ 5–10% show weak CD20+ (should be noted in report)	CD45+, strong PAX5 & OCT2 strong CD20
Classical R-S cell markers (CD15+, CD30+, Fascin+)	+ *occasionally R-S cells are CD15–	–
EMA	–	+ (50%)
EBV (EBER in situ hybridization preferred)	~50% + (esp. MC-HL ~75% +)	–
Background cells	• T cells and mixed inflammatory cells i.e. eosinophils, plasma cells, neutrophils, histiocytes (varies with the subtype). • The appropriate background of inflammatory cells is required for a diagnosis of HL i.e. R-S cells in a background of CLL/SLL is *not* considered HL. • If there are bands of fibrosis, prominent aggregates of R-S cells and patchy necrosis then consider the "syncytial variant" of NSHL.	• Abundant small B cells (CD20+). • T cells (CD3+, CD57+) surround LP cells forming "T-cell rosettes." • Expanded nodular dendritic cell meshworks (CD21 & CD23 positive).
Differential Diagnosis	• Angioimmunoblastic T-cell lymphoma: prominent vascular proliferation, partial effacement of nodal architecture, no true R-S/Hodgkin cells (CD30+ cells are immunoblasts and lack CD15) • ALCL: Hallmark cells, neoplastic cells are CD30+, CD15–, ALK+ (often) and fascin +	• T-cell/histiocyte rich large B-cell lymphoma (THRLBCL): few small B-cells in the background, lacks nodular architecture, T-cell "rosettes" are not present. It may be difficult to distinguish THRLBCL from NLPHL on core biopsies. Neoplastic cells in both THRLBCL and NLPHL show variable EMA+.

Typical immunostain panel for HL: CD30, CD15, CD20, CD3, EBV (EBER in situ hybridization preferred); if initial panel is non-diagnostic add CD45 and Pax-5

Typical immunostain panel for NLPHL: CD30, CD15, CD20, CD3, EMA, CD57, CD21 (or CD23), EBV (EBER in situ hybridization preferred)

DDx of Plasma Cell-Rich Neoplasms				
	Plasma Cell Neoplasm (Myeloma, Plasmacytoma)	**Lymphoplasmacytic lymphoma (LPL)[2]**	**Marginal zone lymphoma (MZL)[2]**	**Plasmablastic Lymphoma[3]**
CD20, PAX5, CD45	– (5%+)	+	+	–
CD79	+	+	+	+/– (50–85%)
CD38, CD138, MUM1	+	+ (may be patchy)	+/–	+
CD43	–/+	–/+	–/+	–
CD56	+/–[1]	–	–	–
Cytoplasmic immunoglobulins	+	+ (patchy); usually IgM	+/–	+/– (50–70%)
EBV, HIV association	–	–	–	+ (EBER in situ hybridization +)
Bone marrow involvement	+	+	–/+	–
Extra-medullary/extra-skeletal sites (visceral organs, lymph nodes, soft tissue)	Rare	+/–	+	+

1) Plasma cell leukemias are often CD56–

2) LPL and MZL may be very difficult to differentiate; in this case a diagnosis of small B-cell lymphoma with plasmacytic differentiation is appropriate.

3) Plasmablastic lymphoma also tends to be CD30+ and have a very high proliferation index (Ki67>90%)

Note: Occasionally other low grade B-cell lymphomas such as FL and CLL/SLL can show plasmacytic differentiation.

Reference: [146–149]

Hematopoietic System: Select Immunoprofiles

Immunoprofiles of Select Hematopoietic Disorders: B-cell and Plasma Cell Neoplasms	
Diagnosis	Immunoprofile
B lymphoblastic lymphoma/leukemia	CD19+, CD22+, PAX5+, CD79a+, TdT+ CD10: usually + but may be –, CD20 variable, CD34 variable, CD45: dim or – Note: expression of sIG (dim), CD13, or CD33 may be seen on flow cytometric analysis *Typical panel: CD45, CD3, CD20, CD19 (or CD79a, CD22 or PAX5), CD10, MPO, CD34, TdT, Ki67*
Burkitt lymphoma t(8;14)(MYC-IGH) t(8;22)(MYC-IGL) t(2;8) (MYC-IGK)	CD45+, pan B-cell markers (CD19/20/22/79a/PAX5)+, CD10+, Bcl6+, Ki67 near 100%, sIg+, Bcl-2–; Oil Red O+. Negative blast markers (TdT–, CD34–). *Typical panel: CD3, CD20, CD10, Bcl-6, Bcl-2, Ki67*
Diffuse large B cell lymphoma, NOS (DLBCL)	CD45+, pan B-cell markers (CD19/20/22/79a/PAX5)+ CD20 reactivity is lost in DLBCL treated with Rituximab (anti-CD20 antibody), but CD19, CD22 and CD79a remain (+). Variable expression of CD10, CD15, Bcl-6 and Bcl-2 Usually sIG+, Ki67 typically >40–50% Based on recent gene expression profiling, two types of DLBCL are now recognized: 1) Germinal center B-cell-like DLBCL (better prognosis) and 2) Non-germinal center (Activated) B-cell-like DLBCL (worse prognosis) A 3-marker algorithm to distinguish the two has been proposed: [150,151] An updated, 5-marker algorithm that incorporates FOXP1 has shown higher accuracy. [152] Note: DLBCLs rarely express CD5, but if CD5 is positive in a high-grade mature B-cell neoplasm then the specimen should be stained for CyclinD1 to rule out the blastoid variant of mantle cell lymphoma. *Typical panel: CD3, CD 20, CD 10, Bcl-6, Bcl-2, CD5, Ki67, MUM1 (if treated with Rituximab add CD79a, PAX5 or CD19), DLBCL lymphoma can be diagnosed on small biopsies using an abbreviated panel of CD3, CD20, and Ki67.*
Blastoid variant of mantle cell lymphoma t(11;14) (CCND1-IGH)	CD45+, pan B-cell markers (CD19/20/22/79a/PAX5)+ CD5+ (rarely –), Cyclin D1+, CD10+/–, sIG+ Note: the blastoid variant of mantle cell lymphoma may be leukemic. If the disease involves the peripheral blood it typically demonstrates a dimorphic population of circulating tumor cells (small mature lymphocytes and blast-like cells). *Typical panel: CD3, CD 20, CD 10, Bcl-6, Bcl-2, CD5, Cyclin D1, Ki67*
Primary mediastinal (thymic) large B-cell lymphoma	CD45+, pan B-cell markers (CD19/20/22/79a/PAX5)+ CD30+ (>80%; weak & heterogenous), MUM1+ (75%), CD23+ (70%) Variable expression of CD10, CD15, Bcl-6 and Bcl-2 Surface Ig – (best evaluated by flow cytometry) *Typical panel: CD3, CD 20, CD 10, Bcl-6, Bcl-2, MUM1, CD30, CD23, Ki67*
B-cell lymphoma, unclassifiable, with features intermediate between DLBCL and Burkitt lymphoma*	CD45+, pan B-cell markers (CD19/20/22/79a/PAX5)+ and a) Immunophenotye consistent with Burkitt (CD10+, Bcl-6+, Bcl-2–, MUM1– or weak) & very high proliferation index by Ki67 immunostain with morphologic features consistent with DLBCL or b) Morphologic features of Burkitt lymphoma with an immunophenotype consistent with DLBCL (i.e. Bcl-2+, Ki67 labeling <90%) Note: Some of these lymphomas may have a *MYC* translocation, but the translocation partner is typically not *IGH* as in Burkitt. Lymphomas that have a *MYC* translocation but otherwise resemble DLBCL should not be placed in this category. *Typical panel: CD3, CD 20, CD 10, Bcl-6, Bcl-2, MUM1, Ki67*
B-cell lymphoma, unclassifiable, with features intermediate between DLBCL and classical Hodgkin lymphoma	CD45+, pan B-cell markers (CD19/20/22/79a/PAX5)+ Bcl-6 +/–, CD10–; usually CD30+, CD15+ Note: Typically has overlapping morphologic features of Hodgkin lymphoma and DLBCL (particularly primary mediastinal large B-cell lymphoma); most frequently presents as a mediastinal mass. *Typical panel: CD3, CD 20, CD 10, Bcl-6, Bcl-2, MUM1, CD30, CD15, CD23, Ki67, EBER*
Plasma cell neoplasms	CD138+, CD38+, MUM1, EMA+, Ig κ or λ light chain restriction; CD79a+ but often negative for other pan-B markers (CD19, 20, 22 , 20), Cyclin D1 +/–, CD43 –/+; CD45 and CK show occasional patchy staining. CD56, c-kit, CD10 or dim CD20 may be aberrantly expressed in neoplastic plasma cells. If frequent mitotic figures, apoptotic cells and prominent nucleoli are seen then rule out plasmablastic lymphoma (EBER+). *Typical panel: CD138, κ, λ*

Hematopoietic System: Select Immunoprofiles – continued

Immunoprofiles of Select Hematopoietic Disorders: T-cell Neoplasms	
Precursor T lymphoblastic lymphoma/leukemia	TdT+, cytoplasmic CD3 usually +, CD7 usually + Often CD4/CD8 double positive or double negative Variable expression of CD2, surface CD3, CD5, CD34, CD10, CD99, CD1a and CD45. Occasionally positive for CD79a, CD33, CD13, c-kit, CD56. *Typical panel: CD3, CD20, CD4, CD8, CD7, CD34, TdT, CD1a, CD99, CD10, Ki67*
Anaplastic large cell lymphoma (ALCL) ALK+ ALCL:t(2;5)(NMP-ALK)	CD45 and CD45RO are variable, usually CD43+ Always CD30+ (intense membranous and paranuclear "target-like" pattern) but almost entirely CD15-negative. At least some T-cell antigens are + (CD2, CD4 or CD5) but CD3 and CD8 are usually absent. Cytotoxic proteins (TIA-1, granzyme, perforin) are often +, CD25+, EMA+/−. ALK+ 60–85% (ALK+ patients are younger and do better than ALK− patients). Primary skin ALCL is ALK− but has a good prognosis; this diagnosis requires clinical correlation. *Typical panel: CD 3, CD 4, CD 5, CD 7, CD 8, CD 20, CD 30, CD15, ALK*
Peripheral T-cell lymphoma, NOS	CD3+, CD4>CD8 (rarely double positive), loss or dim expression of CD5, CD4, CD7 and/or CD8 CD30+/−, CD56+/−, typically T cell receptor βF1+ (T-cell receptor β chain), high proliferation index (Ki67) CD10−, EBV− *Typical panel: CD3, CD20, CD4, CD5, CD7, CD8, CD30, Ki67*
Angioimmunoblastic T-cell lymphoma	Neoplastic T-cells: CD3+, CD4+; may see some loss of CD5 or CD7; at least a subset of the T-cells are CD10+ (and Bcl-6+) Background B-cells and plasma cells are polyclonal & immunoblasts are CD20+, CD30+, CD15− Usually EBV+ (EBER in situ hybridization preferred) Expanded dendritic cell meshworks: CD21+, CD23+ *Typical panel: CD20, CD3, CD4, CD5, CD7, CD8, CD10, CD30, CD15, CD21 (or CD23), EBER*
Hepatosplenic T-cell lymphoma Isochromosome 7q	CD3+, CD56 +/−, CD8+/1, TIA-1+, granzyme B−, CD4−, CD5−, EBV− Usually T cell receptor βF1− (tumor cells are most often of the γδ T-cell receptor type and do not express T cell receptor αβ) although some are αβ type Spleen: diffuse involvement of red pulp and sinusoids Bone marrow: characteristic sinusoidal distribution of tumor cells *Typical panel: CD3, CD20, CD4, CD5, CD6, CD7, CD8, CD56, TIA-1, granzyme B, βF1, EBER*
Cutaneous T-cell lymphoma (Mycosis Fungoides)	T cell antigens (CD3+, CD2+) with abnormal CD4/CD8 ratio (usually CD4>>CD8) and aberrant loss of some T-cell markers (CD7 and/or CD5). Expression of CD30 is associated with histologic transformation. Loss of CD26 is seen on flow cytometric analysis. *Typical panel: CD 3, CD 20, CD 4, CD 8, CD 5, CD 7*

Immunoprofiles of Select Hematopoietic Disorders: Other	
Extranodal NK/T-cell lymphoma, nasal type	NK-cell (CD56+, CD3−) or T-cell (CD56−, CD3+) phenotype; cytoplasmic CD3ε+; cytotoxic proteins+ (e.g. perforin, TIA-1, granzyme B), EBV+, CD45+, CD43+. Negative for CD4, CD5, CD8, CD57. Occasionally positive for CD7 or CD30. *Typical panel: CD45, CD3, CD20, CD4, CD5, CD7, CD8, CD56, CD 57, TIA-1, EBER*
Myeloid sarcoma (granulocytic sarcoma, chloroma)	Most myeloid sarcomas are CD43+. Blast markers (CD34, c-kit, TdT), CD99, and CD45 are variable. *Myeloid (granulocytic) sarcoma:* CD13, CD33, CD15, MPO, c-kit *Monoblastic chloroma:* CD14, CD64, CD11b, lysozyme (typically negative for the blast markers CD34 & c-kit) *Typical panel: CD45, CD43, MPO, Lysozyme, CD34, c-kit; also CD3 & CD20 (to rule out lymphoma)*
Paroxysmal Nocturnal hemoglobinuria (PNH)	Deficiency of glycophosphatidylinositol (GPI)-anchored proteins is best detected by flow cytometry. Red blood cells: loss of CD59 (preferred) and CD55 Monocytes: loss of CD14 & CD55; failure to bind FLAER* Granulocyte: loss of CD16 & CD24; failure to bind FLAER * *Fluorescent aerolysin (FLAER) is a protein that binds specifically to the GPI anchor. Absence of FLAER binding to WBCs is the most sensitive measure of PNH, and can be detected using flow cytometry

Hematopoietic System: Select Immunoprofiles – continued

DDx of Post-transplant lymphoproliferative disorders (PTLD)				
	Definition	Site of involvement	Morphology	Immunophenotype
Early lesions: • Plasmacytic hyperplasia (PH) • Infectious mononucleosis-like (IM)	Lymphoid proliferation WITH architectural preservation of underlying tissue	Typically tonsils and adenoids	Dense polymorphic infiltrate of lymphoid tissue	Polyclonal B-cells & plasma cells. PH is typically EBV+ IM-like are nearly always EBV+
Polymorphic	• Polymorphic lesions that form destructive masses • Do not meet the criteria for a recognized type of high-grade lymphoma	Lymph nodes or extranodal sites	Neoplastic cells show a full range of B-cell maturation; patchy necrosis and mitoses may be present	B-cells:may be polyclonal or rarely monoclonal Nearly always EBV+
Monomorphic	Lymphoma in an allograft recipient that meets the criteria for a recognized type of high-grade lymphoma* (DLBCL, Burkitt, plasma cell neoplasm, T/NK cell or HL)[1]	Lymph nodes or extranodal sites	See criteria for specific lymphomas. "Monomorphic" does not imply cellular monotony but rather indicates that nearly all of the cells are transformed	See criteria for DLBCL, Burkitt, plasma cell neoplasm, T/NK cell or HL. B-cell neoplasms: many cases are CD30+ and EBV+ T-cell neoplasms: ~33% EBV+ HL: nearly all EBV+

* It is important to provide a diagnosis of monomophic PTLD rather than only listing the type of lymphoma because the treatment options differ; i.e. PTLD may respond to decreased immunosupression.

1) Indolent lymphomas (i.e. FL, CLL/SLL, MZL) arising in allograft recipients are not considered PTLD.

Immunostains:

Histiocytic and Dendritic Cell Lesions

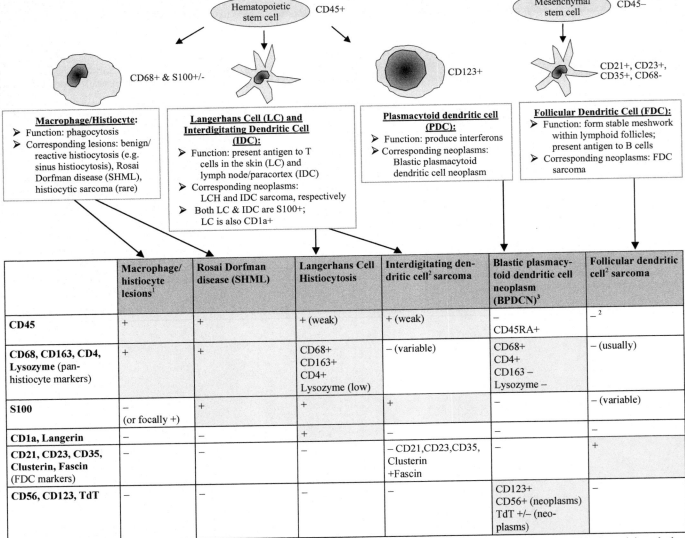

	Macrophage/ histiocyte lesions[1]	Rosai Dorfman disease (SHML)	Langerhans Cell Histiocytosis	Interdigitating dendritic cell[2] sarcoma	Blastic plasmacy-toid dendritic cell neoplasm (BPDCN)[3]	Follicular dendritic cell[2] sarcoma
CD45	+	+	+ (weak)	+ (weak)	– CD45RA+	–[2]
CD68, CD163, CD4, Lysozyme (pan-histiocyte markers)	+	+	CD68+ CD163+ CD4+ Lysozyme (low)	– (variable)	CD68+ CD4+ CD163 – Lysozyme –	– (usually)
S100	– (or focally +)	+	+	+	–	– (variable)
CD1a, Langerin	–	–	+	–	–	–
CD21, CD23, CD35, Clusterin, Fascin (FDC markers)	–	–	–	– CD21,CD23,CD35, Clusterin +Fascin	–	+
CD56, CD123, TdT	–	–	–	–	CD123+ CD56+ (neoplasms) TdT +/– (neo-plasms)	–

1) The group includes both benign proliferations (histiocytosis) and histiocytic neoplasms (histiocytic sarcoma). Ki67 may be helpful in determining whether a histiocytic proliferation is benign or malignant since the proliferation index can be high in true histiocytic malignancies.

2) All above entities, except FDC sarcoma, are CD45+ at least weakly/focally. FDC sarcoma is CD45 (–) because it is non-hematopoietic in origin (see diagram). Dendritic Cells (Interdigitating and Follicular) were formerly known as reticulum cells (no relation to reticular fibers).

3) BPDCN (formerly blastic natural killer cell lymphoma) is extremely rare neoplasm of plasmacytoid dendritic cells; this entity is included with AML and related precursor lesions in the 2008 WHO.

Note: True histiocytic malignancies must be differentiated from hemophagocytic syndromes as well as neoplasms that are rich in histiocytes, including T-cell/histiocyte rich large B-cell lymphoma, lymphoepithelioid peripheral T-cell lymphoma (Lennert lymphoma), histiocyte rich HL, and the lymphohistio-cytic pattern of ALCL.

Typical panel: CD45, CD43, CD68, CD163, S100, CD1a, CD21, CD23, CD20, CD3, CD30, Ki67

Diagram based on: [153]

Hematopathology Abbreviations: ALCL anaplastic large cell lymphoma, ALL acute lymphoblastic lymphoma, BM bone marrow, BPDCN Blastic plasmacytoid dendritic cell neoplasm, CLL/SLL chronic lymphocytic leukemia/small lymphocytic lymphoma, DLBCL diffuse large B cell lymphoma, FDC Follicular Dendritic Cell, FL follicular lymphoma, GC germinal center, HCL hairy cell leukemia, HL Hodgkin lymphoma, IDC Inter-digitating Dendritic Cell, LC Langerhans Cell, LCH Langerhans cell histiocytosis, LGBCL low grade B cell lymphoma, LPL lymphoplasmacytic lymphoma, MALT mucosa-associated lymphoid tissue, MCL mantle cell lymphoma, MPO myeloperoxidase, MZL marginal zone lymphoma, NK natural killer, NLPHL nodular lymphocyte predominant Hodgkin lymphoma, NSHL nodular sclerosing Hodgkin lymphoma, PB peripheral blood, PH plasmacytic hyperplasia, PNH paroxysmal nocturnal hemoglobinuria, PTLD post-transplant lymphoproliferative disorder, R-S Reed Sternberg, SHML sinus histiocytosis and massive lymphadenopathy, sIG surface immunoglobulin, THRLBCL T-cell/histiocyte rich large B-cell lymphoma

Chapter 3 Immunostains: Antibody Index

by Justin Bishop, Amy Duffield, Diana Molavi, Natasha Rekhtman

Common Multipurpose Immunostains at a Glance

β-catenin, nuclear: deep (desmoid) fibromatosis (vs. GIST is negative), tubular adenoma (vs. DALM/dysplasia-associated lesion or mass) is negative), colon cancer (vs. urothelial CA is negative), pancreatic solid-pseudopapillary neoplasm (vs. cytoplasmic staining in pancreatic neuroendocrine tumors), pancreatoblastoma, juvenile nasal angiofibroma, fundic gland polyp, cribriform morular variant of papillary thyroid carcinoma, adamantinomatous craniopharyngioma

Calretinin: mesothelioma and normal mesothelial cells, adenomatoid tumor, cardiac myxoma, sex cord-stromal tumors, adrenocortical tumors

CD5: normal T cells, CLL/SLL, mantle cell lymphoma, thymic carcinoma, expression of CD5 is lost in many T-cell lymphomas

CD10 (CALLA): most B lymphoblastic leukemia/lymphomas, some T lymphoblastic lymphomas, follicular lymphoma, Burkitt, some DLBCL, neoplastic T-lymphocytes in angioimmunoblastic T-cell lymphoma; HCC (canalicular pattern), RCC, pancreatic solid-pseudopapillary neoplasm, sex cord-stromal tumors, endometrial stromal sarcoma

CD30 (Ki1): RS cells in Classical Hodgkin lymphoma, anaplastic large cell (Ki1) lymphoma, embryonal carcinoma, subset of DLBCL (often EBV-related) and mycosis fungoides (associated with transformation)

CD34:
- many soft tissue tumors:
  - vascular tumors (angiosarcoma, Kaposi, hemangiopericytoma)
  - dermatofibrosarcoma protuberans (+) vs. dermatofibroma (–)
  - gastrointestinal stromal tumor (70%+) vs. fibromatosis (–) vs leiomyoma/leiomyosarcoma (–)
  - solitary fibrous tumor (strong/diffuse +) vs. synovial sarcoma (always –) vs. HPC (focally +) in the brain
  - nerve sheath tumors (schwannoma, neurofibroma, MPNST)
  - epithelioid sarcoma (50%+)
  - adipocytic tumors
- Other
  - primitive leukemias (including myeloid, B- and T-cell – more common in B than T ALL)
  - HCC ("sinusoidal capillarization") vs. benign hepatocellular nodules (–)
- **CD34-negative tumors:** carcinomas (except NUT midline carcinomas – about 50%+), melanoma, lymphoma (except ALL/lymphoblastic lymphoma).

CD99/O13 (relatively non-specific marker – expressed in many soft tissue tumors): Ewing sarcoma/PNET, sex cord-stromal tumors; always negative in neuroblastoma, T lymphoblastic lymphoma

c-kit/CD117: GIST (95%), acute myeloid leukemia, seminoma (membranous), thymic carcinoma, melanoma (~30%), mast cell lesions, sclerosing mesenteritis

D2-40: lymphatic endothelium and related endotheliomas, adrenocortical neoplasms, hemangioblastoma, mesothelioma, skin adnexal tumors, dermatofibroma, seminoma, embryonal carcinoma (30%+), follicular dendritic cells and tumors, nerve sheath tumors (!!)

ER/PR: breast, uterus and ovary (endometrioid CA >> serous CA), some skin adnexal tumors, cystic neoplasms with ovarian-type stroma (e.g. MEST/mixed epithelial stromal tumor of the kidney), meningioma (PR), pancreatic solid-pseudopapillary neoplasm (PR), pancreatic neuroendocrine tumor/islet cell tumor (PR)

HMB-45: melanoma (non-desmoplastic), other melanosome-containing tumors: e.g. clear cell sarcoma/melanoma of soft parts, melanotic schwannoma, angiomyolipoma and other PEComas (Perivascular Epithelioid Cell tumor family, which also includes clear cell "sugar" tumor of the lung, lymphangioleiomyomatosis, and rare clear cell tumors in other sites)

Inhibin: adrenocortical neoplasms, sex cord-stromal tumors, trophoblastic tumors, hemangioblastoma, granular cell tumor

Melan-A (A103 clone): melanoma (non-desmoplastic), other melanosome-containing tumors (same as for HMB-45 above), steroid-rich tumors (adrenocortical neoplasms and sex cord-stromal tumors)

Napsin A: lung adenoCA, papillary RCC

PAX8: carcinomas of renal, thyroid, GYN tract

S100:
- *Nerve sheath/glia:* schwannoma (diffuse), neurofibroma (focal), MPNST (focal), granular cell tumor, gliomas;
- *Melanocytes:* melanoma (including desmoplastic), nevi;
- *Soft tissue:* clear cell sarcoma/melanoma of soft parts, synovial sarcoma (30%), chordoma, lipomatous tumors;
- *Histiocytes:* Langerhans cell histiocytosis, Rosai-Dorfman, histiocytic sarcoma, benign histiocytoses;
- *Myoepithelial cells:* myoepithelioma, myoepithelial carcinoma
- *Other:* sustentacular cells in pheochromocytoma/paraganglioma and esthesioneuroblastoma
- Note: S100 is generally negative in carcinomas (except breast – 30%+)

TTF-1: lung (75% of non-mucinous adenocarcinomas), thyroid (all types except anaplastic), SmCC of lung (~95%+), SmCC of many non-pulmonary sites (prostate ~60%+, bladder ~35%+, cervix 20%+); subset (20%) of GYN carcinoma of various type – watch out!!

WT1: Wilms tumor, intraabdominal desmoplastic small round cell tumor, mesothelioma, serous ovarian carcinoma

N. Rekhtman, J.A. Bishop, *Quick Reference Handbook for Surgical Pathologists*,
DOI:10.1007/978-3-642-20086-1_3, © Springer-Verlag Berlin Heidelberg 2011

Alphabetical Antibody Index

by Justin Bishop, Amy Duffield, Diana Molavi, Natasha Rekhtman

Antibody or Antigen (other names)	Cellular Localization	Normal Tissues Stained and Functional Information if Pertinent	What this marker is used to identify and differential diagnoses
4A4 → see p63			
34ßE12 → see Cytokeratins			
α1-Antitrypsin (AAT-1)	cytoplasmic	hepatocytes, histiocytes	• Globules of AAT (which accumulate in the liver in AAT-deficiency); • HCC (HepPar is more specific); • Histiocytic lesions (CD68 is more specific).
A103 → see Melan-A			
ACTINS — **α-Actin** (Smooth Muscle Actin, SMA)	cytoplasmic	smooth muscle, myoepithelial cells, myofibroblasts	• Smooth muscle differentiation (skeletal muscle is negative); • ME cells/differentiation (e.g., myoepithelial carcinoma, layer present in benign or in situ breast lesions/absent in invasive breast carcinoma).
ACTINS — **Muscle Specific Actin** (MSA, ACTIN, HHF-35)	cytoplasmic	smooth, skeletal, and cardiac muscle, myoepithelial cells	• Smooth and skeletal muscle differentiation (less sensitive for smooth muscle than α-Actin).
AE1/AE3 → see Cytokeratins			
AFP (Alpha fetoprotein)	cytoplasmic	fetal liver	• Yolk sac tumor (not specific, also present in some embryonal CA); • HCC except fibrolamellar variant (not specific, HepPar is a better marker); • Hepatoblastoma (particularly helpful as a serum marker, where it is usually very high).
ALK (Anaplastic Lymphoma Kinase, p80)	nuclear, cytoplasmic, membranous	few neuronal cells	• Inflammatory myofibroblastic tumor (~60%, cytoplasmic); • ALCL (~70%); • Lung adenocarcinoma with EML4-ALK rearrangement; • Expression is a result of t(2;5)/NMP-ALK and other ALK translocations. Most commonly ALK is both nuclear and cytoplasmic, but location depends on the type of translocation. Other lymphomas are (–), except rare DLBCL are (+).
AMACR (alpha-methylacyl-CoA reductase) → see Racemase			
Arginase-1	cytoplasmic	normal hepatocytes	• New marker for hepatocellular differentiation. [1]
B72.3	cytoplasmic, membranous	secretory endometrium	• Adenocarcinoma (+) vs. mesothelioma (–) – a second-line marker.
β-catenin	only nuclear staining is significant	cytoplasm of most cells, where it binds to APC (adenomatous polyposis coli) protein. Nuclear staining indicates a mutation in either APC or β-catenin. Endothelial cells serve as a good internal positive control for staining.	• Colon cancer; • Pancreatic solid-pseudopapillary neoplasm; • Craniopharyngioma; • Pancreatoblastoma; • Hepatoblastoma; • Familial adenomatous polyposis (FAP)-associated tumors (e.g., deep [desmoid] fibromatosis, nasal angiofibroma, fundic gland polyps, cribriform-morular variant of papillary thyroid CA); • Tubular adenoma (+) vs. Dysplasia-associated lesion or mass (DALM) (–).
β-HCG → see Human Chorionic Gonadotropin			
BAF47 → see INI1			
Bcl-1 → see Cyclin D1			
Bcl-2 (B cell lymphoma-2)	membranous and cytoplasmic	inhibits apoptosis. Normally present in mantle cells and turns OFF in a germinal center (normal secondary follicles are Bcl-2-negative).	• FL (+) vs. reactive follicles (–). In FL Bcl-2 expression is maintained due to t(14;18)/*Bcl2-IgH*. Bcl-2 is NOT specific for FL (also + in CLL/SLL, MCL, MZL), but Burkitt should be (–). • Synovial sarcoma (~100%) and some CD34+ tumors (SFT, GIST), but specificity is low.
Bcl-6 (B cell lymphoma-6)	nuclear	germinal center cells	• Lymphomas of follicular origin (FL, Burkitt, some DLBCL, "popcorn cells" in LP-HL), neoplastic T-lymphocytes in angioimmunoblastic T-cell lymphoma.

Antibody or Antigen (other names)	Cellular Localization	Normal Tissues Stained and Functional Information if Pertinent	What this marker is used to identify and differential diagnoses
Ber-EP4	membranous	epithelial cells	• Adenocarcinoma in general (similar to EMA); • Lung adenocarcinoma (+) vs. mesothelioma (−).
BG8	cytoplasmic	RBC	• Adenocarcinoma (+) vs. mesothelioma (−) – a second-line marker.
BOB.1 → see OCT2			
Brachyury	nuclear	transcription factor involved in notochord development. Expressed in some normal spermatogonia	• Chordoma; • Hemangioblastoma.
BRST2 → see GCDFP-15			
BSAP (B-cell specific activator protein) → see PAX-5			
CAIX (Carbonic Anhydrase)	membranous	ischemic tissues (expression related to Hypoxia Inducible Factor)	• Clear cell RCC (very sensitive and specific, though focal expression may be seen focally in various tumors in areas of necrosis/ischemia such as in papillary RCC).
CA-125	luminal	many cell types	• Serum marker for monitoring ovarian cancer, but is not specific for ovary by IHC (many other tumors are positive).
CA 19-9 (Carbohydrate antigen 19-9)	cytoplasmic	many cell types	• Serum marker for monitoring pancreatic and GI cancers, but is not specific for these sites by IHC (many other tumors are positive).
Calcitonin	cytoplasmic and extracellular	C cells of the thyroid	• Medullary carcinoma of the thyroid (not entirely specific, can be positive in other NE tumors)
Caldesmon (h-Caldesmon)	cytoplasmic	smooth muscle and myoepithelial cells, negative in myofibroblasts	• Leiomyosarcoma (+) vs. myofibroblastic lesions, such as fibromatosis (−).
CALLA (Common Acute Leukemia Antigen) → See CD10			
Calponin	cytoplasmic	smooth muscle and myoepithelial cells, variable in myofibroblasts	• Same as α-Actin but variable in myofibroblasts
Calretinin (CRT)	cytoplasmic and nuclear	mesothelium, sex-cord stromal cells, some neural and epithelial cells	• Adenomatoid tumor; • Sex-cord stromal tumors; • Adrenocortical tumors; • Cardiac myxoma; • Epithelial mesothelioma (+) vs. adenocarcinoma (−).
CAM 5.2 → see Cytokeratins			
Cathepsin-K	cytoplasmic	Osteoclasts	• Xp11 translocation RCC; • PEComas; • Chordoma.
CD1a	membranous	thymocytes (immature T cells), Langerhans' cells	• Langerhans' cell histiocytosis; • Some T-cell lymphoblastic lymphomas; • Thymoma with admixed thymocytes (CD1a, TdT, CD99+)
CD2	membranous	pan-T cell marker, NK cells	• T- and NK-cell lymphomas and leukemias.
cCD3 – flow cytometry only	cytoplasmic	pan-T cell marker	• Most lineage-specific marker for T-cell differentiation; • (Flow cytometric analysis of cytoplasmic CD3 expression is determined by permeabilizing the cells prior to incubation with the antibody
CD3	membranous, cytoplasmic	pan-T cell marker	• T-cell lymphomas and leukemias (best pan-T cell IHC marker); often lost in ALCL.
CD4 and CD8	membranous	CD4: helper T cells, monocytes CD8: Cytotoxic and suppressor T cells, NK-like T-cells CD4+/CD8+: thymus	• T-cell lymphomas and leukemias (majority of peripheral T cell lymphomas are CD4+); • CD4 is also (+) in monocytic/histiocytic lesions (e.g. monocytic AML); • Large populations of double negative or double positive T-cells are typically neoplastic except in the thymus where these phenotypes are normally seen. A small number of circulating CD4–/CD8– T-cells is normal.

Antibody or Antigen (other names)	Cellular Localization	Normal Tissues Stained and Functional Information if Pertinent	What this marker is used to identify and differential diagnoses
CD5	membranous	T cells and subset of B cells (naïve B cells)	• CD5+ low-grade B cell lymphomas: CLL/SLL and MCL; • CD5+ high grade B cell lymphomas: blastoid MCL, occasional DLBCL; • T-cell lymphomas and leukemias: aberrant loss of pan-T antigens, particularly CD7 and CD5, is a common signature in peripheral T cell lymphomas, such as mycosis fungicides; • Thymic carcinoma (+ in epithelial cells) vs. thymoma (–).
CD7	membranous	T cells; NK cells	• T-ALL (near 100%+ and often very brightly expressed); • MF and other mature T-cell lymphomas (aberrant *loss* of CD7) vs. reactive T-cell proliferations (+); • Aberrant expression in AML is used for flow cytometric monitoring of residual disease; expression of CD7 on myeloid blasts can occasionally be seen in recovering marrow
CD10 (CALLA, Common Acute Leukemia Antigen)	membranous	precursor B & T cells, germinal center B cells, granulocytes, liver canaliculi, myoepithelial cells, endometrial stroma	• CD10 (+) lymphomas: B and T lymphoblastic lymphoma (B>T), FL, Burkitt, some DLBCL; neoplastic cells in angioimmunoblastic T-cell lymphoma; • HCC (+ canalicular pattern) vs. cholangiocarcinoma (–); • RCC; • Pancreatic solid-pseudopapillary neoplasm; • Sex cord-stromal tumors; • Endometrial stromal sarcoma; • ME cells (p63 or SMMHC are better markers); • Atypical fibroxanthoma (+) vs. sarcoma, sarcomatoid carcinoma, and melanoma of the skin (–).
CD11b – a flow marker	membranous	monocytes, granulocytes; NK cells	• Myeloid leukemias with differentiation and NK cell tumors.
CD11c – a flow marker	membranous	myeloid and lymphoid cells	• Hairy cell leukemia.
CD13, CD14, CD33 – flow markers	membranous	myeloid cells (CD13, CD33) and monocytes (CD14, CD33)	• Myeloid leukemias.
CD15	membranous and Golgi (paranuclear dot-like)	monocytes, myelocytes, granulocytes endothelial cells and some carcinomas	• R-S cells in classical HL (occasionally negative in HL, but always negative in NLP-HL); • AML with differentiation, especially granulocytic; • Adenocarcinoma (+) vs. mesothelioma (–).
CD19 CD20 (L26) CD22	cytoplasmic and membranous	pan-B cell markers	• B-cell lymphomas, but plasmacytoma are (–); • B-precursor ALL almost always expresses CD19, but CD22 and CD20 are variable; • CD20 reactivity is lost in DLBCL after Rx with Rituximab (anti-CD20 antibody) but CD19 remains (+).
CD21, CD35	membranous	B cells, follicular dendritic cells (FDC), other	• Follicular dendritic cell network in lymphomas (FL, MCL, NLP-HL, angioimmunoblastic T-cell lymphoma); • Follicular dendritic cell sarcoma (very rare).
CD23	membranous	B cells, follicular dendritic cells (FDC), monocytes	• DDx of CD5+/CD10– low grade B cell lymphomas: SLL/CLL (CD23+) vs. MCL (CD23–); • Follicular dendritic cell network in lymphomas (FL, MCL, NLP-HL, angioimmunoblastic T-cell lymphoma).
CD25 (IL2 receptor)	membranous and cytoplasmic	activated T and B cells	• Hairy cell leukemia; • Adult T-cell leukemia/lymphoma (HTLV-related); • Most ALCLs; • Neoplastic mast cells.
CD30 (Ki-1)	membranous and Golgi (paranuclear dot-like)	activated B (immunoblasts) and T lymphocytes, plasma cells, some non-heme cells	• R-S cells in classical (+) vs. NLP (–) Hodgkin lymphoma; • ALCL (strong staining with characteristic "target-like" membrane and Golgi pattern); • Mycosis fungoides (+/– focally; suggests transformation); • Embryonal carcinoma.
CD31	cytoplasmic and membranous	endothelial cells, megakaryocytes, macrophages, other	• Endothelial differentiation (e.g., angiosarcoma, Kaposi sarcoma); more sensitive and specific than CD34.

Antibody or Antigen (other names)	Cellular Localization	Normal Tissues Stained and Functional Information if Pertinent	What this marker is used to identify and differential diagnoses
CD34	cytoplasmic and membranous	endothelial cells, fibroblasts, and hematopoietic blasts (stem cells)	• Many soft tissue tumors: – vascular tumors (angiosarcoma, Kaposi, hemangiopericytoma); – dermatofibrosarcoma protuberans (+) vs. dermatofibroma (–); – GIST (70%+) vs. fibromatosis (–) vs leiomyosarcoma (–); – solitary fibrous tumor (strong/diffuse +) vs. synovial sarcoma (always –) vs. HPC (focally +) in the brain; – nerve sheath tumors (schwannoma, neurofibroma, MPNST) ; – epithelioid sarcoma (50%+); – adipocytic tumors. • Other – primitive leukemias (including myeloid, B- and T-cell – more common in B than T ALL) ; – HCC ("sinusoidal capillarization") vs. benign hepatocellular nodules (–). • **CD34-negative tumors**: carcinoma (except NUT midline carcinomas – about 50%+), melanoma, lymphoma (except ALL/lymphoblastic lymphoma).
CD38	membranous	immature lymphocytes, plasma cells	• Plasma cell differentiation; • Poor prognosis in CLL/SLL.
CD41, CD42b, CD 61– flow markers	membranous	Megakaryocytes, platelets	• AML with megakaryocytic differentiation (M7).
CD43	membranous	T cells, myelocytes	• Classification of low-grade B-cell lymphomas: aberrant expression in CLL/SLL, MCL, MZL, but not FL; • Normal and malignant T cells, myeloid sarcoma (chloroma) – more sensitive than CD45.
CD44	membranous	normal urothelium (basal layer), also considered a cancer stem cell marker	• Reactive urothelium (+ in basal layer) vs. CIS (– or reduced); • Small cell carcinoma of the prostate. [2]
CD45 (Leukocyte Common Antigen, LCA or CLA)	cytoplasmic, membranous	pan-leukocyte marker (lymphocytes, myeloids, and histiocytes) but absent on plasma cells and nucleated reds	• Screening for hematopoietic origin in an unknown malignancy (part of a standard first-line panel); • Virtually all hematopoietic neoplasms, except some myelomas, R-S cells in classical Hodgkin lymphoma, some lymphoblastic lymphomas, some anaplastic large cell lymphoma, some myeloid sarcomas, and follicular dendritic cell sarcoma.
CD56 (NCAM, Neural Cell Adhesion Molecule)	membranous	neuroendocrine cells, schwann cells, NK cells	• Neuroendocrine neoplasms (e.g. carcinoid). Particularly useful to identify small cell carcinoma, which may be non-reactive for other neuroendocrine markers (SYN, CHR); • Nasal-type NK/T cell lymphoma and other T-cell lymphomas (panniculitis-like T-cell lymphoma, hepatosplenic T-cell lymhoma); • Neoplastic plasma cells; • Aberrant expression in acute myeloid leukemia.
CD57	membranous	neuroendocrine cells, schwann cells, NK-like T cells	• NLP HL (CD57+ T-lymphocyte surround L&H cells forming "rosettes") vs. T-cell rich DLBCL or classical HL (rosettes of CD57 cells absent); • T-cell large granular cell leukemia, neuroendocrine neoplasms and some nerve sheath tumors; • Metanephric adenoma of the kidney.
CD68	cytoplasmic, membranous	lysosomal marker in histiocytes/macrophages/monocytes, granulocytes, others	• Histiocytic differentiation; • Myeloid sarcoma (AML with monocytic differentiation).
CD71 (transferrin receptor) – flow marker	membranous	erythroid cells (not specific)	• AML with erythroid (M6) or megakaryocytic (M7) differentiation; • Aggressive (+) vs. indolent (–) CD10+ B-cell lymphomas (by flow). [3]
CD79a	membranous	B-cells and plasma cells (broader than CD20)	• B-cell neoplasms, including B-ALL and myelomas (myelomas may be negative for all other pan-B markers); • Also (+) in some cases of T-ALL.

Antibody or Antigen (other names)	Cellular Localization	Normal Tissues Stained and Functional Information if Pertinent	What this marker is used to identify and differential diagnoses
CD99 (MIC2, O13)	membranous (more specific reactivity) and cytoplasmic	immature T cells including cortical thymocytes, various epithelial cells, endothelial cells	• PNET/Ewing sarcoma, but expression is NOT specific – many other sarcomas, particularly small round cell tumors of childhood, are also (+). Neuroblastoma is always (–). • B- and T-cell lymphoblastic leukemia/lymphoma (mature lymphomas are negative); • Thymoma: contains admixed immature T cells (CD99+, TdT+); • Sex cord-stromal tumors.
CD103 – a flow marker	cytoplasmic	intestinal epithelial T lymphocytes	• Hairy cell leukemia; • Enteropathy-associated T cell lymphoma.
CD117 → see c-kit			
CD138	membranous	plasma cells squamous epithelium	• Plasma cell differentiation; • Many carcinomas (such as SqCC).
CD141 → see Thrombomodulin			
CD146 (MelCAM)	membranous	intermediate trophoblast, smooth muscle, vascular endothelial cells	• Mesothelioma (+) vs. reactive mesothelial proliferation (–); • Tumors of implantation site intermediate trophoblast: Exaggerated placental site and placental site trophoblastic tumor; • Choriocarcinoma; • Melanoma.
CD163	membranous	member of scavenger receptor cysteine-rich superfamily restricted to the monocyte/macrophage line	• Histiocytic differentiation.
CDX2	nuclear	intestine (from duodenum to rectum)	• Strong/diffuse expression in intestinal carcinomas (more sensitive than villin); • Variable/focal expression in gastric and pancreaticobiliary carcinomas; • Variable in carcinomas with enteric phenotype (e.g. mucinous ovarian CA, intestinal sinonasal adenoCA, adenoCA of urinary bladder); • Appendicial carcinoid tumor; • Yolk sac tumor (40%) [4]
CEA	cytoplasmic	fetal tissues and glandular epithelium (strongest in mucin-secreting glandular tissues)	• Adenocarcinoma (mCEA+) vs. mesothelioma (mCEA–); • HCC (canalicular pCEA) vs. cholangiocarcinoma and metastatic adenocarcinoma (cytoplasmic pCEA); • Adenocarcinoma in general (e.g. lung, colon, pancreas); • Medullary thyroid carcinoma.
c-erB → see HER2			
Chromogranin (CHR, Chromogranin A)	cytoplasmic (granular)	neurosecretory granules in neuroendocrine tissues and neurons	• Neuroendocrine differentiation (pheochromocytoma, carcinoid, pancreatic neuroendocrine tumor/islet cell tumor, small cell CA, Merkel cell CA, etc).
Chymotrypsin → see Trypsin			
c-kit (CD117, stem cell factor receptor)	cytoplasmic and membranous	interstitial cells of Cajal (origin of GIST), germ cells, hematopoietic progenitor cells, mast cells	• GIST (95%+, diffuse staining) vs. leiomyoma and schwannoma (–); • Seminoma (membranous) and intra-tubular germ cell neoplasia; • Mast cell lesions, • Melanoma (30–40%+); • Sclerosing mesenteritis; • Luminal epithelium in salivary gland tumors with epithelial and myoepithelial components; • PEComas; • Thymic carcinoma (+) vs. thymoma (–); • Renal oncocytoma; • Blasts in acute myeloid leukemia.
CLA (common leukocyte antigen) → see CD45			
Clusterin	cytoplasmic	follicular dendritic cells	• Follicular dendritic cell tumors; • Also tenosynovial giant cell tumors, pancreatic NE tumors, and many others.
CyclinD1 (Bcl-1)	nuclear	dividing cells	• MCL and blastoid MCL – t(11;14)/CCND1-IgH. Endothelial cells are normally Cyclin D1 (+), which may be used as an internal control in lymphoma work-up.

Antibody or Antigen (other names)		Cellular Localization	Normal Tissues Stained and Functional Information if Pertinent	What this marker is used to identify and differential diagnoses
CYTOKERATINS	**AE1/AE3** (pan-cytokeratin cocktail)	cytoplasmic	most epithelial cells	• Used in conjunction with Cam5.2 to screen for carcinoma (see "Epithelial Markers" section for details): ID's all carcinomas except HCC, RCC, adrenocortical CA and some high grade NE CA.
	CAM 5.2	cytoplasmic	low-molecular weight keratins (8, 18) present in simple (non-squamous) epithelia	• Used in conjunction with AE1/AE3 to screen for carcinoma, but is negative in SqCC; • Particularly useful to ID carcinomas that are negative for AE1/AE3, most notably HCC (negative for AE1/AE3, CK903 and EMA) and some undifferentiated CA; • Paget's disease (+) vs. Bowen's disease/SqCC in situ (–).
	CK7	cytoplasmic	a specific LMW cytokeratin	• CK7: Barrett's mucosa (+) vs. intestinal metaplasia in gastric cardia (–); • CK20: urothelial CIS (+ in all layers) vs. reactive urothelium (+ in umbrella cell layer only);

	CK20	cytoplasmic	a specific LMW cytokeratin	• CK7 and 20 are used in combination to narrow the differential of carcinoma of unknown origin:
				  – CK7 is generally positive in above-the-diaphragm carcinomas (lung, breast, thyroid) and Gyn organs.
				  – CK20 is generally positive in below-the-diaphragm carcinomas (colon CA), and in Merkel cell CA.
				  – CK7 and CK20 are co-expressed in peri-diaphragmatic organs (pancreas, stomach) and bladder.
				  – Negative for both are simple visceral organs (liver, kidney, prostate). (See 7/20 table for details).

	CK903 (34ßE12, K903)	cytoplasmic	high molecular weight keratin present in stratified epithelia (squamous, urothelial, respiratory) plus myoepithelial and basal cells	• Urothelial (+) vs. prostate (–) carcinoma ; • Prostatic basal cells (loss of staining indicates carcinoma); • Usual duct hyperplasia (+) vs. ductal carcinoma in situ (–); • Metaplastic breast cancer (+).
	CK5/6	cytoplasmic	two specific HMW keratins	• Squamous cell CA (+) and mesothelioma (+) vs. adenoCA (–); • Prostatic basal cells and metaplastic carcinoma (similar to CK903).
Desmin (DES)		cytoplasmic	intermediate filament in smooth, striated, and cardiac muscle	• Smooth and skeletal muscle differentiation in tumors; • Reactive mesothelial cells (+) vs. mesothelioma (–). Low specificity.
D2-40 (Poloplanin)		membranous	novel marker of mesothelial cells, germ cells, lymphatic endothelial cells, FDCs	• Mesothelioma (+) vs. adenocarcinoma (–); • Dermatofibroma (+) vs. dermatofibrosarcoma protuberans (–); • Hemangioblastoma (+) vs. metastatic RCC (–); • Primary skin adnexal tumors (+) vs. metastatic adenocarcinoma (–); • Adrenocortical neoplasms (+) vs. RCC (–); • Lymphatic channels; • Seminoma (100%+) and embryonal carcinoma (30%+); • Nerve sheath tumors: schwannoma and MPNST; • Follicular dendritic cell tumors. References: [5–7]
DPC-4, clone B8 (Deleted in Pancreatic Carcinoma, SMAD4)		nuclear and cytoplasmic	most normal tissues	• Pancreatic carcinoma – 55% of invasive cancer exhibits the loss of expression. Both nuclear and cytoplasmic staining must be negative to count. Loss of expression is fairly specific to pancreas, but is also seen in a subset of colon CA.
DOG1		membranous and cytoplasmic	interstitial cells of Cajal	• GIST (reportedly better sensitivity and specificity than c-kit); • Stains 1/3 of c-kit negative GISTs. Reference: [8]
EBV (Epstein-Barr Virus)	**EBER** (EBV- encoded early RNA)	nuclear	EBV-infected cells	• Most sensitive marker for EBV. ID's all EBV-related tumors. Detected by in situ hybridization.
	LMP-1 (late membrane protein)	membranous	EBV-infected cells	• Less sensitive that EBER. ID's PTLD and AIDS-related lymphomas, variable in NPC, Hodgkin and Burkitt lymphoma.
	EBNA (EBV nuclear antigen)	nuclear	EBV-infected cells	• Least sensitive EBV marker. ID's PTLD and AIDS-related lymphomas only.
E-cadherin (CAD-E)		membranous	breast – normal ductal and lobular cell (functions as adhesion molecule)	• In situ and invasive lobular CA (–) vs. ductal lesions (+); • Loss of expression also seen in gastric signet-ring CA and undifferentiated pancreas carcinoma (note that neoplasms with the loss of E-cadherin are discohesive, which is consistent with its role as adhesion molecule).

Antibody or Antigen (other names)	Cellular Localization	Normal Tissues Stained and Functional Information if Pertinent	What this marker is used to identify and differential diagnoses
EGFR (Epidermal Growth Factor Receptor)	membranous and cytoplasmic	many cell types	• Membranous staining predicts response to Erbitux (a monoclonal antibody) in advanced colon cancer.
EMA (Epithelial Membrane Antigen, MUC1)	cytoplasmic or membranous	epithelial, perineurial, meningothelial cells	• Carcinomas in general, synovial sarcoma, epithelioid sarcoma, chordoma (used in conjunction with CKs); • EMA(+) CK (−) tumors: meningioma, perineurioma, plasma cell neoplasms, ALCL, R-S cells in NLP HL; • Mesothelioma (strong membranous staining) vs. adenocarcinoma (cytoplasmic staining).
Estrogen receptor (ER) and Progesterone receptor (PR)	nuclear	breast, ovary, endometrium	• Hormone-receptor (+) breast CA: favorable prognosis, responsiveness to Tamoxifen; • Metastatic breast cancer; • Tumors of uterus and ovary (cervix is negative); • (+) in few non-mammary/non-GYN tumors: ~5% of lung adenocarcinomas, skin adnexal tumors, cystic neoplasms with ovarian-type stroma (e.g. mixed epithelial stromal tumor), meningioma (PR+), pancreatic solid-pseudopapillary neoplasm (PR+), pancreatic neuroendocrine tumor (PR+).
Factor VIII (Factor VIII-related antigen, vWF)	cytoplasmic	endothelial cells, megakaryocytes, platelets	• Endothelial differentiation – specific but not sensitive; • AML with megakaryocytic differentiation (M7).
Factor XIIIa	cytoplasmic	histiocytes, fibrohistiocytic cells, other	• Dermatofibroma (+) vs. dermatofibrosarcoma protuberans (−); • Histiocytic differentiation (a pan-histiocytic marker, similar to CD68); • Sinonasal glomangiopericytoma (often with peculiar nuclear localization).
Fascin	cytoplasmic	many cell types	• R-S cells in classical HL; • Follicular dendritic cell tumors.
Fli-1 (Friend leukemia integration 1)	nuclear	endothelial cells, many other cell types	• Endothelial differentiation; • Ewing sarcoma/PNET (EWS-Fli-1 translocation) – not specific, present in many tumors.
FMC-7 – flow marker	cytoplasm	B cells	• CD5+ lymphomas: MCL (+) vs. CLL/SLL (−). Expression is opposite of CD23.
Gastrin	cytoplasmic	G cells	• G cell hyperplasia in autoimmune metaplastic atrophic gastritis; • Gastric antrum (+) vs. "antralized" body (−).
GCDFP (Gross Cystic Disease Fluid Protein-15, BRST2)	cytoplasmic	apocrine cells of the breast and sweat glands	• Metastatic breast cancer (~50%+). Staining is notoriously focal. Expression unrelated to grade and ER/PR status. Stains lobular carcinoma best. • Other tumors with apocrine differentiation: tumors of salivary gland (especially salivary duct CA) and skin adenxae.
GFAP (Glial Fibrillary Astrocytic Protein)	cytoplasmic	glial, myoepithelial and schwann cells	• Gliomas (astrocytoma, ependymoma; oligodendroglioma may be focal), myoepithelioma, some schwannomas
GLUT1 (Glucose transporter 1)	membranous	RBCs and many tissues	• Mesothelioma (+) vs. reactive mesothelium (−); • Thymic carcinoma (+) vs. thymoma (−). Among carcinomas, though, not specific for thymus; • Juvenile hemangioma (+) vs. other benign vascular lesions (−).
Glycophorin – flow marker (CD235a)			
Glypican-3 (GPC3)	cytoplasmic, membranous, and canalicular	Embryonic liver, placenta (syncytiotrophoblasts)	• HCC, hepatoblastoma, yolk sac tumor, choriocarcinoma, placental site trophoblastic tumor [9]; • HCC (+) vs. benign hepatic nodules (−).
Granzyme B, Perforin, & TIA-1 (T-cell intracellular antigen)	cytoplasmic	cytotoxic proteins in CD8+ T cells and NK cells	• T- and NK-cell lymphomas
HBME-1	cytoplasmic and membranous	epithelial and mesothelial cells	• Mesothelioma (+) vs. adenocarcinoma – not specific • Thyroid carcinoma (+/−) vs. benign follicular lesions (−/+) – not specific
Hemoglobin A (HbA)	cytoplasmic	RBCs and precursors	• Erythrocytic differentiation
HepPar-1 (Hepatocyte Paraffin 1; OCH1E5)	granular cytoplasmic	mitochondria in normal hepatocytes, small intestinal epithelia	• Hepatocellular differentiation: HCC (90%+), hepatoblastoma, and carcinomas with "hepatoid" phenotype (ovary, testis, stomach)

Antibody or Antigen (other names)	Cellular Localization	Normal Tissues Stained and Functional Information if Pertinent	What this marker is used to identify and differential diagnoses
HER2 (Her2Neu)	membranous and cytoplasmic	growth factor receptor which is only weakly expressed in normal epithelial cells	• To evaluate breast carcinomas: overexpression is a poor prognostic sign, but can be treated with Herceptin (only membranous reactivity counts); • Increasingly used to evaluate stomach and GE junction adenocarcinomas, too; • Generally not used to ID metastatic breast cancer because HER2 is overexpressed in several non-mammary carcinomas, such as lung and GYN tract
HHF-35 → see Actins			
HLA-DR (MHC lass II)	membranous	antigen presenting cells	• Most myeloid leukemias (+) vs. acute promyelocytic leukemia (–).
HMB45 (Human Melanoma, Black)	cytoplasmic	immature melanocytes (negative in mature melanocytes such as those present at the base of normal nevi)	• Epithelioid (but not desmoplastic) melanoma and other melanosome-containing tumors, including clear cell sarcoma/melanoma of soft parts, melanotic schwannoma, angiomyolipoma and other PEComas; • Melanoma (+) vs. nevus (–). Nevus shows progressive diminution of HMB45 as cells mature toward the base; • Metastatic melanoma (+) vs. benign nevus inclusion (–) in a lymph node.
hMLH1, hMSH2, hMSH6 → see under MLH1 (human *mutL* homolog 1 and human *mutS* homolog 1 and 6) – genes encoding mismatch repair proteins MLH1, MSH2, MSH6			
HNF-1beta (Hepatocyte nuclear factor)	nuclear	hepatocytes	• Clear cell carcinoma of gynecologic tract.
HSD3B1	cytoplasmic	IT and ST	• All trophoblastic tumors.
hSNF5 → see INI1			
Human Chorionic Gonadotropin (hCG beta chain)	cytoplasmic	syncytiotrophoblasts	• Choriocarcinoma; • Syncytiotrophoblastic giant cells in seminoma (better prognosis than chorio) and some carcinomas.
Human Placental Lactogen (hPL)	cytoplasmic	trophoblasts (syncytiotrophoblasts and intermediate trophoblasts)	• Syncytiotrophoblastic tumors (choriocarcinoma), tumors of intermediate trophoblasts (placental site tumors), moles
IgG4	cytoplasmic	Subset of plasma cells	• Increased number of positive plasma cells in a spectrum of inflammatory, sclerosing diseases including autoimmune pancreatitis, chronic sclerosing sialadenitis (Kuttner's tumor), and sclerosing mesenteritis (though criteria for what qualifies as "increased" are not uniform).
Immunoglobulin Kappa & Lambda Light Chains	surface cytoplasmic	B cells (surface) Plasma cells (cytoplasmic)	• Restricted kappa or lambda staining indicates a monoclonal population of B or plasma cells; double negative B-cells are neoplastic (typically seen in mediastinal diffuse large B cell lymphoma); • Surface staining in B-cell neoplasms is best assessed by flow cytometry; cytoplasmic staining in plasma cells can be assessed by immunohistochemistry or flow cytometry.
Inhibin (INH)	cytoplasmic	granulosa cells, Sertoli cells, adrenal cortical cells, trophoblasts, other	• Adrenocortical neoplasms; • Sex cord-stromal tumors (granulosa cell, Sertoli and Leydig, fibrothecomas); • Trophoblastic tumors; • Hemangioblastoma; • Granular cell tumor.
INI1 (hSNF5/BAF47)	nuclear	expressed in normal tissues (product of tumor suppressor gene on 22q11.2)	• Loss of expression (due to mutation) in atypical teratoid/rhabdoid tumor, rhabdoid tumor of the kidney (and other sites), epithelioid sarcoma, medullary carcinoma of the kidney, epithelioid MPNST (50%), subset of myoepithelial carcinomas of soft tissue. Reference: [10]
K903 → see Cytokeratins			
Ki-1 → See CD30			
Ki67 (MIB-1)	nuclear	any proliferating cell	• To gauge mitotic activity for prognosis; • Burkitt lymphoma (100% positivity); • Cytoplasmic reactivity in hyalinizing trabecular adenoma, sclerosing hemangioma of lung.
KP1 → see CD68			

Antibody or Antigen (other names)	Cellular Localization	Normal Tissues Stained and Functional Information if Pertinent	What this marker is used to identify and differential diagnoses
Langerin	membranous and cytoplasmic	Langerhans cells	• Langerhans cell histiocytosis [11]
LMP-1 (late membrane protein) → See EBV			
LCA (Leukocyte Common Antigen) → See CD45			
Leu7 → See CD57			
LeuM1 → See CD15			
Lysozyme (muramidase)	cytoplasmic	monocyte/ macrophage/histiocyte, salivary gland	• Histiocytic differentiation; • Myeloid sarcomas with monocytic differentiation.
Mammaglobin	cytoplasmic	breast epithelium, sweat glands	• Tumors with apocrine differentiation: breast cancer (~50%+), sweat gland tumors, and salivary gland tumors (similar to GCDFP); • Also positive in tumors of female genital tract (ovary, endometrium, cervix); • More sensitive but less specific for ID of metastatic breast cancer than GCDFP. References: [12,13]
MART-1 (Melanoma Antigen Recognized by T cells, N2-7C10 clone)	cytoplasmic	melanocytes	• Melanoma (mainly epithelioid), more sensitive than HMB45. Recognizes same protein as Melan-A antibody.
Mast Cell Tryptase (MCT)	cytoplasmic	mast cells	• Mast cells.
Melan-A (A103 clone)	cytoplasmic	melanocytes	• Epithelioid (but not desmoplastic) melanoma and other melanosome-containing tumors (same as for HMB-45 above). More sensitive than HMB45; • Steroid cell tumors (adrenocortical, Sertoli/Leydig and granulosa cell tumors).
MelCAM (Melanoma Cell Adhesion Molecule) → see CD146			
Mesothelin	membranous	mesothelial cells	• Serous ovarian carcinoma; • Mesothelioma; • Pancreatic CA (also a target for immunotherapy).
MITF (Microphthalmia Transcription Factor)	nuclear	melanocytes	• Melanoma and melanocytic tumors, also angiomyolipoma (but can also stain macrophages!)
MLH1, MSH2, MSH6, PMS2 (*mutL* homolog 1, *mutS* homolog 2 and 6, postmeiotic segregation increased 2)	nuclear	DNA mismatch repair (MMR) proteins are present in most normal cells. Mutation and consequent loss of expression leads to microsatellite instability (MSI).	• Loss of MMR proteins is due to germline mutations affecting MMR genes in Lynch syndrome (see page 111) vs. due to promoter hypermethylation in 10–15% of sporadic colorectal CA (see page 123). • Because of different distribution of affected genes in Lynch syndrome vs. sporadic tumors, the loss of MSH2, MSH6, or PMS2 is nearly diagnostic of Lynch syndrome (germline mutation), whereas the loss of MLH1 is more commonly sporadic. • Tumors with defective MMR/MSI-high have distinctive histology and clinical behavior. (See pages 34 and 117).
MOC31	membranous	most epithelial cells	• Adenocarcinoma in general; • Hepatic adenocarcinoma (primary or metastatic) vs. HCC.
MUC1 → see EMA			
MUC2	cytoplasmic	normal colon and stomach	• Barrett's mucosa (+) vs. intestinal metaplasia of gastric cardia (–); • Intraductal papillary mucinous neoplasm (IPMN) (+) vs. pancreatic intraepithelial neoplasia (PanIN) (–).
MUC18 → see CD146			
MUM1(IRF4) (multiple myeloma 1; interferon regulatory factor 4)	nuclear and cytoplasmic	various hematolymphoid cells (particularly plasma cells) and melanocytes	• Plasma cell neoplasms; • Subtyping of diffuse large B cell lymphomas; • Epithelioid melanoma (a recent addition to other melanocytic markers).
Muramidase → see Lysozyme			

Antibody or Antigen (other names)	Cellular Localization	Normal Tissues Stained and Functional Information if Pertinent	What this marker is used to identify and differential diagnoses
Muscle Specific Actin (MSA) → See Actins			
Myeloperoxidase (MPO)	cytoplasmic	enzyme granules in myeloid cells	• AML and myeloid sarcoma (chloroma).
Myogenin (MGN) and **MyoD1**	nuclear	transcription factors in regenerating, but not normal, skeletal muscle	• Skeletal muscle differentiation (rhabdomyoma, rhabdomyosarcoma).
Napsin A	cytoplasmic (granular)	pneumocytes and renal tubular cells	• Lung adenocarcinoma. Also positive in some renal cell carcinoma (especially papillary), focal in small % of thyroid carcinomas. Similar sensitivity for lung adenocarcinoma as TTF-1.
NCAM (Neural Cell Adhesion Molecule) → See CD56			
NeuN	nuclear	neurons	• Neuronal/ganglion cell tumors.
Neurofilament Sm311 (pan-NF), Sm32 (cell body), Sm31 (axons)	cytoplasmic	neurons	• Neuronal/ganglion cell tumors (gangliocytoma), neuroblastic tumors (neuroblastoma, medulloblastoma, Merkel cell CA) and some neuroendocrine tumors (pheo). SYN is best for this purpose; • Brain infiltration: Sm31 may be used to highlight normal axons to help identify permeation of normal brain parenchyma by a glioma or meningioma.
Neuron-Specific Enolase (NSE)	cytoplasmic	neuroectodermal and neuroendocrine cells	• Neural and neuroendocrine differentiation but not very specific (NOT the same as nonspecific esterase, an enzyme assay for heme path). Sensitive for neuroblastoma.
NUT (<u>N</u>uclear protein in <u>T</u>estis)	nuclear	Germ cells in testis and ovary	• NUT midline carcinoma.
O13 → see CD99			
OCT2 (BOB.1)	nuclear	transcription factor in B cells	• R-S cells in NLP (+) vs. classic HL (– or weak); • B cell lymphomas
OCT4 (OCT3/4)	nuclear	not expressed in normal, differentiated cells	• Seminoma/dysgerminoma, intratubular germ cell neoplasia, and embryonal carcinoma
p16	nuclear and cytoplasmic	cell with inactivated pRb (due to cells high-risk HPV or other means)	• Cervical high grade squamous intraepithelial lesion (+) vs. immature metaplasia (–) • Endocervical adenoCA (+/diffuse) vs. endometrial CA (– or patchy); • Metastatic SqCC of the tonsil, cervix, anus (i.e., HPV-driven cancers) but not specific; • Only strong, diffuse nuclear and cytoplasmic positivity counts when used as a surrogate for HPV. • Serous CA of GYN tract (robustly +) vs. endometrioid CA (–) – analogous to p53, and unrelated to HPV
p53	nuclear	tumor suppressor gene, not expressed at high levels in normal cells	• Overexpression serves as a negative prognostic marker in various tumors (p53 accumulates because it is not being degraded properly; abnormal p53 is also unable to function as a tumor suppressor); • Serous carcinoma of GYN tract (robustly +) vs. endometrioid carcinoma (– or focal); • Dyplasia-associated lesion or mass (DALM)(+) vs. sporadic tubular adenoma (–); • Urothelial flat carcinoma in situ (+) vs. reactive urothelium (–); • Fallopian tube intraepithelial carcinoma; • High grade lymphomas.
p57	nuclear	trophoblasts	• Complete mole (–) vs. incomplete mole (+) and hydropic fetus (+). *p57 gene is paternally imprinted and is normally transcribed entirely from a maternal allele (absent in complete mole).*
p63 (4A4)	nuclear	tumor suppressor gene related to p53. marker of squamous epithelia, basal and myoepithelial cells	• Breast myoepithelial cells (loss of staining indicates a carcinoma). Endothelium and myofibroblasts are negative – cleaner stain than actin and smooth muscle myosin heavy chain; • Prostate basal cells (loss of staining indicates a carcinoma); • Used in a manner similar to HMWCK for sarcomatoid/metaplastic carcinomas, Squamous cell carcinoma (but less specific – can be positive in lymphomas and sarcomas, for example).
p80 → see ALK			

Antibody or Antigen (other names)	Cellular Localization	Normal Tissues Stained and Functional Information if Pertinent	What this marker is used to identify and differential diagnoses
p120 (p120 catenin)	membranous and cytoplasmic	E-cadherin-binding protein in breast epithelium	• Lobular carcinoma in cases with equivocal E-cadherin: ductal carcinoma (membranous p120) vs. lobular carcinoma (strong cytoplasmic p120). If E-cadherin is absent, the cytoplasmic pool of p120 increases.
P501S → see Prostein			
P504S → see Racemase			
Parafibromin	nuclear	protein product of tumour suppressor gene *HRPT2*, expressed in normal tissues	• *Loss* of expression seen in parathyroid carcinoma and parathyroid adenomas of the Hyperparathyroidism-Jaw Tumor Syndrome. Reference: [14]
PAX2 (paired box gene 2)	nuclear	renal epithelium and tissue of Mullerian origin (but not thyroid)	• Renal cell carcinoma (clear cell, papillary), oncocytoma, nephrogenic adenoma; • Superior to CD10 and RCC in specificity and sensitivity; • Minority (about 30%) of Mullerian carcinomas. References: [15,16]
PAX5 (BSAP, B-cell-specific activator protein, paired box gene 5)	nuclear	B-cell specific transcription factor (plasma cells are negative)	• B-cell differentiation including lymphoblasts (used as a novel pan B-cell marker); • R-S cells in NLP HL (+) vs. classic HL (weak).
PAX8 (paired box gene 8)	nuclear	normal thyroid follicles, renal epithelial cells (all segments of renal tubules), tissue of Mullerian origin, lymphocytes	• Pan-RCC (all types, broader than PAX2 – clear cell, papillary, chromophobe, medullary, collecting duct); • Thyroid carcinoma (follicular origin; most anaplastic carcinomas; usually negative in medullary); [17,18] • Pan-Mullerian carcinomas (ovarian+uterine serous+endometrioid); • Pancreatic neuroendocrine tumors.
PE10 → see Surfactant protein A			
Perforin → see Granzyme B			
Placental Alkaline Phosphatase (PLAP)	cytoplasmic	placenta	• Germ cell tumors (does not stain spermatocytic seminoma), intratubular germ-cell neoplasia, trophoblastic tumors.
PNL2	cytoplasmic	melanocytes	• Melanocytic lesions (a new melanocytic marker); reactivity is similar to HMB45.
Podoplanin → see D2-40			
POU5F1 → see OCT4			
PMS2 (postmeiotic segregation increased 2) → see under MLH1			
ProExC	nuclear	cocktail against 1) topoisomerase II alpha, and 2) minichromosome maintenance 2, proteins upregulated in cervical CA	• New marker that is similar to Ki67 and used together with p16 and/or Ki67 or in some combination for differentiating HPV-related lesions from mimickers in the GYN tract.
Progesterone receptor (PR) → see Estrogen receptor			
Prostein (P501S)	cytoplasmic (perinuclear dots pattern)	prostatic epithelium	• Metastatic prostate cancer. Relatively new marker that has a similar sensitivity as PSA [19]
PSA (Prostate Specific Antigen)	cytoplasmic	prostatic epithelium but also salivary gland	• Metastatic prostate cancer (sensitivity 80%); • PSA reactivity is also present in benign and neoplastic salivary gland duct epithelium (pleomorphic adenoma, mucoepidermoid CA), periurethral glands of women, anal glands of men, and glandular urothelium (cystitis glandularis, urachal remnants, urothelial adenocarcinoma); [20] • PSA is more specific but less sensitive than PSAP.
PSAP or PAP (Prostate Acid Phosphatase)	cytoplasmic	prostatic epithelium	• Metastatic prostate cancer; • (+) in carcinoids and some bladder adenocarcinomas. Be careful not to mistake rectal carcinoid for prostate CA!
PSMA (Prostate Specific Membrane Antigen)	cytoplasmic, membranous	prostatic epithelium, urothelium	• Metastatic prostate cancer – in contrast to PSA and PSAP, expression does not decrease with tumor grade.

Antibody or Antigen (other names)	Cellular Localization	Normal Tissues Stained and Functional Information if Pertinent	What this marker is used to identify and differential diagnoses
Racemase (P504S; AMACR; alpha-methylacyl-CoA reductase)	cytoplasmic	prostatic carcinoma and PIN (normal prostate is negative)	• Prostate cancer (+) vs. adenosis and other benign mimics (−); – False positive: 20% adenosis, nephrogenic adenoma; – False negative: 20% adenoCA, 65% foamy CA, 65% atrophic CA, 75% pseudohyperplastic CA; • Not specific for prostate; also (+) in other carcinomas such as lung, breast, papillary RCC, and clear cell adenoCA of bladder.
RCC (Renal Cell Carcinoma marker, gp200/RTA)	cytoplasmic	proximal renal tubules	• Renal cell carcinoma (poor sensitivity and specificity); • RCC (+) vs. oncocytoma (−).
SALL4	nuclear	embryonic stem cells	• Germ cell tumors (pan-germ cell tumor marker); • Some leukemias.
S100 (Solubility in 100% ammonium sulfate)	nuclear and cytoplasmic	schwann cells/glia, melanocytes, histiocytes, dendritic and Langerhans cells, myoepithelial cells, other mesenchymal cells	• *Schwann cells/glia* (schwannoma – diffuse, neurofibroma – focal, MPNST – focal, granular cell tumor, gliomas; *melanocytes* (melanoma, including desmoplastic, nevi); *soft tissue* (clear cell sarcoma/melanoma of soft parts, synovial sarcoma – 30%, chordoma, lipomatous tumors); *histiocytes* (benign histiocytoses, Rosai Dorfman, Langerhans cell histiocytosis, Langerhans cell sarcoma, some histiocytic sarcomas, interdigitating cell sarcoma); *myoepithelial cells* (myoepithelioma), *other* (sustentacular cells in pheochromocytoma/paraganglioma); • Negative in carcinomas, except 30% of breast cancers are S100-positive; • Not used to screen lymph nodes for metastatic melanoma because normal dendritic cells are (+).
SF1 (steroidogenic factor 1)	nuclear	transcription factor	• Sex cord-stromal tumors.
Sm311, Sm32, Sm31 → see Neurofilament			
SMAD4 → see DPC4			
Smooth Muscle Actin (SMA) → see α-Actin			
Smooth muscle myosin heavy chain (SMMHC)	cytoplasmic	myoepithelial cells, blood vessels, myofibroblasts	• Myoepithelial layer in breast to rule out invasive breast cancer.
Smoothelin	cytoplasmic	terminally-differentiated smooth muscle	• Bladder muscularis propria (strong) vs. muscularis mucosae (negative or weak) in assessing depth of invasion in bladder carcinoma.
SOX2 (sex determining region of Y chromosome-related high mobility group box2)	nuclear	fetal CNS tissue	• Embryonal carcinoma; • PNET in teratoma. [21]
SOX9	nuclear	normal cartilage – acts as master regulator of chondrogenesis	• Cartilagenous differentiation, but not specific.
SOX10	nuclear	melanocytes, Schwann cells, myoepithelial cells	• Melanoma; • Clear cell sarcoma; • Nerve sheath tumors; • Pheochromocytoma/paraganglioma (sustentacular cells); • Carcinoid tumors (about 50%). Reference: [22]
SOX11	nuclear	CNS (not well known yet)	• New marker for mantle cell lymphoma.
Spectrin	membranous	RBCs and precursors	• AML with erythroid differentiation (M6)
Surfactant protein A (PE10)	membranous and cytoplasmic	pneumocytes	• Complements TTF-1 in identification of lung carcinomas (but Napsin A is a much more sensitive marker for this role)
Synaptophysin (SYN; secretogranin)	cytoplasmic	neuroendocrine cells, neuronal cells, neuro-muscular junction, Merkel cells	• Neuroendocrine neoplasms (e.g. carcinoid, pheochromocytoma, pancreatic neuroendocrine tumor/islet cell tumors, small cell carcinoma, Merkel cell carcinoma, medullary carcinoma of thyroid), primitive neuroectodermal tumors (neuroblastoma, medulloblastoma, PNET/Ewing), and neuronal tumors (ganglioglioma); • Adrenocortical tumors and pancreatic solid-pseudopapillary tumor (these are SYN +, CHR−).
Syndecan-1 → see CD138			
Synuclein	Lewy bodies	brain	• Lewy bodies in Parkinson's disease and Lewy body dementia.
Tau (AT8)	cytoplasm	brain	• Neurofibrillary tangles in Alzheimer's disease.

Antibody or Antigen (other names)	Cellular Localization	Normal Tissues Stained and Functional Information if Pertinent	What this marker is used to identify and differential diagnoses
TdT (Terminal deoxytransferase)	nuclear	immature B and T lymphocytes	• Precursor B and T leukemia/lymphoma (+) vs. lymphoma of mature cells, including Burkitt (−). Myeloid blasts are generally TdT-negative but can occasionally be (+); • Thymoma (admixed immature T cells are TdT, CD1a, CD99+).
TFE3	nuclear	transcription factor, reactivity in normal tissue extremely rare	• Xp11-translocation RCC; • Alveolar soft part sarcoma; • Subset of renal angiomyolipomas [23]
TFEB	nuclear	transcription factor, reactivity in normal tissue extremely rare	• (6;11)-translocation RCC.
Thyroglobulin (TGB)	cytoplasmic	thyroid follicles	• Carcinomas of thyroid follicular origin (papillary and follicular, medullary CA is negative).
Thrombomodulin (CD141)	cytoplasmic and membranous	endothelial (cytoplasmic) and mesothelial (membranous) cells	• Urothelial carcinoma, mesothelioma (second-line), some vascular tumors.
TIA-1 → see Granzyme B			
TLE1	nuclear	transcription factor whose gene was discovered to be upregulated in gene expression profiles of synovial sarcoma	• Synovial sarcoma (can be focal in schwannoma, SFT).
Transferrin → see CD71			
TTF-1 (Thyroid Transcription Factor 1)	nuclear	transcription factor in lung and thyroid	• Thyroid carcinoma (follicular, papillary, and medullary); • Lung adenoCA (80%+) vs. extra-pulmonary adenoCA (−, with the exception of 20% of gynecologic carcinomas of various types); • Poorly differentiated lung adenoCA (80%+) vs. SqCC (−); • Lung adenoCA (+) vs. mesothelioma (−); • Lung carcinoid (50+, usually weak) vs. extra-pulmonary well-differentiated neuroendocrine tumors • Small cell carcinoma: lung (90%+), and extra-pulmonary (overall 44%) – prostate (58%), bladder (34%), cervix (20%); [24,25] • HCC (+) for cytoplasmic TTF-1.
Trypsin and Chymotrypsin	cytoplasmic	pancreatic acinar cells	• Pancreatic acinar cell carcinoma (+) vs. neuroendocrine tumor and adenocarcinoma (−).
Uroplakin	cytoplasmic	urothelium	• Urothelial carcinoma – specific, but not very sensitive.
Villin	cytoplasmic ("brush border" pattern)	enterocytes	• Intestinal differentiation in carcinoma of unknown primary (but expression is also present in any tumor with "enteric" differentiation; see under CDX2). Similar specificity but lesser sensitivity than CDX2.
Vimentin	cytoplasmic	most mesenchymal cells including fibroblasts, endothelium, smooth muscle	• Sarcoma, lymphoma, and melanoma (+) vs. carcinoma and glioma (−) – historical use. • Clear cell RCC (+) vs. chromophobe RCC and oncocytoma (−) • Bladder muscularis mucosa (+) vs. muscularis propria (−) – used in conjunction with smoothelin, which has the opposite pattern • Because of wide reactivity currently used mainly to confirm "immunoviability" of tissue.
vWF (von Willebrand factor) → see Factor VIII			
WT1 (Wilms Tumor 1)	nuclear	tumor suppressor gene in developing nephrons, nephrogenic rests and adult glomerular podocytes. Also stains normal and neoplastic mesothelium	• Mesothelioma (+) vs. adenocarcinoma (−); • Wilms tumor; • Desmoplastic small round cell tumor; • Ovarian serous carcinoma (80%+).

Abbreviations: ALCL anaplastic large cell lymphoma, ALL acute lymphocytic leukemia, AML acute myeloid leukemia, CLL/SLL chronic lymphocytic leukemia/small lymphocytic lymphoma, DLBCL diffuse large B cell lymphoma, FL follicular lymphoma, GIST gastrointestinal stromal tumor, HL Hodgkin lymphoma, MCL mantle cell lymphoma, MZL marginal zone lymphoma, NLP nodular lymphocyte predominant, R-S Reed-Sternberg, SFT solitary fibrous tumor

Chapter 4 Special Stains

by Justin Bishop, Jennifer Broussard, Natasha Rekhtman

Quick Primer on Mucins

- Mucins (aka mucoproteins or mucopolysaccharides) are large glycoproteins which are the chief components of mucus. Note that these are biochemically distinct from lipids and do not react with a lipid stain Oil-Red-O.

- Mucins are secreted by epithelial cells for protection and lubrication such as in the mucosal surfaces of the GI and respiratory tracts. This type of mucin is known as "epithelial mucin", and it may be produced in abundance (or focally) by some adenocarcinomas.

- Stromal tissues also contain mucopolysaccharides, which impart resilience to connective tissue. Stromal mucins are biochemically distinct from epithelial mucins in that they consist chiefly of hyaluronic acid. In contrast, hyaluronic acid is absent from epithelial mucins. By convention, stromal mucins are referred to as "myxoid" material. Many types of sarcoma secrete myxoid substances (such as myxoid chondrosarcoma) and various tissues may undergo myxoid change as a degenerative process (such as heart valves). Epithelial mucin and stromal myxoid substances are usually readily distinguishable by H&E – mucin is thick and stringy, whereas myxoid material is not. But in some situations they may look similar, and then special stains can be used to distinguish the two, although this is rarely used for diagnostic purposes. See table and diagram below.

- Epithelial mucins come in two varieties, acidic and neutral:
  - **Acid mucins** are present in goblet cells and esophageal submucosal glands. They are **Alcian Blue (AB)-positive** (**blue color**). Most adenocarcinomas elaborate acid mucins.
  - **Neutral mucins** are present in gastric foveolar cells, duodenal Brunner glands and prostate glands. They are **PAS-positive** (**pink color**). Unlike acid mucins, neutral mucins do not react with mucicarmine, AB or colloidal iron.

- Acid mucins are further subdivided into 2 groups (not of major diagnostic importance):
  - **Sialomucins** are the simplest form; they are present in small and large bowel.
  - **Sulfomucins** are the more complex sulfated forms, which are present only in the large bowel.

	Composition	Location	Mucicarmine (pink)	PAS (pink)	AB[1] (blue)	Hale's colloidal iron
Epithelial mucin	Acid mucins, sialated (Sialomucins)	Small and large bowel, salivary glands	+	+	+ (pH 2.5 only)	+
	Acid mucins, sulfated (Sulfomucins)	Large bowel	+	+	+ (pH 2.5 and 0.5)	+
	Neutral mucin	Gastric foveolar cells, prostate	–	+	–	–
Stromal mucin[2] (myxoid material)	Hyaluronic acid (among others)	Myxoid sarcomas, Mesothelioma, Skin in lupus and granuloma annulare	–	–	+ (removed by hyaluronidase digestion)	+

1) The pH of AB can be adjusted to specifically recognize sialomucins (react at pH 2.5, but not 0.5) vs sulfomucins (react at either pH). Only standard pH (2.5) is used for routine applications, wherein all types of mucin are recognized.
2) Note that stromal mucins are detected by AB and Hale's colloidal iron only, whereas mucicarmine and PAS are negative! In addition, sensitivity to digestion with hyaluronidase distinguishes stromal mucins (hyaluronidase-sensitive) from epithelial mucins (hyaluronidase-resistant).

- Because of distinct biochemical composition, various types of mucin can be distinguished by special stains:

    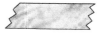

Epithelial (acid) mucin: Mucicarmine+, PAS+, AB+ (Hyaluronidase-resistant)	**Epithelial (neutral) mucin:** PAS+, Mucicarmine–, AB–	**Myxoid Material ("Stromal mucin"):** Negative for mucicarmine and PAS, AB+ (Hyaluronidase-sensitive)

- Distinct types of mucin are utilized in the following differentials:
  1. distinction of <u>mesothelioma</u> (hyaluronic acid-rich; AB+/hyaluronidase-sensitive) from <u>adenocarcinoma</u> (epithelial mucin-rich; AB+/ hyaluronidase-resistant);
  2. diagnosis of <u>intestinal metaplasia</u> in Barrett's esophagus or stomach (see table below for details): native gastric epithelium has neutral mucin (PAS-positive/pink), whereas metaplastic intestinal epithelium has acid mucin (AB-positive/blue). Furthermore, some experts have suggested that sulfomucins portend a poorer prognosis than sialomucins in these metaplasias, but this suggestion is controversial.
  3. distinction of <u>mucinous carcinoma</u> (mucicarmine+) from <u>myxoid sarcoma</u> (mucicarmine–). This application is mainly of historic interest because immunostains can easily resolve this differential.

References: [1-3]

Abbreviations: PAS Periodic Acid Schiff's, AB Alcian Blue

N. Rekhtman, J.A. Bishop, *Quick Reference Handbook for Surgical Pathologists*, DOI:10.1007/978-3-642-20086-1_4, © Springer-Verlag Berlin Heidelberg 2011

Special Stains at a Glance

CARBOHYDRATES: Glycogen and mucosubstances	
Stain [color]	Background and key applications
Mucicarmine [deep rose to red]	• stains **epithelial mucin** (stromal myxoid substances, as in myxoid sarcomas, are mucicarmine–) • used to ID intracytoplasmic mucin; this is a rapid and cheap method to diagnose adenocarcinoma • also used to ID other mucin-producing tumors (e.g. mucoepidermoid carcinoma)
Periodic Acid Schiff's, PAS [pink]	• stains **glycogen** and **mucin**; also stains basement membranes and fungi • used to ID glycogen-rich lesions (e.g. acinar carcinoma, pancreatic serous cystadenoma) • certain tumors are PAS+ (e.g. Ewing sarcoma/PNET, rhabdomyosarcoma are + versus lymphoma is –), but this feature is rarely utilized diagnostically in lieu of advances in immunohistochemistry • used to ID ASPS, which contains PAS+ intracytoplasmic crystals
PAS with Diastase Digestion, PAS/D	• diastase (D) enzyme digests glycogen yielding a negative PAS reaction; in contrast, mucin is resistant to digestion and PAS remains positive • used to differentiate glycogen (PAS/D^{Sensitive}) from mucin (PAS/D^{Resistant})
Alcian Blue, AB [blue, dah!]	• stains **acid mucin** (goblet cells) and stromal mucins (myxoid sarcomas) • staining properties are pH-dependent (see above)
PAS/Alcian Blue, PAS/AB	• "pan-mucin" stain: reacts with both neutral (PAS+) and acid (AB+) mucins; routine stain on GI biopsy service • used to ID intestinal metaplasia with goblet cells (*AB+/deep blue*) in esophagus (Barrett's mucosa) and stomach • used to ID gastric mucin cell metaplasia (*PAS+/pink*) in small bowel (seen in chronic peptic duodenitis and IBD) • aids in the diagnosis of adenocarcinoma: PAS/AB may be used in conjunction with or in place of mucicarmine to demonstrate intracytoplasmic mucin
AB with Hyaluronidase Digestion	• used to differentiate adenocarcinoma (AB+/hyaluronidase digest resistant) from hyaluronic acid-rich mesothelioma (AB+/ hyaluronidase digest sensitive)
Hale's colloidal iron [light blue]	• mucin stain with iron as a reagent (this is NOT a stain for iron!) • used to distinguish renal chromophobe carcinoma (positive) from oncocytoma (negative) • also used to identify intradermal mucin (as in granuloma annulare)

CONNECTIVE TISSUE	
Masson's Trichrome ("three colors")	• can be used to differentiate collagen [blue] from smooth muscle [red] • routine stain in evaluation of medical liver and kidney

Movat's Pentachrome ("five colors")	• primarily used to evaluate lung disease:
	  – loose collagen (mucopolysaccharide-rich) is blue-green: indicates a subacute process (e.g. BOOP structures)
	  – dense collagen/fibrosis is yellow: indicates chronicity (e.g. usual interstitial pneumonia)
	• can aid in evaluation of vessels and pleura (stains elastic fibers)

Reticulin	• reticulin pattern can aid in DDx of certain neoplasms:
	  – meningioma (reticulin-negative) vs HPC (reticulin-positive) (see neuropath section)
	  – loss of reticulin network differentiates well diff HCC from hepatic adenoma (see liver section) and normal pituitary from adenoma
	  – lymphomas – fine reticulin network
	• used to evaluate bone marrow (to r/o reticulin fibrosis)

Elastic (VVG or Verhoerff's Van Gieson)	• used to assess the invasion of elastica in the visceral pleura in staging of pulmonary carcinomas • also used to evaluate vessels

OTHER COMMON APPLICATIONS	
Fat (lipids)	Oil red O [red], Sudan black B [black]; tissue must be fresh or frozen, not fixed!
Melanin	Fontana-Masson [black]
Calcium	Von Kossa [black]
Iron	Prussian blue [blue]
Amyloid	• Congo Red (dense salmon pink in direct light; apple green birefringence in polarized light), Crystal violet, Sirius Red, Thioflavin T (amyloid fluoresces in UV light) • Also used are immunostains for Ig κ and λ light chains (primary amyloidosis), amyloid A protein (secondary amyloidosis), β$_2$ Microglobulin (dialysis-associated amyloidosis), Transthyretin (hereditary amyloidosis), other

4 Special Stains: Special Stains at a Glance.

Special Stains at a Glance: Microorganisms

GENERAL	

Fungi	• **GMS (Grocott's Methenamine Silver)** [black]
	  – demonstrates all fungi, including *Pneumocystis*
	  – also stains *Actinomyces*, *Nocardia*, and some encapsulated bacteria
	• **PAS & PAS/LG** (PAS/Light Green is preferred for dermatophytes) [red]
	• **Mucicarmine (& AB):** capsule of *Cryptococcus* [red (& blue)]
	• **Fontana-Masson:** melanin pigment in *Cryptococcus* and pigmented filamentous fungi [black]

Bacteria	• **Brown and Brenn (or Brown and Hopps modification):** demonstrates Gram – [red] and Gram + [blue] bacteria • **Gram-Weigert:** demonstrates Gram + bacteria [blue to purple] and PCP [blue to purple] but not Gram – bacteria! • **Warthin Starry:** demonstrates spirochetes (*Treponema*), *Helicobacter*, *Chlamydia*, and *Legionella* [black]
Acid-Fast Organisms	• **Kinyoun's** (a variant of **Ziehl-Neelsen**): routine AFB stain [red]; detects all Mycobacteria, including MAI • **Auramine/Rhodamine** (fluorescent stain): more sensitive than Kinyoun's • **Fite:** demonstrates delicate acid fast organisms (*Nocardia*, *M.leprae*) [red] • **Feulgen:** stains microbial DNA [magenta] • **Gram-Weigert:** acid fast organisms are gram +, but sensitivity is low

SELECT MICROORGANISMS	
Pneumocystis	GMS is best [black]; Gram-Weigert [blue to purple], Giemsa [intracystic trophozoites are purple]
Nocardia	Fite [bright red], Brown-Hopps [blue], Gram-Weigert [blue], GMS [black]
Histoplasma	GMS [black], Giemsa [reddish blue]
Cryptococcus	GMS [black], Mucicarmine [capsule red], Alcian Blue [capsule blue], PAS [cell wall red], Fontana-Masson [black], India Ink (on CSF samples; historic use)
Spirochetes	Warthin Starry [black], Dieterle [dark brown-black]
Actinomyces	Brown-Hopps [blue], Gram-Weigert [blue], GMS [black]
Helicobacter Pylori	Diff Quick [dark blue], Giemsa [dark blue], Warthin-Starry [black]
Tropheryma whippelii (Whipple's disease)	PAS highlights filamentous organisms [pink]; AFB negative; also, an immunostain for *Tropheryma Whippelii* is available (DDx: MAI is chunky on PAS, AFB+)
Leishmania	Giemsa [reddish blue], GMS-negative, PAS-negative
Entamoeba	PAS [pink cytoplasm]

Alphabetical Index of Special Stain

by Jennifer Broussard, Natasha Rekhtman, Justin Bishop

Stain	What this stain is used to identify and comments	How it stains
Acid-Fast Bacteria (AFB, Kinyoun's, Ziehl-Neelsen)	• Acid-fast bacilli (Mycobacteria) include *M. tuberculosis* (TB), *M. leprae* (leprosy), and atypical/non-tuberculous mycobacteria (*M. avium-intracellulare* complex – MAC or MAI). • AFB detects TB and MAI. *M. leprae* requires FITE. • Other organisms detected by AFB: *Cryptosporidium*, *Isospora* and hooklets of Cysticerci. • Kinyoun's = modified Ziehl-Neelsen. • Note: "Acid-fast" refers to the organism's ability to retain the red dye in the presence of acid (meaning it is "color-fast" or "holds on tight to color"). Some delicate organisms (*Nocardia, M. leprae*) are "weakly Acid Fast": they get decolorized by strong acids in standard AFB stains (Kinyoun's) but are able to retain the dye when treated with weaker acids in modified acid-fast stain (Fite).	Acid-fast bacilli: bright red Background: blue
Alcian Blue (AB)	• **Acid mucin** (goblet cells) and stromal mucins (myxoid sarcomas) • Staining properties are pH-dependent (see mucin primer above for details)	Acid mucins/mucosubstances: blue Nuclei: reddish pink
Alcian Blue with Hyaluronidase Digestion	• Hyaluronidase digests hyaluronic acid but not mucin, and is used to differentiate adenocarcinoma with mucin (AB+/hyaluronidase digest [resistant]) from hyaluronic acid-rich mesothelioma (AB+/ hyaluronidase digest [sensitive])	Digested areas: unstained Undigested areas: blue Nuclei: reddish pink
Auramine-Rhodamine	• Acid fast bacteria. Supposed to have higher sensitivity than AFB, but you have to use a fluorescent microscope.	Acid-fast organisms: reddish-yellow fluorescence Background: black
Bilirubin (Hall's Bilirubin Stain)	• Bilirubin (the principal bile pigment, and a normal product of red cell degradation) • Excessive amounts of bile pigment in the liver may be found in cases of hepatic or extra-hepatic biliary obstruction.	Bile pigment: green Muscle and cell cytoplasm: yellow Collagen: red
Brown & Hopps (Brown & Brenn)	• Gram-negative and Gram-positive bacteria in tissue.	Gram-positive bacteria: blue Gram-negative bacteria: red Nuclei: red Background: yellow
Congo Red (CR)	• Amyloid deposits in tissue sections.	Amyloid: red to pink (direct light); apple-green (polarized light) Nuclei: blue Need to cut sections slightly thicker (8um) for optimal birefringence
Copper	• Copper deposits left in the liver, such as in Wilson's disease.	Copper deposits: bright red to orange
Cresyl Violet	• Nerve cells and glia.	Nerve cell nucleus: pale blue Nissl bodies: dark blue Astrocytes: pale blue Oligodendroglia: very dark blue
Crystal Violet	• Carbohydrates. • May be used to highlight amyloid.	Amyloid: blue-purple All other tissue elements: blue
Dieterle	• Spirochetes, *Legionella*, and other bacteria. • Melanin granules, chromatin, formalin pigment and some foreign material also stain.	Spirochetes, *Legionella*, etc: black to dark brown; Background: pale yellow to tan
Diff Quick (Diff Quik®, Rapid Romanowsky)	• *H. pylori*. • A modified Giemsa stain. • Routine stain for air-dried smears in cytopathology.	*H. pylori*: dark blue Nuclei: blue Cytoplasm: pink
Elastic van Gieson (EVG) → see Verhoeff's Van Gieson		
Feulgen	• DNA in tissue. • Often used for ploidy studies. • Also used to identify AFB.	Nuclei: magenta Background: green

Stain	What this stain is used to identify and comments	How it stains
Fite	• *M. tuberculosis* (TB) PLUS delicate acid-fast organisms - *Mycobacterium leprae* (leprosy) and *Nocardia*. • Uses a weaker acid than other AFB stains. • More user-friendly than AFB because the background tissue architecture is visible.	Acid-fast bacilli: red Background: blue
Fontana-Masson	• Argentaffin granules and melanin. • Cryptococcus and other melanin-producing fungi.	Melanin, argentaffin cells: black Nuclei: red
Giemsa	• *H. pylori*. • Also differentiates hematopoietic cells, and is used in blood smears.	*Helicobacter*, bacteria: dark blue Cell nuclei: blue Connective tissues: pink Red blood cells: salmon pink Starch and cellulose: sky blue
Giemsa– Bone Marrow	• Differentiation of cells present in hematopoietic tissue. • Also used for the demonstration of some microorganisms.	Nuclear chromatin: dark blue Cytoplasm of lymphocytes and monocytes: pale blue Neutrophil granules: purple Eosinophil granules: pink/orange Basophil granules: purple/black Nucleoli: blue Erythrocytes: pink Connective tissue: pink to light purple Mast cell granules: ark purple
Gram-Weigert	• Gram-positive bacteria. • *Pneumocystis jirovecii* (formerly *P. carinii* or PCP) • Does not stain Gram-negative bacteria, so often ordered with Brown and Hopps.	Gram-positive Bacteria: blue-purple Background: pink
Grimelius – Pascual's Modified	• Argentaffin cells will have a positive reaction with the argyrophil techniques, but the argyrophil cells will not react with the argentaffin techniques. • This procedure was used for the differentiation of carcinoid tumors (mostly of historical interest)	Argyrophilic cells: black Nuclei: red Background: yellow to gold
Grocott's (or Gomori's) Methenamine Silver (GMS)	• Fungi, including *Pneumocystis jirovecii* (formerly *P. carinii* or PCP). • Also stains elastic fibers, suture material, calcifications, and others.	Fungi: black Background: green
Hale's Colloidal Iron	• A mucin stain with iron as a reagent (this is NOT a stain for iron!). • Used to ID intradermal mucin (as in granuloma annulare). • Chromophobe RCC (+) vs. oncocytoma (-).	Cytoplasm of chromophobe RCC, stromal mucins: Light blue Nuclei: Red
Hall's Bilirubin Stain → see Bilirubin		
Iron	• Ferric iron in tissue sections. • Small amounts of iron are found normally in spleen and bone marrow. Excessive amounts are present in hemochromatosis (deposits in the liver and pancreas), and hemosiderosis (deposits in the liver, spleen, and lymph nodes).	Iron (hemosiderin): blue Nuclei: red Background: pink
Kinyoun's → see Acid Fast Bacteria		
Leder	• Neutrophils, mast cells and their precursors.	Cytoplasm of neutrophilic myeloid cells and mast cells: red Nuclei: blue Erythrocytes: pale pink to colorless
Luxol Fast Blue	• Myelinated fibers.	Myelinated fibers: blue Neutrophils: pink Nerve cells: purple
Masson's Trichrome ("three colors")	• Collagen (+) vs. smooth muscle (-) in tumors • Collagen in diseases such as cirrhosis. • Reinke crystals in Leydig cell tumor. • Routine stain for liver and kidney biopsies.	Nuclei: black Cytoplasm, muscle, erythrocytes: red Collagen: blue
Melanin Bleach	• When melanin pigment is present in large amounts, cell detail may be obscured. • Also the ability to be bleached serves as an identifying factor for melanin.	If the pigment is melanin it will not be present on the slide that was bleached.

Special Stains

Special Stains

Stain	What this stain is used to identify and comments	How it stains
Miller's Elastic	• Elastic fibers.	Elastic fibers, nuclei and mast cells: blue-black Muscle: yellow Collagen: red

Movat's Pentachrome ("five colors")	• Connective tissue stain that demonstrates many entities: nuclei, elastin, collagen, ground substance, mucin, muscle and fibrin.
	• Can aid in evaluation of vessels and pleura (stains elastic fibers)
	• Primarily used to evaluate lung disease:
	  – loose collagen (mucopolysaccharide-rich) is blue-green: indicates a subacute process (e.g. organizing fibroplasia in organizing pneumonia)
	  – dense collagen/fibrosis is yellow: indicates chronicity (e.g. usual interstitial pneumonia)
		Nuclei: black
		Elastic fibers: black
		Collagen (established): yellow
		Ground substance/mucin/subacute fibroblastic tissue: blue to green
		Muscle: red
		Fibrinoid: intense red

Mucicarmine	• **Epithelial mucin** (stromal myxoid substances, as in myxoid sarcomas, are mucicarmine–) • Demonstration of intracytoplasmic mucin is a rapid and cheap method to diagnose adenocarcinoma and other mucin-producing tumors (e.g. mucoepidermoid carcinoma). • (See mucin primer above for details)	Mucin: deep rose Nuclei: black Other tissue elements: yellow
Oil Red O	• Fat or lipids. • Requires FRESH (UNFIXED) tissue. • Fat occurring in an abnormal place, such as fat emboli that may develop after either a bone fracture or an injury that crushes a fatty body area or fat accumulation in the liver (steatosis). • Certain tumors (e.g. liposarcoma, sebaceous carcinoma, lipid vacuoles in Burkitt lymphoma) • Hemangioblastoma (+) vs. RCC (-)	Fat: red Nuclei: blue

Periodic Acid Schiff's (PAS)	• Glycogen, neutral mucin, basement membranes, and fungi.
	• A routine stain for liver and kidney biopsies.
	• Can be difficult to read because of high background.
	• Has applications in tumor diagnosis:
	  – glycogen-rich tumors: acinar carcinoma, pancreatic serous cystadenoma
	  – Alveolar soft parts sarcoma – contains PAS+ intracytoplasmic crystals
	  – Ewing sarcoma/PNET and rhabdomyosarcoma (+) versus lymphoma (PAS–) this is rarely utilized diagnostically in lieu of advances in immunohistochemistry
		Mucin, glycogen, fungus: pink
		Nuclei: blue

PAS/AB (Periodic Acid Schiff's /Alcian Blue)	• Both acid (AB) and neutral (PAS) mucins.
	• A routine stain for GI biopsies with many applications:
	  – Intestinal metaplasia with goblet cells (*AB+/deep blue*) in esophagus (Barrett's mucosa) and stomach.
	  – Gastric mucin cell metaplasia (*PAS+/pink*) in small bowel (seen in chronic peptic duodenitis and inflammatory bowel disease)
	  – Adenocarcinoma at any site: PAS/AB may be used in conjunction with or in place of mucicarmine to demonstrate intracytoplasmic mucin
		Acid mucosubstances (AB+): blue
		Neutral polysaccharides (PAS+): pink

PAS/Diastase (PAS/D)	• Fungus. • Diastase enzyme digests glycogen yielding a negative PAS reaction whereas mucin is resistant to digestion and PAS remains positive. • Used to differentiate glycogen (PAS/D^{Sensitive}) from mucin (PAS/D^{Resistant})	Glycogen: pink by PAS and absent by PAS/D. Mucin: Pink by PAS and PAS/D Note: If slide is over digested, the tissue must be recut. Over digestion has the appearance of lace; there is no tissue left.
PAS Light Green	• Fungus. • Does not stain mucin or basement membranes.	Fungus: pink Background: green
PAS/Methenamine Silver (PAS/MS)	• Basement membrane. • Especially suitable for demonstrating fine glomerular basement membranes in thin sections.	Basement membrane: black Nuclei: blue Background: pink
PTAH (Phostphotungstic Acid-Hematoxylin)	• Muscle cross-striations and fibrin. • Nemaline rods, present in some skeletal muscle diseases, may also be demonstrated by the method. • Truly oncocytic neoplasms, wherein PTAH stains mitochondria.	Cross-striations, fibrin, glial fibers: blue Neurons: pink Mitochondria: Blue Nuclei: blue Collagen: red-brown Elastic fibers: purplish

Stain	What this stain is used to identify and comments	How it stains
Reticulin	• A silver impregnation technique that demonstrates reticulin fibers, which form a support function of the body and are abundant in liver, spleen, and kidney. • The reticulin framework is characteristically lost in some tumors (e.g., HCC, pituitary adenoma). • Reticulin fibers also form characteristic patterns in relationship to certain tumor cells (positive in sarcoma and lymphoma, negative in carcinoma and glioma).	Reticular fibers: black Nuclei: red
Sirius Red	• Amyloid.	Amyloid: rose red Nuclei: blue Background: pale pink
Sudan Black	• Fat. • Like Oil Red O, tissue must be fresh.	Fat: blue-black Nuclei: red
Thioflavin S	• Amyloid. • A fluorescent stain.	Amyloid: fluorescent green Background: black
Toluidine Blue	• Mast cells. Their cytoplasm contains metachromatic granules composed of heparin and histamine.	Mast cells: violet Background: blue
Verhhoeff's Van Gieson (VVG or Elastic Van Gieson, EVG)	• Useful in demonstrating atrophy of elastic tissue in cases of emphysema, and the thinning and loss of elastic fibers in vascular diseases. • Also used to confirm invasion of elastic fibers in the visceral pleura for lung cancer staging • Also used to evaluate vessels	Elastic fibers and nuclei: black Collagen: red Other tissue elements: yellow
Von Kossa	• Deposits of calcium in any area of the body. • May discriminate between urate crystals and true calcium, which appear similar histologically, to make the diagnosis of chondrocalcinosis (pseudo-gout).	Calcium salts: black Nuclei: red Cytoplasm: pink
Warthin Starry	• Spirochetes, *H. pylori*, *B. henselae* (cat scratch), and *Legionella* in tissue.	Bacteria: black Nuclei and red blood cells: brown. Background: pale yellow
Ziehl–Neelsen→ see Acid Fast Bacteria		

Special Stains

Chapter 5 Grading (and Classification) Systems

by Justin Bishop, Amy Duffield, Diana Molavi, Natasha Rekhtman

Grading Systems

Grading of Adenocarcinoma, NOS	
	Fraction of tumor composed of glands
Well differentiated (Grade 1)	> 95%
Moderately differentiated (Grade 2)	50% – 95%
Poorly differentiated (Grade 3)	< 50%

- Applies mainly to adenocarcinomas of the gastrointestinal tract (esophagus, stomach, bowel, anus).

- Undifferentiated (Grade 4) CA applies to carcinomas that are so poorly differentiated that they cannot be identified as adenocarcinoma vs. SqCC vs. other. Small cell and large cell neuroendocrine carcinomas are usually classified as grade 4.

- For colon cancer, AJCC recommends a two-tiered system: low-grade (WD+MD) versus high-grade (PD).

- Grade is assigned based on the least differentiated area.

- Note that this is a "rule of thumb" and more detailed grading systems (incorporating other features such as cytologic pleomorphism, necrosis, mitoses, etc) are either available or being developed. However the loss of glandular architecture is a general hallmark of poor differentiation.

References: [1,2]

Grading of Squamous Cell Carcinoma (SqCC), NOS		
	Nuclear pleomorphism and mitoses (including atypical mitoses)	Keratinization and intercellular bridges
Well differentiated (Grade 1)	Absent	Abundant
Moderately differentiated (Grade 2)	Intermediate	Intermediate
Poorly differentiated (Grade 3)	Abundant	Nearly absent

- Applies to SqCC of any site: head and neck, lung, abdominal organs (esophagus, bladder), skin, etc.

- There is no widely accepted quantitative definition of grading in SqCC. As a "rule of thumb", WD SqCC are said to closely resemble normal squamous epithelium, whereas PD SqCC are those in which squamous origin can be barely discerned.

- It is generally emphasized that the grade should be assigned based on nuclear features rather than degree of keratinization, although the two almost always go together. Nevertheless, the degree of keratinization is usually expressed by designating a SqCC as "keratinizing" vs. "non-keratinizing" separately from the grade.

- HPV-related SqCC of the oropharynx should not be graded. [3]

- As for adenocarcinoma, grade is assigned based on the least differentiated area.

- In contrast to adenocarcinoma, grade does not appear to be a strong predictive factor in SqCC, particularly of the head and neck.

Reference: [4,5]

Breast

Elston* Grading of Infiltrating Breast Cancer

Parameter	Point Score	Final Score (add point scores in rows 1, 2 and 3) and corresponding grade
1) Tubule formation (% composed of tubules) • >75% • 10–75% • <10%	1 2 3	
2) Nuclear Pleomorphism [1] • mild • moderate • severe	1 2 3	**3–5 points → Grade I** (well-differentiated) **6–7 points → Grade II** (moderately-differentiated) **8–9 points → Grade III** (poorly-differentiated)
3) Mitoses per 10 HPF (HPF = 40X objective or 400X field) [2] Field diameter [3] 0.44 mm 0.52 mm 0.59 mm • <5 <8 <9 • 6–11 8–15 10–19 • >12 >16 >20	1 2 3	

1) Mild pleomorphism: uniform nuclei, size similar to normal duct cells.
   Moderate and severe pleomorphism: increasing severity of nuclear enlargement, hyperchromasia, clumped (vesicular) chromatin and prominent nucleoli.

2) Mitotic count should be performed at the peripheral edge of a tumor, which is the most mitotically active site.

3) The actual size of 400X field is microscope-dependent, and should be measured with stage micrometer. For a table with conversion between field size, mitotic count and point score see reference [6] or http://www.cancerscreening.nhs.uk/breastscreen/publications/nhsbsp58.html (see NHSBSP 58 pages 79–80).

• Lobular carcinoma is always given 3 points for lack of tubule formation. It is still usually Elston grade 1 or 2, as nuclei generally get 1–2 points and mitotic count gets 1 point. Ductal carcinoma is more commonly Elston grade 2 or 3. Tubular cancer is by definition grade 1.

* "Elston grade" is mercifully short for "Elston-Ellis modification of Scarff-Bloom-Richardson" grading system (or Nottingham combined histological grade).

References: [1,6,7]

Nuclear Grading of Ductal Carcinoma in Situ (DCIS)

	Nuclear Size	Mitoses per 10 HPF	Nuclear Pleomorphism [1]	Necrosis [2]
Grade 1	<1.5 rbc or normal duct cell	<1	mild	–
Grade 2	1–2 rbc	1–2	moderate	+ (central necrosis)
Grade 3	>2.5 rbc	>2	severe	+++ (comedonecrosis)

1) Nuclear pleomorphism is graded as described above for invasive lesions.

2) Note that the term comedonecrosis is reserved for grade 3 lesions; necrosis in grade 2 lesions is referred to as "central necrosis".

Note: LCIS is not graded (it is by definition grade 1).

Reference: [1,6]

Grading of Phyllodes Tumor

	Stromal cellularity	Stromal overgrowth (4X field is all stroma)	Stromal pleomorphism	Infiltrative Border	Mitoses/10 HPF
Benign	mild	–	minimal	usually –	0–1
Borderline/low grade malignant	moderate	–	mild	+/–	2–5
Malignant	marked	+ (required for Dx)	marked	+	>5–10*

* WHO criteria is >10 mitoses/10 HPF

References: [1,8]

Grading Systems

Genitourinary Tract: Prostate and Kidney

<table>
<tr><td colspan="3">Gleason Grading of Prostate Cancer
(see http://pathology2.jhu.edu/gleason/patterns.cfm for tutorial)</td></tr>
<tr><td colspan="3">The Gleason system is a five-tier system based entirely on architectural pattern; nuclear features are not factored in. The grade is reported as a sum of the most prevalent (primary) and second most prevalent (secondary) pattern to obtain a "combined Gleason grade" or "Gleason score". For example, a tumor with primary Gleason pattern 3 and secondary Gleason pattern 4 is reported as Gleason grade 3+4=7. Note that in this example 3 and 4 are "Gleason patterns" and 7 is a "Gleason score".</td></tr>
<tr><td>Gleason Pattern 1</td><td><ul><li>non-infiltrative nodule</li><li>round to oval back-to-back glands</li><li>exceedingly rare diagnosis, usually seen on TURP specimens</li></ul></td><td rowspan="5"></td></tr>
<tr><td>Gleason Pattern 2</td><td><ul><li>fairly well circumscribed nodule, but minimal infiltration is allowed</li><li>glands are more loosely arranged and not as uniform as those in pattern 1</li><li>usually but not always in transition zone</li></ul></td></tr>
<tr><td>Gleason Pattern 3</td><td><ul><li>clearly infiltrative pattern (unlike patterns 1 & 2)</li><li>glands vary in size and shape</li><li>all glands are distinct, such that one can draw a mental circle around each gland</li><li>PIN-like ductal adenocarcinoma</li></ul></td></tr>
<tr><td>Gleason Pattern 4</td><td><ul><li>glands are no longer separate as seen in patterns 1–3 (one cannot draw a mental circle around each gland): glands are fused, poorly defined, cribriform, or glomeruloid</li><li>all cribriform glands are now considered pattern 4</li><li>ductal adenocarcinoma (except PIN-like variant, which is graded as pattern 3)</li></ul></td></tr>
<tr><td>Gleason Pattern 5</td><td><ul><li>cells in solid sheets, rosettes, cords or single cells with virtually no glandular differentiation</li><li>nests of tumor with central "comedonecrosis" are also classified as pattern 5</li></ul></td></tr>
<tr><td>Not Graded</td><td><ul><li>small cell prostate carcinoma</li><li>adenocarcinoma with Paneth cell-like differentiation (by criteria, would be graded 5+5, but behaves like 3+3)</li></ul></td><td></td></tr>
<tr><td colspan="3">Because clinical decisions are based primarily on the total Gleason score, two recent modifications to the traditional Gleason grading have been proposed to better convey the severity of disease:
1. "5% cut-off rule": If lower-grade pattern occupies <5% of the tumor, it can be ignored. For example, a 4+3=7 in traditional Gleason grading should be diagnosed as 4+4=8.
2. When three Gleason patterns (e.g. 3, 4, 5) are present, the Gleason score is derived by adding the most prevalent and the highest grades (this applies only to needle biopsies, but not resections).
Abbreviations: PIN prostatic intraepithelial neoplasia, TURP transurethral resection of the prostate

References: http://pathology2.jhu.edu/gleason/patterns.cfm, [9]
Illustration by Jennifer Brumbaugh; reprinted from Journal of Urology 2010 (183): 433-440; Epstein JI; An update of the Gleason grading system; with permission from © Elsevier 2010.</td></tr>
</table>

<table>
<tr><td colspan="2">Grading of Prostatic Intraepithelial Neoplasia (PIN)</td></tr>
<tr><td>LGPIN (low grade prostatic intraepithelial neoplasia)</td><td>darker nuclei (stand out at low power)</td></tr>
<tr><td>HGPIN (high grade prostatic intraepithelial neoplasia)</td><td>nucleoli visible at 20X</td></tr>
</table>

Reference: [10]

<table>
<tr><td colspan="4">Fuhrman Nuclear Grading of Renal Cell Carcinoma</td></tr>
<tr><td></td><td>Nuclei</td><td>Nucleoli</td><td>other</td></tr>
<tr><td>Grade 1</td><td>small, round, uniform</td><td>absent</td><td></td></tr>
<tr><td>Grade 2</td><td>larger, crinkly nuclear membrane</td><td>absent-inconspicuous</td><td></td></tr>
<tr><td>Grade 3</td><td>large, very crinkly</td><td>conspicuous (visible at 10X)</td><td></td></tr>
<tr><td>Grade 4</td><td>pleomorphic, clumped chromatin</td><td>prominent</td><td>Sarcomatoid (spindly) features</td></tr>
</table>

- Tumors are graded by the worst area, however focal.
- Grading is applied to clear cell and papillary RCC (although grading of papillary RCC is controversial).
- Collecting duct carcinoma is Fuhrman grade 3–4.
- Sarcomatoid RCC is by definition Fuhrman grade 4.
- Chromophobe RCC is generally not graded.
- Oncocytoma is benign and therefore not graded.

Reference: [11]

Genitourinary Tract: Bladder and Wilms Tumor

The WHO (2003)/ISUP Consensus Classification of Non-invasive (In Situ) Papillary Urothelial Neoplasms (see www.pathology.jhu.edu/bladder for tutorial)					
	Urothelial thickness	Cellular disorganization: loss of polarity, crowding	Pleomorphism[4]	Mitoses	Fusion & branching of papillae (soft feature)
Papilloma	Normal (<7 layers)	Absent (perfectly orderly, identical to normal)	Absent	Absent	None
PUNLMP[1]	Increased	Absent (perfectly orderly, identical to normal)	Absent	Rare, basal	Rare
LGTCC[2]	Increased	Minimal	Mild	Occasional, at any level	Occasional
HGTCC[3]	Increased	Prominent	Moderate-Severe	Frequent, at any level	Frequent

1) **PUNLMP** (Papillary urothelial neoplasm of low malignant potential): cells may be uniformly enlarged but they are identical to each other in all fields and are perfectly oriented (orderly).
2) **LGTCC** (Low-grade TCC or papillary urothelial carcinoma): overall low-power appearance is orderly but there is distinctive variation of architectural and/or cytological features.
3) **HGTCC** (High-grade TCC or papillary urothelial carcinoma): distinctive pleomorphism and loss of polarity/crowding. Necrosis and cellular discohesion, when present, are specific to HGTCC.
4) Pleomorphism refers to nuclear enlargement, hyperchromasia, variation in size and shape, and prominence of nucleoli. Nuclear grooves, a feature of normal urothelium, are preserved in PUNLMP but are lost in carcinomas (low-grade and high-grade).

"5% rule": Grade is assigned based on the highest-grade area, unless it is <5% of the tumor (presence of a small higher-grade area may be mentioned in a note).

Reference: [12]

The WHO (2003)/ISUP Consensus Classification of Flat In Situ Urothelial Neoplasms (see www.pathology.jhu.edu/bladder for tutorial)	
Dysplasia	Some features of CIS are present, but fall short of the threshold for CIS (cytology similar to LGTCC). Uncommon diagnosis.
Carcinoma in situ (CIS)	Nucleomegaly (nuclei are **5X** the size of stromal lymphocytes versus normal urothelium is 2–3X), pleomorphism, crowding, loss of polarity (cytology similar to HGTCC).

Reference: [12]

Abbreviations: TCC transitional cell carcinoma, ISUP International Society of Urological Pathology

Wilms tumor: Criteria for Anaplasia (unfavorable histology)
1) Nucleomegaly (at least 3X enlargement). 2) Nuclear hyperchromasia. 3) Atypical mitoses.
Note: Anaplasia predicts resistance to chemotherapy rather than inherent aggressiveness.

Reference: [11]

Head and Neck

Grading of Thyroid Carcinomas	
Well differentiated[1]	Papillary carcinoma[2] Follicular carcinoma[3] • Widely invasive • Encapsulated
"Moderately differentiated"	(None)[4]
Poorly differentiated (Insular)	Insular, solid, or trabecular architecture + no papillary nuclear features + one of these three: convoluted nuclei, elevated mitoses ($\geq$3/10 HPF), or necrosis.[5]
Undifferentiated (Anaplastic)	Minimal or no thyroid differentiation. Includes squamoid, pleomorphic/giant cell, and spindled variants

1) Medullary carcinoma has a significantly worse prognosis than papillary or follicular carcinoma and is not really graded. As a result, when you hear the term "well differentiated thyroid cancer," it usually refers to just the papillary and follicular types.

2) Tall cell, columnar cell, and diffuse sclerosing variants have a worse prognosis and should be mentioned in the report.

3) In widely invasive there is often no capsule to evaluate because the cancer has pretty much blown past it. Some authorities recommend limiting the term "minimally invasive" to cases that have capsular invasion only. [13] For angioinvasive follicular carcinomas, the approximate number of invasive foci should be reported (if <3, the prognosis is good).

4) Some regard the high risk variants of papillary CA as well as widely invasive follicular CA as "moderately differentiated" thyroid carcinoma. [14] We do not use this designation at JHH or MSKCC (thanks to Nora Katabi for helpful discussions).

5) The criteria listed above are from the Turin proposal. [15] However, at MSKCC the criteria are less strict, requiring only elevated mitoses (>4/10 HPF) *or* necrosis. [16] Regardless of what criteria are used to diagnose poorly differentiated carcinoma, the presence of the high-grade features or elevated mitoses and necrosis in a follicular or papillary carcinoma should be mentioned.

Grading of Salivary Gland Carcinomas			
Low Grade	Intermediate Grade	High Grade	Variable Grade
Acinic Cell Carcinoma Polymorphous Low Grade Adenocarci-noma Basal Cell Adenocarcinoma Epithelial-Myoepithelial Carcinoma	Adenoid Cystic Carcinoma [1] Myoepithelial Carcinoma	Salivary Duct Carcinoma Large Cell Carcinoma	Mucoepidermoid Carcinoma (see table below) Adenocarcinoma, NOS [2] Carcinoma-ex-Pleomorphic Adenoma [3]

1) Although adenoid cystic carcinoma is generally considered an intermediate grade carcinoma, tumors with solid areas (especially >30%) behave worse (more like high grade).

2) Adenocarcinoma, NOS is graded low, intermediate, or high based on cytological and architectural features.

3) The type of carcinoma arising in the mixed tumor should be graded as if would if it had arisen *de novo*.

Reference: [17]

Mucoepidermoid Carcinoma, AFIP Grading System		
Histopathological Feature	Point Value	Total Point Score (add points in Point Value column) and Corresponding Tumor Grade
Cystic component <20%	2	
Neural invasion	2	0–4 → **Low-grade**
Necrosis	3	5–6 → **Intermediate-grade**
> 4 mitoses per 10 HPF	3	> 7 → **High-grade**
Anaplasia	4	

References: [17,18]

Evaluation of Autoimmune Sialiadenitis (Sjögren's Disease) in Labial Biopsy		
Grade	Amount of inflammation (lymphocytes, plasma cells, histiocytes)	Likelihood of Sjögren's disease
0	absent	nondiagnostic
1	slight infiltrate	nondiagnostic
2	moderate infiltrate (less than 1 focus* per 4 mm^2)	nondiagnostic
3	one focus per 4 mm^2	suggestive
4	more than one focus per 4 mm^2	diagnostic

* "Focus" is defined as an aggregate containing at least 50 lymphocytes, plasma cells, or macrophages.

References: [19,20]

Grading Systems

Pancreas

Grading of Pancreatic Intraepithelial Neoplasia (PanIN) and Pancreatic Cystic Mucinous Neoplasms (IPMN and MCN)					
Terminology for PanIN	Cytology	Architecture	Illustration	Terminology for IPMN (WHO 2010)	Terminology for MCN (WHO 2010)
PanIN-1A	small bland cuboidal basally-located nuclei	flat	PanIN-1A	IPMN-low grade dysplasia (formerly adenoma)	MCN- low grade dysplasia
PanIN-1B		papillary	PanIN-1B		
PanIN-2	moderate pleomorphism (↑N/C ratio, prominent nucleoli) stratified nuclei some rising to luminal surface	usually papillary	PanIN-2	IPMN-moderate dysplasia (formerly borderline)	MCN-moderate dysplasia
PanIN-3	severe pleomorphism (as in carcinoma) loss of nuclear polarity dystrophic goblet cells (goblet cells with flipped polarity – nuclei oriented toward the lumen and mucinous cytoplasm toward the basement membrane) atypical mitoses	papillary or micropapillary, luminal budding, fusion of micropapillae, cribriforming + necrosis (even with bland cytology complex architecture supports PanIN3)	PanIN-3	IPMN-severe dysplasia	MCN-severe dysplasia

Rule of thumb: Think of how you would grade dysplasia in a colon adenoma, and then add a grade: normal mucinous epithelium (small basal nuclei) in the colon = mild dysplasia in the pancreas, low-grade dysplasia (typical adenoma) in the colon = moderate dysplasia in the pancreas [pearl from Dr. Ralph Hruban, used with permission]

The key distinguishing features of PanIN vs IPMN vs MCN are:
- PanIN – usually <5 mm, radiologically occult
- IPMN – grossly visible (usually >1 cm), associated with pancreatic duct (main or branch), mucin extrusion at the papilla
- MCN – almost exclusively women, not connected to pancreatic duct, associated with ovarian-type stroma

References: http://pathology.jhu.edu/pancreas/professionals/panin-illustrations.html [21-24]
Illustration by Thom Graves, updated by Jennifer Brumbaugh, Reproduced with permission.

Abbreviations: PanIN Pancreatic Intraepithelial Neoplasia, IPMN Intraductal Papillary Mucinous Neoplasm, MCN Mucinous Cystic Neoplasm

Esophagus

	Architectural Atypia*	Cytologic Atypia**	Surface maturation	Inflammation
Grading of Dysplasia in Barrett's Mucosa				
NFD (reactive)	None	None	Present	Variable
IFD	Minimal	Mild	Present	Frequent
LGD	Mild	Moderate	Absent	Minimal
HGD	Prominent	Severe (loss of nuclear polarity)	Absent	Minimal

* **Architectural Atypia** = glandular crowding and complexity (budding, branching, contour irregularity, papillary projections into lumen)
* **Cytologic Atypia** = ↑N/C ratio, hyperchromasia, ↑nucleoli, stratified nuclei, loss of mucin
Abbreviations: HGD high grade dysplasia, IFD indefinite for dysplasia, LGD low grade dysplasia, NFD negative for dysplasia,

Reference: [25]

Liver Biopsy

Grading and Staging of Chronic Viral Hepatitis

Grade = Lymphocytic Inflammation and "necrosis*" (indicates "activity")
- Portal inflammation
- Peri-portal inflammation/necrosis (= interface activity=piecemeal necrosis*)
- Lobular inflammation/necrosis

Stage = Fibrosis (indicates "chronicity")
- Portal fibrosis
- Bridging fibrosis (early → established)
- Cirrhosis

* Note that "necrosis" does not manifest as necrotic debris in the setting of viral hepatitis, but rather as replacement of hepatic parenchyma by lymphocytes.
There are multiple scoring systems in use to quantify the above parameters. These are nicely reviewed (with diagrams) in reference [26].

Criteria	Description
Criteria for Acute Liver Allograft Rejection	
1) **Portal Inflammation**	Lymphocytes with admixed neutrophils and eosinophils involving portal tracts
2) **Ductulitis**	Lymphocytes involving bile ducts with evidence of bile duct damage
3) **Endotheliolitis**	Subendothelial and perivenular lymphocytes involving portal and/or hepatic venules

The diagnosis of rejection requires at least two of the three above criteria. The severity of rejection is further qualified as "mild, moderate or severe" based on intensity of inflammation and the number of involved structures.

Reference: [27]

Sarcoma Grading (not for the Faint of Heart!)

Reviewer: Meera Hameed

There are two main systems, the NCI system and the French Federation of Cancer Centers (FNCLCC or "French") system. However, most organizations have now endorsed the French system, which is what we use at JHH and MSKCC.

French Grading System for Soft Tissue Sarcomas	
Parameter	**Point Score**
1) Tissue differentiation (how closely the tumor resembles the tissue from which it arose) **SEE TABLE BELOW** • Tumors closely resembling normal mesenchymal tissue (i.e. difficult to distinguish from a benign tumor). Ex. Well-differentiated leiomyosarcoma. • Tumors of a definite histologic type. Ex. Myxoid liposarcoma. • Tumors that are embryonal, poorly differentiated, or of uncertain histologic type	1 2 3
2) Mitoses • 0–9/10 HPF • 10–19/10 HPF • ≥20/10 HPF	1 2 3
3) Tumor Necrosis • No necrosis at all • <50% • ≥50%	0 1 2
	Final Score (combined point score) and corresponding grade
	2–3 points = Grade 1 — Low grade **4–5 points = Grade 2** — High grade **6–8 points = Grade 3**

• A high power field is = 0.1744 mm^2
• Sectioning the tumor at least 1 section/2 cm is recommended

Reference: [28]

For the most commonly encountered sarcomas (assuming you know what type it is!), the differentiation score can simply be looked up in this table:

Histology-Specific Tumor Differentiation Scores	
Sarcoma	**Score**
Adipocytic	
Myxoid liposarcoma	2
Round cell liposarcoma	3
Pleomorphic liposarcoma	3
Dedifferentiated liposarcoma	3
Fibrous/Fibrohistiocytic	
Well differentiated Fibrosarcoma	1
Conventional Fibrosarcoma	2
Poorly differentiated Fibrosarcoma	3
Myxofibrosarcoma (Myxoid MFH)	2
Pleomorphic MFH/undifferentiated/ pleomorphic sarcoma	3
Giant cell/Inflammatory MFH	3
Smooth muscle	
Well differentiated leiomyosarcoma	1
Conventional leiomyosarcoma	2
Poorly differentiated/pleomorphic/ epithelioid leiomyosarcoma	3
Other/Unknown	
Well differentiated chondrosarcoma	1
Synovial sarcoma	3
Mesenchymal chondrosarcoma	3
Extraskeletal osteosarcoma	3
Extrarenal rhabdoid tumor	3
Undifferentiated sarcoma	3
Abbreviation: MFH malignant fibrous histiocytoma	

Modified from [28]

But unfortunately it's not that simple. In practice, some of the sarcomas are high grade or low grade by definition. Also, the French Federation of Cancer Centers Sarcoma Group "doesn't recommend" grading a few of the common sarcomas. This is really confusing, since most of the "differentiation charts" include these sarcomas that they don't recommend grading …

So basically, for these tumors, you *can* go through the fun process of grading them by counting up the points, but it would be a waste of time because 1) for some sarcomas you will always get to a certain grade (i.e. they are either high grade or low grade by definition) or 2) applying a grade would be misleading because the actual prognosis doesn't match it.

Sarcomas For Which Grading is Generally Not Recommended or Not Necessary	
Sarcoma	**Reason**
Alveolar and embryonal rhabdomyosarcoma (except for botryoid and spindle cell variants)	Grade 3 by definition
Ewing sarcoma/PNET	Grade 3 by definition
Angiosarcoma	Grade 3 by definition by definition, except in superficial lesions like the breast or skin
Desmoplastic small round cell tumor	Grade 3 by definition
Extrarenal rhabdoid tumor	Grade 3 by definition
Extraskeletal osteosarcoma	Grade 3 by definition
Pleomorphic liposarcoma	Grade 3 by definition
Mesenchymal chondrosarcoma	Grade 3 by definition
Infantile fibrosarcoma	Grade 1 by definition. (Has a good prognosis, but if grade strictly applied, would be high)
Angiomatoid MFH	Tumors of intermediate malignancy that are low grade by definition
DFSP	
Atypical lipomatous tumor/well-differentiated liposarcoma	
MPNST	Grading does not seem to predict metastasis
Extraskeletal myxoid chondrosarcoma	Grade does not predict outcome. Would be low grade based on histology, but mets late in 40% of cases.
Alveolar soft parts sarcoma	Considered by many experts to be "ungradable," but usually managed as high grade sarcomas. Would often meet histologic criteria for low grade, but often metastasize long-term (within 10–20 years).
Clear cell sarcoma	
Epithelioid sarcoma	
"Low grade" fibromyxoid sarcoma	
Abbreviations: DFSP dermatofibrosarcoma protuberans, MFH malignant fibrous histiocytoma	

References: [29–33]

Neuroendocrine and Neuroectodermal Neoplasms

Pulmonary Neuroendocrine Neoplasms, WHO 2004 Classification				
	Mitoses per 10 HPF	Necrosis	Ki67 (Mib1)*	5 year survival
Typical carcinoid (=low grade)	<2	absent	<2%	>90%
Atypical carcinoid (=intermediate grade)	2–10	focal	<20% (mean 10%)	60%
Neuroendocrine carcinoma (small cell and large cell type) (=high grade)	>10	extensive	20–100% (mean for small cell >80%)	Small cell – 5% Large cell – 35%

HPF (high power field) = field diameter with a 40X objective (0.2 mm²)
* Ki67 is not part of the WHO 2004 criteria, but it is very helpful in small crushed biopsies where distinction of carcinoid tumors and small cell carcinoma can be difficult.
Carcinoid tumorlet is defined by size of ≤0.5cm.

References: [34,35]

Gastroenteropancreatic Neuroendocrine Neoplasms, WHO 2010 Classification			
	Mitoses per 10 HPF	Ki67	Morphology
Neuroendocrine tumor, Grade 1 (=low grade)	<2	<3%	look like carcinoid of any site
Neuroendocrine tumor, Grade 2 (=intermediate grade)	2–20	3–20%	look like carcinoid of any site
Neuroendocrine carcinoma (small cell and large cell type), Grade 3 (=high grade)	>20	>20%	look like small cell or large cell neuroendocrine carcinomas of any site

- This system attempts to unify the classification of all neuroendocrine neoplasms of the GI tract and pancreas. It parallels the 3 categories applied in the lung but note that criteria are different (in lung mitotic cut-point for high-grade is lower, Ki67 is not part of criteria whereas necrosis is part of criteria).

- Grading requires a mitotic count in at least 50 HPF (with 1 HPF = 0.2mm²) and a Ki67 index as a percentage of 500–2000 cells counted in "hot spots". Get your coffee ready!!

- If the mitotic rate and Ki67 index differs, use the higher of the two.

- Other terminology applied to neuroendocrine neoplasms is *well-differentiated* NE neoplasm (grade 1+2) vs *poorly differentiated* NE neoplasm (grade 3). For clinical management distinguishing these two groups is what is most important.

- "Micro" neuroendocrine proliferations are considered benign and include pancreatic neuroendocrine microadenoma (≤0.5 cm) and gastric carcinoid (ECL cell) tumorlet (≤0.5 cm).

- In addition to the above grading system, other important prognostic features for GI NETs include:
  - Anatomic location: bad (colon, esophagus), good (appendix, rectum), intermediate (small bowel, stomach).
  - For gastric NETs – clinical setting: tumors arising in the setting of hypergastrinemia (Zollinger-Ellison syndrome/MEN1, or autoimmune metaplastic atrophic gastritis/Pernicious anemia) have excellent prognosis, whereas sporadic tumors are aggressive.
  - Size and depth of invasion which are a part of staging system.

- For pancreatic NETs, additional feature associated with prognosis is the type of hypersecretory syndrome:
  - Insulinoma – better prognosis (may be related to earlier detection due to symptoms).
  - Glucagonoma – worse prognosis.

References: [22,36]

Abbreviations: NE = neuroendocrine, NET = neuroendocrine tumor

Grading Systems

Neuroblastoma, Revised Shimada Grading System (not graded if metastatic or post-treatment)			
Designation		Histology	Prognosis
Ganglioneuroma, maturing	Stroma-rich[1,2] (schwannian stroma >50%)	no microscopic nodules of NB cells	FH
Ganglioneuroblastoma, intermixed		microscopic nodules of NB cells present	FH
Ganglioneuroblastoma, nodular		macroscopic (gross) nodules of NB cells present	UH/FH
Undifferentiated neuroblastoma	Stroma-poor (schwannian stroma <50%)	no ganglion cells; no neuropil	always UH (any age)
Poorly differentiated neuroblastoma		<5% ganglion cells; neuropil present	UH if age >1.5yrs or MKI[3] >4% otherwise FH
Differentiating neuroblastoma		>5% ganglion cells; neuropil present	UH if any of the following: • age >5yrs or • age 1.5–5yrs plus MKI>2% or • age <1.5yrs plus MKI>4% otherwise FH

1) Schwannian stroma consists of spindle cells, which resemble schwannoma or neurofibroma. In contrast, neuropil consists of fibrillary processes similar to the kind seen in ependymoma.
2) Stroma-rich neuroblastomas generally have >50% ganglion cells, but this feature is not a criterion in grading of ganglioneuroblastoma.
3) MKI (mitotic karyorrhexic index): percentage of mitotic and karyorrhexic cells based on a 5000 cell count (2% is 100 of 5000 cells and 4% is 200 of 5000 cells). A 900-cell count is sometimes mercifully applied (2% is 19 of 900 cells and 4% is 36 of 900 cells).
Sample sign-out: "Neuroblastoma, Stroma Poor, Differentiating, Low MKI"

Abbreviations: FH favorable histology, MKI mitotic karyorrhexis index, NB neuroblast, UH unfavorable histology

Reference: [37]

Olfactory Neuroblastoma/Esthesioneuroblastoma, Hyams Grading System				
	Grade 1	Grade 2	Grade 3	Grade 4
Mitotic activity	Absent	Present	Prominent	Marked
Nuclear pleomorphism	Absent	Moderate	Prominent	Marked
Necrosis	Absent	Absent	+/– Present	Common
Fibrillary matrix	Prominent	Present	Minimal	Absent
Rosette type	Homer Wright	Homer Wright	Flexner-Wintersteiner	Flexner-Wintersteiner

The four-tiered system may be simplified into low grade (Hyams grades I and II) and high grade (Hyams grade III and IV).

Reference: [38]

Central Nervous System

Reviewer: Jason Huse

Meningioma, WHO Grading System	
Grade I	lack of the higher grade features
Grade II (atypical) [1]	Any one of the three criteria: 1) ≥ 4 mitoses/10 HPF or 2) brain invasion or 3) at least 3 of the following features: • sheet-like growth (i.e. loss of lobular architecture) • prominent nucleoli • hypercellularity • small cell features • foci of spontaneous necrosis
Grade III (anaplastic/ malignant) [2]	Frankly malignant cytology (like that of a carcinoma, melanoma, or MFH) or > 20 mitoses/10 HPF

1) Clear cell and chordoid meningioma are always Grade II.
2) Papillary and rhabdoid meningioma are always Grade III.

Note: Bone invasion does not raise the grade.

Reference: [39]

Grading Systems

Gliomas, WHO Grading System	
Astrocytomas [1]	**Grade II (low grade):** lack of the higher grade features **Grade III (anaplastic/malignant):** ↑mitoses[2], ↑cellularity, ↑atypia; no MVP or necrosis **Grade IV (glioblastoma):** glomeruloid MVP and/or palisaded necrosis are the two defining features (usually both features are present but at least one is minimally required for diagnosis); plus ↑↑mitoses, ↑↑cellularity, ↑↑atypia
Pilocytic astrocytoma [1]	**Grade I:** always
Subependymal Giant Cell Astrocytoma (SEGA) [1]	**Grade I:** always
Pleomorphic xanthoastrocytoma (PXA)	**Grade II:** most cases **PXA with anaplastic features:** ≥ 5mitoses/10 HPF, often with MVP and/or necrosis
Oligodendroglioma	**Grade II:** most cases (more mitoses tolerated than for grade II astrocytoma) **Grade III (anaplastic):** ↑↑mitoses, ↑cellularity, ↑atypia; MVP and/or necrosis may be present
Ependymoma [3]	**Grade II:** most cases **Grade III:** mitoses, ↑cellularity, MVP &/or necrosis (usually supratentorial)

1) Grade I is assigned to a group of "special" astrocytomas, which are discrete/non-infiltrative (pilocytic astrocytoma, SEGA). Unlike diffuse astrocytomas, Grade I astrocytomas usually do not progress to higher grades.
2) The minimal mitotic count needed to upgrade astrocytoma from grade II to III is controversial. By WHO criteria, even a single mitosis is sufficient, but some experts require a higher number. In borderline cases, Ki67 of >3–4% may be used to support the diagnosis of grade III. [40]
3) Clear cell ependymoma and myxopapillary ependymoma are by definition Grade I.

MVP = microvascular proliferation

Reference: [39]

Neuroradiology 101
Contrast-enhancing CNS lesions: 1) Discrete (non-infiltrative) tumors: pilocytic astrocytoma, PXA, ependymoma, meningioma, schwannoma. 2) Infiltrative gliomas enhance only when high grade (all grade IV and some grade III astrocytomas and oligodendrogliomas). 3) Lymphoma, metastases, inflammatory and infectious lesions. **Non contrast-enhancing CNS lesions**: Low-grade infiltrative gliomas (grade II) and some grade III astrocytomas and oligodendrogliomas. <div align="right">Reference: [40]</div>

Gynecologic Tract
Reviewer: Anna Yemelyanova

Endometrioid Carcinoma, FIGO Grading	
	% solid growth
GRADE 1 (well differentiated)	<5%
GRADE 2 (moderately differentiated)	5–50%
GRADE 3 (poorly differentiated)	>50%

- Squamoid areas are not counted as solid growth.
- Presence of severe nuclear atypia (grade 3 nuclei) raises the grade by one.
- FIGO = International Federation of Gynecology and Obstetrics

Reference: [41]

Smooth Muscle Neoplasms of the Uterus			
	Mitoses per 10 HPF	Atypia	Coagulative Necrosis
Leiomyoma or Cellular leiomyoma (increased cellularity)	<4–10	−	−
Atypical leiomyoma (aka symplastic, pleomorphic or bizarre)	<10	+	−
Mitotically active leiomyoma	>5	−	−
Leiomyosarcoma (diagnosis requires at least 2 of 3 features)	>10	+	+

References: [42–44]

Epithelioid Smooth Muscle Neoplasms of the Uterus			
	Mitoses per 10 HPF	Atypia	Coagulative Necrosis
Epithelioid Leiomyoma	<5	Minimal	−
Epithelioid STUMP[1]	<5	Moderate-severe	−
Epithelioid Leiomyosarcoma	>5[2]	Moderate-severe	+[2]

1) STUMP – smooth muscle tumor of uncertain malignant potential; aka Atypical Epithelial Smooth Muscle neoplasm
2) Presence of either >5 mitoses/10 HPF or necrosis qualifies for the diagnosis of leiomyosarcoma

Reference: [44]

Grading of Immature Ovarian Teratomas	
	Fields occupied by immature neuroepithelial elements
GRADE I	<1 LPF (4X objective)
GRADE II	1–3 LPF
GRADE III	>3 LPF

Rule of thumb: grade I – if immature areas are hard to find, grade III – easy to find.

Reference: [42]

Dating of Endometrium
by Diana Molavi

Proliferative endometrium cannot be dated. The first secretory change occurs, on average, on day 16 or so of a 28 day cycle. This change is the appearance of clear secretory vacuoles at the base of the epithelial cells, below the nuclei. When you see just a few of these in a generally proliferative endometrium, it is called interval endometrium. Beyond that day, specific histologic criteria are:

From day 16 to day 20, the glands are the most helpful feature.

Day 16	subnuclear vacuoles, pseudostratified nuclei
Day 17	subnuclear vacuoles, but with an orderly row of nuclei
Day 18	vacuoles above and below nuclei (the "piano key" look)
Day 19	vacuoles diminishing, only above nuclei; orderly row of nuclei, no mitoses
Day 20	peak secretions in lumen and ragged luminal border, vacuoles rare

From day 21 to 28, the glands stay pretty much the same – they are exhausted, and appear low columnar with orderly nuclei, no mitoses, and ragged luminal edges. They may also have degenerative apical vacuoles – tricky to discern from day 19–20. After day 21, the stroma is the key.

Day 21	stromal edema begins, secretion continues
Day 22	peak stromal edema with naked nuclei
Day 23	spiral arteries become prominent
Day 24	periarteriolar cuffing with predecidua (stromal cells around the arteries begin to get plump pink cytoplasm, creating a pink halo around the vessels)
Day 25	predecidual change under the surface epithelium
Day 26	decidual islands coalesce, polys begin to infiltrate stroma
Day 27	lots of polys in a solid sheet of decidua, with focal necrosis and hemorrhage
Day 28	prominent necrosis, hemorrhage, clumping, and breakup

Grading and Staging of Infections in the Placenta		
STAGE (reflects duration)		
	Chorioamnionitis (maternal neutrophils involving the membranes)	**Funisitis** (fetal neutrophils migrating from fetal vessels into umbilical cord and/or chorionic plate)
Stage I	**Subchorionitis** (neutrophils line up beneath the chorion) and chorionitis (neutrophils involve the chorion)	**Umbilical phlebitis** (neutrophils in the wall of umbilical vein) or **chorionic vasculitis** (neutrophils in the wall of vessels located in the chorionic plate)
Stage II	**Chorioamnionitis:** neutrophils extend into the amnion	**Umbilical arteritis:** neutrophils in the wall of umbilical arteries
Stage III	**Necrotizing chorioamnionitis:** above plus reactive amnion or necrosis or amnionic basement membrane thickening or band-like inflammation	**Necrotizing funisitis:** neutrophils extend into Wharton's jelly and form microabscesses or band-like inflammation
GRADE (reflects severity)		
Grade I	mild-moderate	
Grade II	severe (such as subchorionic microabscesses)	

Note that chorioamnionitis represents a maternal response to infection, whereas funisitis – fetal response to infection. Funisitis usually develops later than chorioamnionitis.

References: [45,46]

Grading Systems

Hematopoietic System

by Amy Duffield

Follicular Lymphoma, WHO Grading System	
Grade	**Number of centroblasts per HPF**[1]
Grade 1*	0–5
Grade 2*	6–15
Grade 3**	>15
3A	Residual centrocytes present
3B	Centroblasts form solid sheets with no residual centrocytes
Pattern	**Proportion of follicular pattern**[2]
Follicular	>75%
Follicular and diffuse	25–75%
Focally follicular/predominantly diffuse	<25%
Diffuse	0

1) HPF = high power field (40X objective). Number should be based on the average of 10-field-count.
2) The relative proportions of follicular & diffuse areas should be provided in the pathology report.
*   Grades 1 & 2 are both clinically indolent. Distinction between the two is not encouraged and low grade FL is best reported as "Grade 1–2 of 3."
** Grade 3 (A or B) lymphomas with a diffuse pattern are reported as "1. Diffuse large B-cell lymphoma (_%). 2. Follicular lymphoma, grade 3 (A or B) (_%)."

Reference: [47]

Diagnostic Criteria for Plasma Cell Disorders, 2009 Update	
MGUS	Requires all 3: 1. Serum monoclonal protein <3g/100 ml 2. Clonal bone marrow plasmacytosis, but <10% 3. Absence of end-organ damage and bone lytic lesions[1] Note: Since clinical and laboratory data are frequently not available with the bx, <10% clonal bone marrow plasmacytosis is typically signed out as "plasma cell dyscrasia."
Smoldering multiple myeloma	Requires both: 1. Serum monoclonal protein (IgA or IgG) >3g/100 ml *AND/OR* clonal bone marrow plasmacytosis ≥10% 2. Absence of end-organ damage or myeloma-related symptoms[1] Note: Since clinical and laboratory data are frequently not available with the bx, ≥10% clonal bone marrow plasmacytosis is typically signed out as "plasma cell myeloma."
Multiple Myeloma	Requires all 3: 1. Clonal bone marrow plasmacytosis (typically >10%, but a minimal % is not designated in the setting of symptomatic myeloma) 2. Serum and/or urine M protein (except in patients with a non-secretory myeloma) 3. Evidence of end-organ damage[1], hyperviscosity, amyloidosis or recurrent infections Note: Since clinical and laboratory data are frequently not available with the bx, ≥10% clonal bone marrow plasmacytosis is typically signed out as "plasma cell myeloma."
Waldenstrom's Macroglobulinemia	Requires both: 1. IgM monoclonal gammopathy of any concentration 2. Lymphoplasmacytic lymphoma with bone marrow involvement
Solitary plasmacytoma of bone	Requires all 4: 1. Biopsy-proven solitary clonal plasma cell lesion of bone 2. No evidence of bone marrow plasmacytosis 3. Normal skeletal survey and spine/pelvis MRI 4. Absence of end-organ damage or other clinical features of myeloma[1]
Extraosseous plasmacytoma	Requires all 3: 1. Biopsy-proven solitary clonal plasma cell lesion of extraosseus tissue (often in the upper respiratory tract) 2. No evidence of bone marrow plasmacytosis 3. Absence of end-organ damage or other clinical features of myeloma[1] Notes: Approximately 20% of patients have a small M-protein. Extraosseus plasmacytoma must be distinguished from a lymphoma with prominent plasmacytic differentiation.
Primary amyloidosis	Requires all 4: 1. Presence of amyloid-related compromised organ function[2] 2. Amyloid depositions in tissue that bind Congo red and exhibit birefringence 3. Evidence that the amyloid is light-chain restricted (except for rare disease caused by heavy chains) 4. Evidence of an underlying plasma cell or lymphoplasmacytic neoplasm (e.g. M protein, clonal plasma cells in bone marrow)
Osteosclerotic myeloma	Monoclonal plasma cell disorder with fibrosis and osteosclerotic changes of the bony trabeculae * Patients with lymphadenopathy often show changes consistent with the plasma cell variant of Castleman's disease * Osteosclerotic myeloma is often a component of POEMS[3] syndrome

1) End-organ damage = "CRAB" (hypercalcemia, renal insufficiency, normochromic normocytic anemia, and/or bone marrow lesions that can be attributed to the plasma cell proliferative disorder).
2) For example, renal, liver, heart, GI, or peripheral nerve involvement
3) POEMS = polyneuropathy, organomegaly, endocrinopathy, monoclonal protein, skin changes

Reference: [48]

Myelodysplastic Syndromes, WHO Classification				
MDS class	% Blasts in the Blood	% Blasts in the Marrow	Key features	Clinical
Refractory cytopenias with unilineage dysplasia (RCUD) [1]	<1%	<5%	Isolated unilineage dysplasia Uni- or bicytopenia (see note below) <15% of erythroid precursors are ring sideroblasts Note: Pancytopenia with unilineage dysplasia is considered MDS, unclassifiable (MDS-U)	~2% progress to AML
Refractory Anemia with Ring Sideroblasts [2] (RARS)	None	<5%	Anemia, eythroid dysplasia only and ≥15% ring sideroblasts in the bone marrow *May be associated with thrombocytosis (RARS-T); RARS-T is a provisional entity in the 2008 WHO	1–2% progress to AML
Refractory Cytopenia with Multilineage Dysplasia (RCMD) (formerly RAEB-T)	<1%	<5%	Cytopenia(s) Dysplasia in ≥10% of the cells in ≥2 myeloid lineages (This a high risk disease but lacks the increased blasts seen in RAEB)	~10% progress to AML; prognosis dependent on cytogenetics
Refractory Anemia with Excess Blasts 1 (RAEB-1)	<5%	5–9%	Cytopenia(s) Significant dysplasia in ≥2 myeloid lineages No Auer rods	~25% progress to AML
Refractory Anemia with Excess Blasts 2 (RAEB-2)	5–19%	10–19%	Cytopenia(s) Significant dysplasia in ≥2 myeloid lineages Presence of Auer rods qualifies as RAEB-2 regardless of blast count	~33% progress to AML
MDS associated with isolated del(5q)	<5%	<5%	Anemia (often macrocytic) Normal or increased platelet count Normal or increased small hypolobated megakaryocytes	Good prognosis; middle-aged women
MDS, Unclassified	≤1%	<5%	• Disease meets the criteria for RCUD or RCMD, but with 1% blasts in blood • Pancytopenia with unilineage dysplasia and no increase in blasts OR • Persistent cytopenia(s), no increase in blasts, unequivocal dysplasia in <10% of cells in ≥1 myeloid lines plus a cytogenetic abnormality seen in MDS	Unknown

1) Includes Refractory Anemia, Refractory Neutropenia, and Refractory Thrombocytopenia

2) Ring sideroblasts (RS) are defined as red cell precursors with sideroblastic granules encircling ≥1/3 of a nucleus (iron stain). Ring sideroblasts may be seen in many myelodysplastic syndromes including high grade disease, and the presence of RS does not necessarily imply RARS

3) Characteristics of Dysplasia:
- *Erythroid dysplasia (dyserythropoiesis)*: multinucleation, nuclear budding, intranuclear bridging, karyorrhexis, megaloblastoid change (nuclear to cytoplasmic asynchrony i.e. nucleus too big or immature for the degree of cytoplasmic maturity), ring sideroblasts, cytoplasmic vacuolization. Best appreciated on the bone marrow aspirate.
- *Myeloid dysplasia (dysgranulopoiesis)*: cytoplasmic hypogranulation, nuclear hypolobation (pelgeroid or pseudo Pelger-Huët cells), and small size. Best appreciated on the peripheral smear.
- *Megakaryocytic dysplasia:* hypolobated megakaryocytes and micromegakaryocytes, megakaryocytes with multiple widely separated nuclei. Often best appreciated on the bone marrow biopsy.

Reference: [47]

Grading Systems

Grading Systems

	Classification	Definition & key features	Clinical
Acute Myeloid Leukemia NOS, WHO Classification[1]			
MYELOID	**AML, minimally differentiated** *(FAB: M0)[2]*	≥20% of marrow nucleated cells are blasts. Blasts: medium size with round nuclei, agranular cytoplasm and lack Auer rods; i.e. no morphologic evidence of myeloid differentiation. *Typical immunophenotype: CD34+, c-kit+, CD38+, HLA-DR+, CD13+, CD33+/–, MPO +/– TdT+/–, CD11b–, CD15–, CD14–, CD64–*	Infants & older adults;; marrow failure ; +/– leuko-cytosis; poor prognosis
	AML without maturation *(FAB: M1)[2]*	≥20% of marrow nucleated cells are blasts. Blasts are ≥90% of non-erythroid cells and most have not matured past the myeloblast stage. Blasts: some morphologic features of myeloid differentiation (scattered granules & Auer rods). *Typical immunophenotype: CD34+/–, c-kit+, HLA-DR+/–, CD13+, CD33+, MPO +, CD11b+/–, CD15–, CD14–, CD64–*	Adults; marrow failure; +/– leuko-cytosis; poor prognosis
	AML with maturation *(FAB: M2)[2]*	≥20% of marrow nucleated cells are blasts. At least 10% of myeloid cells have matured past the mye-loblast stage (i.e. promyelocytes, myelocytes, granulocytes). Monocytic cells comprise <20% of the non-erythroid cells. [excludes AML with t(8;21) which often has CD19+ blasts] Blasts: +/– azurophilic granules and frequent Auer rods. *Typical immunophenotype: CD34+/–, c-kit+/–, HLA-DR+/–, CD13+, CD33+, CD11b+, CD15+, CD14–, CD64–, aberrant expression of CD7+/–*	All age groups; marrow failure with variable WBC count; moderate prognosis
	Acute promyelocytic leukemia with t(15;17)(q22;q12); PML-RARA NOT AML, NOS *(FAB: M3)[2]*	**APL has t(15;17) & is an "AML with recurrent genetic abnormalities," not "AML, NOS."** Abnormal promyelocytes dominate Hypergranular variant (M3): blasts with abundant granules & Auer rods that may obscure nuclei Microgranular variant (M3v): blasts have bi-lobed nuclei; granules are inconspicuous *Typical immunophenotype: CD34dim/–, HLA-DR+/–, c-kit dim/+, CD13+, CD33 bright, CD11b–, CD15–, CD14–, CD64+* *M3v: CD34+, HLA-DR dim/+, c-kit dim, CD13+, CD33 bright, CD2+/– & CD56 +/–*	Adults in mid-life; associated with DIC; Rx with all trans retinoic acid (ATRA); good prognosis
MYELO/MONOCYTIC FEATURES	**Acute myelomonocytic leukemia (AMML)** *(FAB: M4)[2]*	≥20% of marrow nucleated cells are blasts (including promonocytes). Non-erythroid cells contain >20% monocytes & monocytic precursors and >20% neutrophils & neutrophilic precursors. The peripheral blood may contain high numbers of monocytic cells. [excludes AML with inv(16) and t(16;16); previously FAB M4Eo] Monoblasts: round nuclei, delicate chromatin, large prominent nucleoli, basophilic chromatin, scattered fine granules, pseudopod formation Promonocytes: convoluted nuclei, less basophilic cytoplasm, fine scattered granules & vacuoles *Typical immunophenotype shows more than one blast population :* *A) CD34+/–, c-kit+/–, HLA-DR+, CD13+/–, CD33+/–, CD15+/–, CD7–/+* *B) CD4+, CD14+, CD11b+, CD15+, CD64+, CD68+,CD163, lysozyme+*	Older adults; bone marrow failure with variable white count; moderate prognosis
	Acute monocytic/ monoblastic leukemia *(FAB: M5)[2]*	≥20% of marrow nucleated cells are blasts (monoblasts + promonocytes) and >80% of non-erythroid cells are of the monocyte lineage (monoblasts + promonocytes + monocytes) Monoblasts & promonoblasts: see AMML above Acute monoblastic leukemia (M5a): majority of monocytic cells are monoblasts (≥80%). Acute monocytic leukemia (M5b): the majority of the monocytic cells are promonocytes. *Typical immunophenotype: CD34–/+, c-kit+/–, HLA-DR+, CD13+, CD33bright, CD4, CD11b+, CD15+, CD14+, CD64+, MPO +/–, CD68+, CD163+, lysozyme+, may show aberrant expression of CD7 or CD56*	Monoblastic: young people; Monocytic: adults; soft tissue infiltration & bleeding disorders; moderate prognosis
ERYTHOID	**Acute erythroid leukemia** *(FAB: M6)[2]*	Erythroid/myeloid (or erythroleukemia, M6a): ≥50% erythroid precursors in the marrow and ≥20% myeloid blasts in the non-erythroid population Pure erythroid leukemia (M6b): >20% of marrow nucleated cells are blasts and ≥80% are blasts com-mitted to the erythroid lineage with no significant myeloblast population. Erythroblasts: deeply basophilic cytoplasm, prominent nucleoli, cytoplasmic vacuoles *Typical immunophenotype: CD34–, c-kit+/–, HLA-DR–, CD71+, spectrin+, CD41&CD61 +/–*	Rare (<5% AML); poor prognosis
MEGAKARYOCYTIC	**Acute megakaryoblastic leukemia** *(FAB: M7)[2]*	≥20% of marrow nucleated cells are blasts and >50% of non-erythroid cells are megakaryocytic lineage [excludes AML with t(1;22), inv(3) or t(3;3)]. Associated with marrow fibrosis. Megakaryoblasts: large with cytoplasmic blebs/pseudopods and zones of basophilic cytoplasm Differential diagnosis: • Acute panmyelosis with myelofibrosis: acute onset, severe constitutional symptoms, no splenomegaly, marked marrow fibrosis, CD34+ blasts lack megakaryocytic markers • AML with myelofibrosis: blasts lack megakaryocytic markers • High grade MDS (RAEB-2) with fibrosis: less abrupt onset, <20% blasts, often has chromosomal abnormalities associated with MDS: del5q, del7q, –5 or –7 • Myeloid leukemia associated with Down syndrome: typically children less than 5 years old, associ-ated with mutations of GATA1, very favorable prognosis *Typical immunophenotype: CD34–, HLA-DR–,CD45–, CD13+/–, CD33+/–, MPO–,CD7+/–, one or more megakaryocytic markers are + (CD41, CD61 and /or CD42b)*	Adults & children, bone marrow failure, marrow often shows dyspla-sia, poor prognosis. Associated with mediastinal germ cell tumors in young males often with i(12p)

1) These leukemias do not have a recurrent genetic abnormality
2) The FAB classification (i.e. "M7") is no longer in use and should not be incorporated into the pathologic diagnosis; however, this classification scheme is widely used in informal discussion and it is helpful to be familiar with the nomenclature.

Reference: [47]

Myeloproliferative Disorders, WHO Classification				
	Peripheral Blood	Marrow	Key features	Clinical
Chronic Myelogenous Leukemia (CML) Chronic Phase: CP Accelerated Phase: AP Blast Phase: BP	CP: leukocytosis; <2% blasts. AP: persistent or increasing leukocytosis or thrombocytosis; ≥ 20% basophils; 10–19% blasts. BP: ≥ 20% blasts or extramedullary blast proliferation.	CP: <5% blasts AP: 10–19% blasts BP: ≥ 20% blasts	Hypercellular marrow with markedly increased myeloid:erythroid ratio, small megakaryocytes with hypolobated nuclei, increased reticulin fibrosis **Philadelphia chromosome t(9;22) is required for diagnosis**	Very good prognosis if disease is responsive to tyrosine kinase inhibitors
Polycythemia Vera (PCV) Polycythemic phase: PCV Post-polycythemic myelofibrosis: pPVMF	PCV: Hemoglobin >18.5 g/dL in men, >16.5 g/dL in women* pPVMF: anemia, leukoerythroblastosis *Serum erythropoietin level should be low	PCV:<5% blasts pPVMF: >10% blasts suggests transformation to MDS; ≥ 20% is AML	PCV: Hypercellular marrow with proliferation of erythroid, granulocytic and megakaryocytic lineages (panmyelosis) & atypical megakaryocytes of varying sizes pPVMF[1]: Marked fibrosis +/− osteosclerosis **JAK2 mutation is required for diagnosis**	Median survival >10 years; most patients die or thrombosis or hemorrhage. 2–3% progress to AML
Primary myelofibrosis (PMF) Prefibrotic stage Fibrotic stage	Anemia, leukoerythroblastosis May also see leukocytosis or thrombocytosis early in disease	Prefibrotic: <5% blasts Fibrotic: <10% blasts. 10–19% blasts suggests accelerated phase; ≥20% is AML	Prefibrotic: Hypercellular marrow with increased neutrophils and atypical megas Fibrotic[1]: Significant reticulin or collagen fibrosis, extramedullary hematopoiesis (often within marrow sinusoids), osteosclerosis ~50% have *JAK2* mutations; del(13)(q12-22) or der(6)(1;6)(q21-23;p21.3) suggest PMF	Frequent splenomegaly ~5–30% progress to AML
Essential Thrombocythemia (ET) Thrombocythemic phase: ET Post-ET myelofibrosis: post-ET MF	ET: Sustained platelet count of $\geq 450 \times 10^9$/L Post-ET MF: anemia, leukoerythroblastosis	<5% blasts	ET: Normocellular or moderately hypercellular bone marrow; proliferation of megakaryocytic lineage; large megas with deeply lobulated & hyperlobulated nuclei, no increased fibrosis Post-ET MF[1] (relatively rare): increased marrow fibrosis 40–50% have *JAK2* mutations	Indolent; mortality often due to thrombosis or hemorrhage. <5% progress to MDS or AML
Systemic Mastocytosis	Serum tryptase often exceeds 20 ng/mL	Multifocal dense infiltrates of mast cells (≥15 mast cells/ aggregate) <5% blasts	Dense mast cell infiltrates can involve multiple organs. >25% of mast cells in the infiltrate may be spindled or mast cells may express CD2 and/or CD25. Associated with KIT mutations (codon 816)	Variable
Chronic eosinophilic leukemia	Eosinophila ($\geq 1.5 \times 10^9$/L) Blasts are >2% but <20%	Blasts are >5% but <20%	Hypercellular marrow due to eosinophilic proliferation with increased myeloblasts; dysplasia in other cell lineages and occasional marrow fibrosis. **No** evidence of BCR-ABL or t(5:12), **No** rearrangements of PDGFRA, PDGFRB or FGFR1.[2]	Good prognosis Middle-aged women

1) It may be impossible to differentiate the fibrotic stages of PCV, PMF and ET based on pathologic features of the bone marrow biopsy. These cases are best signed out descriptively.

2) Myeloid and lymphoid neoplasms with eosinophilia and abnormalities of PDGFRA, PDGFRB or FGFR1 are considered separately in the 2008 WHO

Reference: [47]

Grading Systems

Classification of Post-transplant Lymphoproliferative Disorders				
	Definition	Site of involvement	Morphology	Immunophenotype
Early lesions: • Plasmacytic hyperplasia (PH) • Infectious mononucleosis-like (IM)	Lymphoid proliferation WITH architectural preservation of underlying tissue	Typically tonsils and adenoids	Dense polymorphic infiltrate of lymphoid tissue	Polyclonal B-cells & plasma cells. PH is typically EBV+ IM-like are EBV+
Polymorphic	• Polymorphic lesions that form destructive masses • Do not meet the criteria for a recognized type of high-grade lymphoma	Lymph nodes or extranodal sites	Neoplastic cells show a full range of B-cell maturation; patchy necrosis and mitoses may be present	B-cells:may be polyclonal or rarely monoclonal Nearly always EBV+
Monomorphic	Lymphoma in an allograft recipient that meets the criteria for a recognized type of high-grade lymphoma* (DLBCL, Burkitt, plasma cell neoplasm, T/NK cell or HL)[1]	Lymph nodes or extranodal sites	See criteria for specific lymphomas. "Monomorphic" does not imply cellular monotony but rather indicates that nearly all of the cells are transformed	See criteria for DLBCL, Burkitt, plasma cell neoplasm, T/NK cell or HL. B-cell neoplasms: many cases are CD30+ and EBV+ T-cell neoplasms: ~33% EBV+ HL: nearly all EBV+

* It is important to provide a diagnosis of monomophic PTLD rather than only listing the type of lymphoma because the treatment options differ; i.e. PTLD may respond to decreased immunosupression.
1) Indolent lymphomas (i.e. FL, CLL/SLL, MZL) arising in allograft recipients are not considered PTLD.

Hematopathology Abbreviations: ALCL anaplastic large cell lymphoma, AML acute myeloid leukemia, AMML acute myelomonocytic leukemia, CLL/SLL chronic lymphocytic leukemia/small lymphocytic lymphoma, CML chronic myelogenous leukemia, DIC disseminated intravascular coagulation, DLBCL diffuse large B cell lymphoma, ET essential thrombocythemia, FAB French-American-British, FL follicular lymphoma, HL Hodgkin lymphoma, MCL mantle cell lymphoma, MDS myelodysplastic syndrome, MGUS monoclonal gammopathy of undetermined significance, MPO myeloperoxidase, MZL marginal zone lymphoma, NK natural killer, PCV polycythemia vera, PMF primary myelofibrosis, PTLD post-transplant lymphoproliferative disorder, RAEB refractory anemia excess blasts, RARS refractory anemia with ringed sideroblasts, RCMD refractory cytopenia with multilineage dysplasia, RCUD refractory cytopenia with unilineage dysplasia, RS ringed sideroblasts, WBC white blood cell

Grading Systems

Transplant Pathology

Grading of Lung Allograft Rejection, 2007 update International Society for Heart and Lung Transplantation (ISHLT) system [reported as, for example, ISHLT A0Bx]	
Grade of rejection	**Histologic features**
Acute rejection	
Grade A0 (no rejection)	
Grade A1 (minimal rejection)	Infrequent, scattered perivascular lymphocytes forming a ring 2–3 cells thick
Grade A2 (mild rejection)	More frequent perivascular lymphocytes readily seen at low power (4X objective), cuffing the vessels and expanding the perivascular interstitium
Grade A3 (moderate rejection)	Lymphocytes extend into alveolar septae and airspaces
Grade A4 (severe rejection)	Diffuse interstitial lymphoid infiltrate with diffuse alveolar damage, hemorrhage, and/or necrosis
Bronchial/bronchiolar inflammation	
Grade B0 (no airway inflammation)	
Grade B1R (low grade)	Mononuclear cells within the submucosa of bronchioles without evidence of epithelial damage or intraepithelial infiltration (combines former B1 and B2 categories)
Grade B2R (high grade)	Mononuclear cells are increased in number, and are larger and accompanied by more eosinophils and plasmacytoid cells (but not many neutrophils, which would make you think infection). Also there is epithelial damage (e.g. necrosis, metaplasia) and intraepithelial lymphocytes
Grade Bx (ungradable)	No evaluable bronchial tissue
Chronic rejection (obliterative bronchiolitis)	
Grade C0	Bronchiolar obliteration absent
Grade C1	Bronchiolar obliteration via fibrosis present. Often subtle and/or focal (a trichrome stain can be helpful).
Chronic vascular rejection	
Grade D	Thickening of arteries and veins, similar to the coronary artery disease seen in transplanted hearts. Not applicable to transbronchial biopsies.

At least 5 pieces of alveolated lung parenchyma each containing bronchioles and >100 air sacs are defined as sufficient to rule out rejection by ISHLT criteria.

Reference: [49]

Grading of Acute Graft-versus-Host Disease (GVHD) in Intestinal (usually rectal) Biopsy	
GRADE I	rare apoptotic cells (approximately >3 per crypt; normal is ≤1 per crypt)
GRADE II	loss of individual crypts
GRADE III	loss of two or more contiguous crypts
GRADE IV	complete loss of crypts; mucosal ulceration (neuroendocrine cells are relatively spared from the damages of GVHD and they may appear as little nests)

Chemotherapy-related changes may be indistinguishable (best not to biopsy <20d post-BMT).

Reference: [50,51]

Grading of Acute Graft-versus-Host Disease (GVHD) in Skin Biopsy	
GRADE I	vacuolization of the basal layer
GRADE II	above + dyskeratotic/necrotic keratinocytes
GRADE III	above + subepidermal clefting
GRADE IV	above + separation of epidermis

Drug reaction looks virtually indistinguishable from GVHD and must be ruled out on clinical grounds. A soft feature that favors GVHD is dyskeratotic cells on hair follicles. Lymphocytes are either absent or minimal in GVHD (unlike drug reaction). Eosinophils favor drug reaction.

Reference: [52]

Grading Systems

The Good the Bad and the Ugly:
Prognostic Features in Neoplasms with Difficult-to-Predict Behavior

Adrenocortical Neoplasms

The only definitive criteria for malignancy are distant metastasis and/or local invasion, but various histologic criteria have been devised to predict an aggressive phenotype (Weiss criteria are listed below; see [53] and [54] for other point-system criteria).

- **Weiss criteria** for histologic assessment of malignancy in adrenocortical neoplasms: [55,56]
    1. >5 mitoses per 50 HPF*
    2. Atypical mitoses*
    3. Venous invasion*
    4. Sinusoidal invasion
    5. Capsular invasion
    6. Nuclear pleomorphism (equivalent to Fuhrman nuclear grade III and IV)
    7. Clear cells representing <25% of tumor cells (>75% are of tumor cells are eosinophilic)
    8. Diffuse architecture (>33% of tumor)
    9. Necrosis

Malignant tumors have > 3 of the above criteria, whereas all benign tumors have < 2. In addition, the asterisked criteria are found exclusively in malignant tumors.

- Other criteria:
    - Weight **>100g** (occasionally >50g); size **>5cm** [57]
    - Ki67 >5–20% [58]
    - Broad fibrous bands [53]
    - Hemorrhage and calcifications [54]

According to some reports, the criteria for malignancy in pediatric tumors should have a higher threshold [58]

Pheochromocytoma

10% of cases are malignant. The only definitive criterion for malignancy is distant metastasis. Local invasiveness is not an unequivocal malignant feature. Aggressive behavior is impossible to predict based on any histologic features, but the following features have been associated with malignancy:

- Large tumor size (mean size 383g for malignant vs. 73g for benign)
- Capsular invasion and extension into adjacent soft tissue
- Vascular invasion
- Confluent tumor necrosis (may occur in benign)
- Expanded large nests (more than 3 times the normal "zellballen" size) and diffuse growth
- Increased cellularity
- Increased mitoses (>3 mitoses per 10–20 HPF)
- Atypical mitotic figures
- Tumor cell spindling
- Profound nuclear atypia with hyperchromasia and macronucleoli (may occur in benign)
- Predominantly small tumor cell size
- ↑Ki67 and p53 (controversial)

References: [58–60]

Solitary Fibrous Tumor (SFT)

Proposed histologic criteria for malignancy in pleural SFT include [61]:
- high cellularity (crowded, overlapping nuclei)
- > 4 mitoses per 10 HPF
- pleomorphism
- hemorrhage
- necrosis

Resectability is the single most important indicator of clinical outcome (regardless of "histologic malignancy"). Size >10cm also predicts worse outcome. These criteria have also been applied to extra-pleural SFT [62]

Reference: [63]

5 Grading Systems: Prognostic Features in Neoplasms with Difficult-to-Predict Behavior.

97

The Good the Bad and the Ugly – continued

Gastrointestinal Stromal Tumor (GIST), AFIP Risk Stratification Scheme					
Tumor Parameters		**Risk of Poor Outcome by Site**			
Size (cm)	Mitotic Rate	Stomach	Jejunum/Ileum	Duodenum	Rectum
≤2	≤5 per 50HPF	None	None	None	None
>2–5		Very low	Low	Low	Low
>5–10		Low	Moderate	High	High
>10		Moderate	High		
≤2	>5 per 50HPF	None	High	Insufficient data	High
>2–5		Moderate		High	
>5–10		High			
>10					

Although there are other similar schemes, the AFIP system was adopted by the AJCC staging manual as well as the National Comprehensive Cancer Network for their Clinical Practice Guidelines. [64]

Reprinted with modification from Semin Diagn Pathol. 2006;23:70-83; Miettinen M, Lasota J; Gastrointestinal stromal tumors: pathology and prognosis at different sites [65], with permission from © Elsevier 2006.

Parathyroid Neoplasms

The only definitive criteria for malignancy are distant metastasis and/or local invasion. Features that have been associated with malignant behavior include:
- Thick fibrous bands (present in 90% of carcinomas but low specificity)
- Thick capsule
- Infiltrative growth
- Capsular invasion * (present in 2/3 of carcinomas)
- Vascular invasion *
- Perineural invasion
- Tumor necrosis
- >5 mitoses per 50 HPF or Ki67 >6%
- Atypical mitotic figures
- Diffuse, marked pleomorphism (may occur in benign)
- Large size (mean size 3 cm, mean weight 12 g)
- Complete loss of parafibromin immunoexpression (also seen in adenomas of the hyperparathyroidism-jaw tumor syndrome) [66]

* Vascular and capsular invasion are assessed using the same criteria as those applied to thyroid follicular carcinoma: vascular invasion should be present within or beyond the tumor capsule and capsular invasion should be completely penetrating.

Reference: [67]

Sertoli and Leydig Cell Tumors

- size > 5 cm
- > 5 mitoses per 10 HPF
- necrosis
- moderate to severe nuclear pleomorphism
- vascular invasion

Generally, all features are present concurrently in the malignant tumors. Overall ~10% of neoplasms are malignant.

Reference: [11]

Criteria for "Micro-entities" in Various Organs

Diagnosis	Size Criteria
Breast metastases to lymph nodes	Isolated tumor cells: <0.2 mm (or <200 cells) Micrometastasis: ≥0.2 mm but <2 mm
Lung, atypical adenomatous hyperplasia (AAH)	≤0.5 cm (+ low-grade cytology, though not all experts agree on an arbitrary size cutoff between AAH and BAC)
Lung, carcinoid tumorlet	≤0.5 cm
Gastric microcarcinoid (ECL cell)	<0.5 cm
Pancreatic neuroendocrine microadenoma (formerly islet cell microadenoma)	<0.5 cm
Pituitary microadenoma versus macroadenoma	≤1 cm versus >1 cm (this is generally a clinical distinction)
Renal cell papillary adenoma	≤0.5 cm
Thyroid papillary microcarcinoma	≤1 cm
Thyroid micromedullary carcinoma	≤1 cm

Criteria for Micro-Invasion in Various Organs

Site	Size Criteria for micro-invasion
Breast	<1 mm (some experts use 2 mm)
Cervix, squamous cell carcinoma (stage IA1)	≤3mm deep and ≤7 mm horizontal extent (controversial) Diagnosed by microscopy only, i.e. no grossly visible lesion in a specimen with negative margins
Ovary, serous borderline tumor	<3–5mm or <10 mm^2
Ovary, mucinous borderline tumor	<3–5 mm or <10 mm^2 (WHO)
Salivary gland, carcinoma ex-mixed tumor	≤1.5 mm beyond the tumor capsule (minimally invasive)
Upper aerodigestive tract	1–2 mm below the basement membrane
Lung (minimally invasive adenocarcinoma arising in BAC)	≤5 mm focus of invasion in a lepidic tumor (BAC) that is ≤3cm in overall size (new proposal) [68]

Abbreviations: BAC bronchioloalveolar carcinoma

Chapter 6   Potpourri of Quick Morphologic References

by Natasha Rekhtman and Justin Bishop

Tumor Differentials 101

Differentials 101: Generic Tumor Types (main tumor-types seen in ALMOST any organ)		
Tumor Type	*Key Features*	*Key immunostains*
Carcinoma	The hallmarks of epithelial cells are cohesiveness (cells stick together), distinct cell borders and usually abundant cytoplasm (cell resembling this description are called "epithelioid"). Main types of carcinoma are listed below:	Epithelial markers (CK, EMA) +
	Squamous cell carcinoma (SqCC): The two hallmark features are 1) **Keratinization**, manifesting as keratin pearls/squamous eddies or isolated cells with glassy salmon-pink cytoplasm/dyskeratotic cells: 2) **Intercellular bridges** – these are desmosomes as seen in the prickle cell layer of the epidermis:	
	Adenocarcinoma • Easy! All you need is gland formation, however focal. Don't be fooled by neuroendocrine or neuroblastic rosettes, though! Also, some tumors can become discohesive and mimic true glands (e.g., acantholytic SqCC). • Intracellular mucin is another hint. Detection of mucin may be aided by a mucicarmine stain.	
	Papillary carcinoma • Papillary carcinomas may be squamous, transitional or glandular, depending on the covering epithelium. Fibrovascular cores are a defining feature. • Note that papillary morphology applies to both to in situ and invasive lesions (curiously, in situ lesions do not usually invade as papillary carcinomas – for example, IPMN usually invades as a colloid CA, etc). • DDx: ovarian serous CA, lung, kidney, thyroid, cholangiocarcinoma. • Beware – not all that is papillary is a carcinoma (e.g. mesothelioma, myxopapillary ependymoma, papillary meningioma)! • **Micropapillary CA** is a variant of papillary CA, which is defined by the absence of fibrovascular cores in the papillae (also typical are clear halos around papillae). DDx includes ovary (micropapillary CA), bladder, breast, lung, and salivary gland. Behavior is typically aggressive.	
Neuroendocrine (NE) neoplasm	This umbrella category encompasses NE neoplasms that are either low grade (e.g. carcinoid) or high grade (e.g. small cell carcinoma, Merkel cell carcinoma). Both types share a set of defining "NE features": • NE cytology: overall nuclear uniformity/monotony (even when high grade), stippled evenly distributed "salt and pepper" chromatin; absence of prominent nucleoli is key (although there are exceptions) • NE architecture: nests, trabeculae, ribbons, rosettes (subtle in high-grade lesions)	NE markers (SYN, CHR, CD56); CK expression is type-dependent
Small cell carcinoma	Unless otherwise specified, this term implies small cell NE carcinoma, also known as "oat cell carcinoma" (note that there are small cell variants of melanoma and some carcinomas). • Despite the name, small size (<3 lymphocytes) is not the only defining feature. • Other key defining features are nuclear molding, very high N/C ratio, lots of mitoses, apoptotic bodies, and geographic necrosis. • Crush artifact with DNA streaming and DNA deposition in vessels ("Azzopardi phenomenon") are characteristic. • NE nature is evidenced by uniform distribution of chromatin (despite high grade), inconspicuous nucleoli, and occasional presence of trabeculae and rosettes.	NE markers (sometimes focal); CK + (frequently focal)
Melanoma	• Can look like anything: epithelioid, spindle cell, small cell, pink cell, clear cell, etc (remember – melanoma is a "great imitator" in pathology!) • Prominent cherry-red nucleoli are characteristic. • Presence of melanin pigment is diagnostic, but melanin may be difficult to distinguish from hemosiderin and many melanomas are amelanotic.	Melan-A+, HMB45+, S100+
Lymphoma	• Sheets of cells, ranging from normal lymphocyte-like (e.g. chronic lymphocytic leukemia) to large epithelioid cells (e.g. diffuse large B cell lymphoma). • Large cell lymphoma may be histologically indistinguishable from poorly differentiated carcinoma or melanoma. • General signature of lymphomas is cellular discohesion (cells fall apart) and clefting (indented) nuclei.	CD45+
Sarcoma	• Most commonly composed of spindle or stellate cells, but can also look epithelioid, small cell, clear or highly pleomorphic. • Look for specific features of muscle, vascular, neural or adipocytic differentiation (see below).	vimentin, actin (muscle), S100 (neural), CD34 (vascular)
Undifferentiated neoplasm	• When all else fails (no histologic clues and negative immunostains); diagnosis of exclusion.	negative or uninformative

In general, these generic tumors have the similar morphology irrespective of the organ of origin, and the origin of metastasis cannot be determined without immunostains or clinical history. However, adenocarcinomas of some organs do have a distinctive morphology, most notably:
- colon: tall pseudostratified nuclei and "dirty, garland necrosis"
- prostate: low-grade nuclei with prominent nucleoli forming rosette-like structures
- breast: nests (rather than glands), relatively bland cytology
- adenocarcinoma with squamous differentiation: endometrioid, pancreas, lung (not prostate, colon, breast – with rare exceptions)

Quick Morphologic References

N. Rekhtman, J.A. Bishop, *Quick Reference Handbook for Surgical Pathologists*, DOI:10.1007/978-3-642-20086-1_6, © Springer-Verlag Berlin Heidelberg 2011

Differentials 101: Tumors by Cell Type	
Tumor Type	Differential
Epithelioid tumors (plump cohesive cells)	DDx includes "carcinoma-melanoma-lymphoma-sarcoma" (the "Big 4"): 1) Carcinoma: look for evidence of glandular or squamous differentiation, however focal. Associated CIS/dysplasia seals the deal. 2) Melanoma: look for melanin pigment and cherry-red nucleoli. Associated melanoma in situ cinches the diagnosis. 3) Lymphoma: diffuse large B cell, anaplastic large cell (a hint of cellular discohesion is a clue). 4) Sarcoma: think of epithelioid sarcoma, epithelioid angiosarcoma, epithelioid MPNST, epithelioid GIST, other. Other: histiocytic neoplasms, leukemic infiltrate (chloroma), germ cell tumors, epithelioid mesothelioma. Diagnosis usually requires immunostains. Typical initial panel includes CK for carcinoma, S100 for melanoma and CD45 for lymphoma.
Large pink cell tumors	Defined as polygonal cells (non-spindle, non-small cell) with bright pink cytoplasm. DDx includes all of the "Big 4": 1) Many carcinomas, most notably HCC (look for bile pigment and lipid vacuoles), RCC (look for nested pattern and prominent vascularity), adrenocortical tumors; also consider SqCC and urothelial CA. 2) Melanoma: commonly has abundant pink cytoplasm. 3) Lymphoma: ALCL. 4) Sarcoma: ASPS, pleomorphic rhabdomyosarcoma (and rhabdoid tumors), angiomyolipoma. Cytoplasmic granularity in pink cell tumors may be due to • mitochondria – oncocytic neoplasms of the salivary gland or kidney, Hurthle cell neoplasms of the thyroid • lysosomes – granular cell tumor • zymogen granules – acinic cell CA of the salivary gland, acinar cell CA of the pancreas • NE granules – carcinoid tumor.
Clear cell (CC) tumors	First think carcinoma, but certain types of soft tissue tumors (e.g. CC sarcoma, PEComa) and very rarely melanoma and lymphoma can be clear. The first-line differential is CC-RCC (most common), seminoma (look for admixed lymphocytes), adrenocortical carcinoma, and CC-HCC (uncommon). Complete list of CC neoplasms is vast (almost any carcinoma can have clear cell change, at least focally). Classic examples are: • Head and neck: oncocytic and Hurthle cell neoplasms (these are particularly prone to clear cell change), parathyroid, salivary gland neoplasms (e.g. myoepithelial tumors, oncocytic tumors, acinic cell and mucoep carcinomas), • Lung: CC/sugar tumor, CC squamous cell carcinoma, • Gyn tract: CC adenocarcinoma, • Soft tissue: CC sarcoma/melanoma of soft parts.
Spindle cell tumors	First think sarcoma (e.g. muscle, neural, vascular), but remember that there are spindle-cell variants of both melanoma and carcinoma! Look for clues to differentiation in mesenchymal spindle cell neoplasms: Cytological clues to differentiation in spindle cell tumors: • Smooth muscle: "box car" or "cigar"-shaped (blunt-ended) nucleus with clear perinuclear vacuoles (fascicles intersect at right angles) • Skeletal muscle: pink cytoplasmic inclusions with cross-striations and "strap cells" (rhabdomyoblasts) • Fibroblast: bipolar or stellate nucleus with pointy ends • Myofibroblast: pointy ends like fibroblast but the nucleus is more plump • Nerve sheath (schwannian): "club-" or "bullet"-shaped nuclei (pointed at one end), typically wavy • GIST (pericyte): nucleus is intermediate between smooth muscle (box-car) and Schwann cell (pointed). Nuclei can be ridiculously long. Architectural clues to differentiation in spindle cell tumors: • Vascular channels or slit-like spaces with RBC's = vascular differentiation (e.g. angiosarcoma) • Wagner-Meissner's bodies = neural differentiation (e.g. MPNST)
Small round blue cell tumors	Defined as patternless sheets of small round blue cells (duh!). Cells are blue because they have very little cytoplasm. Subtle morphologic hints may be present but generally diagnosis requires immunostains +/– molecular studies, cytogenetics (and EM if desperate). DDx is age-dependent (see below).

Differentials 101: Tumors by Architectural Pattern (see Glossary for definitions)	
Pattern	Differential Diagnosis
Hemangiopericytoma (HPC)-like pattern (branching staghorn-like vessels)	hemangiopericytoma (prototype), synovial sarcoma (particularly monophasic), solitary fibrous tumor, mesenchymal chondrosarcoma, nasopharyngeal angiofibroma, MPNST, meningioma, thymoma, myofibromatosis, endometrial stromal sarcoma, infantile fibrosarcoma
Storiform pattern (cartwheel-like arrangement of cells)	Dermatofibrosarcoma protuberans (prototype), dermatofibroma, malignant fibrous histiocytoma (less prominent), focally in many other soft tissue lesions
Nested pattern (packets of cells with intervening stroma)	pheochromocytoma/paraganglioma (prototype), RCC, urothelial carcinoma, granular cell tumor, melanoma, other
Alveolar pattern (nests with central discohesion)	Alveolar soft parts sarcoma and alveolar rhabdomyosarcoma (prototypes), nested neoplasms may appear alveolar (e.g. RCC)
Herringbone pattern (fascicles alternating at acute angles)	fibrosarcoma (prototype), MPNST, synovial sarcoma, leiomyosarcoma, also melanoma (particularly of the head and neck!)
Basaloid tumors (resembling basal cell carcinoma)	basal cell carcinoma (prototype), basaloid SqCC, HPV-related SqCC, adnexal tumors, adenoid cystic carcinoma, other
Nuclear palisading in spindle cell tumors	schwannoma (prototype), smooth muscle tumors, GIST
Perinuclear vacuoles	smooth muscle tumors, GIST
Biphasic tumors (epithelial and stromal components)	Malignant: sarcomatoid carcinomas/carcinosarcomas (including bladder, lung, uterus, etc.), phyllodes tumor, biphasic synovial sarcoma, mesothelioma, pulmonary blastoma, biphasic Wilms tumor, other Benign: fibroadenoma (breast), adenofibroma (gyn tract), cystic neoplasms with ovarian-type (spindly/ER+) stroma (mucinous cystic neoplasm of pancreas, mixed epithelial stromal tumor of kidney, other), benign mixed tumor (salivary)

Potpourri of Differentials

Tumors with prominent lymphocytes	medullary carcinoma (breast and GI), seminoma, lymphoepithelioma (LE) and LE-like carcinomas, thymoma, inflammatory myofibroblastic tumor, follicular dendritic cell sarcoma, clear cell carcinoma of ovary (may look just like dysgerminoma).
Tumors with prominent neutrophils	Hodgkin lymphoma, neutrophil-rich anaplastic large cell lymphoma, inflammatory MFH, inflammatory leiomyosarcoma, inflammatory liposarcoma, anaplastic carcinoma of the thyroid, anaplastic carcinoma of the pancreas, sarcomatoid renal cell carcinoma, medullary carcinoma of kidney
Tumors with prominent eosinophils	classical Hodgkin lymphoma, Langerhans cell histiocytosis, granulocytic sarcoma (chloroma), glassy cell carcinoma of the cervix
Tumors with prominent mast cells	synovial sarcoma, neurofibroma (absent in schwannoma), spindle cell lipoma, myxoid liposarcoma, hemangiopericytoma, hairy cell lymphoma (particularly in bone marrow), other (anything myxoid often has accompanying mast cells)
Tumors with extravasated erythrocytes	Kaposi sarcoma, nodular fasciitis, inflammatory myofibroblastic tumor
Tumors associated with granulomas	classic associations – seminoma, Hodgkin lymphoma, lymphomatoid granulomatosis, also some carcinomas (e.g., reaction to keratin in SqCC)
Intranuclear inclusions	papillary thyroid carcinoma, HCC, melanoma, meningioma, adrenocortical carcinoma, pheochromocytoma, bronchioloalveolar carcinoma, other
Hyaline globules	relatively non-specific, but classic associations are yolk sac tumor, Kaposi sarcoma, solid-pseudopapillary tumor of the pancreas, hepatocellular carcinoma, clear cell carcinoma of GYN tract
Psammoma bodies	papillary carcinomas (papillary thyroid CA, serous ovarian CA, papillary CA of the lung, papillary RCC), metanephric adenoma, meningioma (and normal meninges), mesothelioma (and benign mesothelial proliferations in peritoneum), duodenal somatostatinoma
Tumors with melanin pigment	melanoma (#1, 2, and 3 in the differential), clear cell sarcoma/melanoma of soft parts, Bednar's tumor (pigmented dermatofibrosarcoma protuberans), other neural crest-derived tumors occasionally produce melanin (e.g. melanotic schwannoma, melanotic medulloblastoma)
Mucinous and myxoid tumors	Mucin production is a common feature of carcinomas and soft tissue tumors. Soft tissue mucins are referred to as "myxoid material" to distinguish them from biochemically distinct epithelial mucin. Mucin production is vanishingly rare in melanoma and lymphoma. **Common sites of mucinous (colloid) CA**: bowel, appendix, pancreas, lung, breast. Generally indolent behavior (except colon). **DDx of myxoid soft tissue tumors:** almost ANY soft tissue tumor can be myxoid, at least focally. Major players are intramuscular myxoma, myxoid malignant fibrous histiocytoma (myxofibrosarcoma), myxoid liposarcoma, fibromyxoid sarcoma, myxoid chondrosarcoma, neurofibroma (myxoid change common), nodular fasciitis and abdominal fibromatosis (sometimes myxoid), chondromyxoid fibroma (bone). **Other myxoid tumors:** pleomorphic adenoma, chordoma (midline extra-axial), myxopapillary ependymoma (filum terminale)
Tumors with squamoid morules (have nuclear/mutated β-catenin)	endometrioid carcinoma (low-grade), craniopharyngioma, cribriform-morular variant of papillary thyroid CA, solid pseudopapillary tumor of pancreas, pulmonary blastoma/well-differentiated fetal adenocarcinoma of the lung, colon adenocarcinomas/ adenomas

Benign Mimics of Malignancy 101 – watch out!

Pleomorphic tumors that are actually NOT high grade (degenerative-type atypia)	classically, endocrine and NE neoplasms ("NE atypia"), schwannomas ("ancient change"), renal oncocytoma, pleomorphic xantroastrocytoma (PXA), atypical fibroxanthoma (AFX), uterine leiomyomas ("symplastic" change), pleomorphic hyalinizing angiectatic tumor (PHAT). A clue to degenerative nature of atypia is smudgy chromatin and absence of atypical mitoses.
Perineural invasion in benign lesions	breast sclerosing adenosis, endometriosis, vasitis nodosa, Leydig cell tumors, benign vascular tumors, prostate "benign perineural involvement" (tumor apposed but not surrounding a nerve), pyloric gland metaplasia in gall bladder
Benign tumors which may have isolated vascular invasion	pleomorphic adenoma [1,2], pheochromocytoma/paraganglioma, granular cell tumor [3]
Benign tumors which may invade bone (bone invasion ≠ malignancy)	meningioma, pituitary adenoma, inverted Schneiderian papilloma (extension into bone occurs as a result of pressure erosion, and by itself is not an indication of malignancy)
Benign inclusions in lymph nodes	Müllerian (endometriosis, endosalpingiosis, endocervicosis), nevus (intracapsular location), salivary gland, thyroid (somewhat controversial), mesothelial, breast (heterotopic tissue or benign mechanical transport due to procedure or massage; usually from papillary lesions), hemangioma
Benign tumors that can metastasize (!)	salivary pleomorphic adenoma, uterine leiomyoma, chondroblastoma and giant cell tumor of bone, meningioma, sclerosing hemangioma of lung [4]

Differentials 101: Small Round Blue Cell Tumors (SRBCT) of Adulthood					
Diagnosis	Age/Clinical	Location	Histologic Clues	Key immunostains	Cytogenetics
Lymphoma	Any age (type-dependent)	Lymph nodes and any extra-nodal site	No molding (cells are disco-hesive)	CD45+, CD20 (B cell) or CD3 (T cell)	Various translocations
Small cell NE carcinoma	Older adults, ectopic hormones, early mets	Any organ	Molding, no nucleoli, "salt and pepper" chromatin, prominent necrosis NE architecture: rosettes, trabeculae (usually subtle)	CK+, NE markers+, TTF-1+ (lung and some non-lung), Neurofilament–, CK20– (opposite to MCC)	
Merkel cell carcinoma (MCC)	60–70 yo	Dermis Head and extremities	Molding, "dusty" vesicular chromatin Rosettes and trabeculae (occasionally)	CK+, NE markers+, always TTF-1–, Neuro-filament+, CK20+ (punctate) Merkel cell polyomavi-rus antigen+	
Desmoplastic small round cell tumor (DSRCT)	Mean age 21, M:F = 4:1; rare tumor	Serosal cavities (perito-neum, pleura)	Angulated nests of SRBC in desmoplastic stroma	WT1+, CK+, EMA+, NSE+, desmin+/actin–	t(11;22) EWS-WT1
Synovial sarcoma, poorly differenti-ated	Any age, typically young adults; mean age 26; 20% <20yo	Extremities/para-articular (not joints), head and neck, almost any other site	High grade SRBCT Immunostains (+/– cytoge-netics) required for diagnosis	CK+, EMA+, calponin+, most CD99+	t(X;18) SYT-SSX
Olfactory neuroblastoma (esthesioneuro-blastoma)	Bimodal peaks: age 15 and 55	Roof of nasal fossa (cribri-form plate)	Similar to abdominal neuro-blastoma: fibrillar rosettes and fibrillar stroma (neu-ropil); ganglion cells gener-ally absent	NE markers+ (SYN most sensitive), CK can be focal but EMA always –, sustentacular S100	
Small Cell Osteosarcoma	Bimodal age peaks: 20's and 50's	Around knee (distal femur, proximal tibia)	Tumor osteoid required for diagnosis		
Mesenchymal chondrosarcoma	Typical range 10–40yo (peak 20's and 30's)	Axial skeleton	Chondroid differentiation required for diagnosis	Sox9+ Focally desmin+ in 50% [5–7]	t(9;22) EWS-CHN
Cellular myxoid/round cell liposarcoma	Peak incidence in the 30's	Soft tissue of extremities (thigh) or retroperitoneum	Cytoplasmic vacuoles (lipo-blasts) at least focally Chicken-wire vessels	S100 (immunos gener-ally not used)	t(12;16) TLS-CHOP t(12;22) EWS-CHOP
DDx also includes Ewing sarcoma/PNET (young adults, see below), small cell melanoma (adults, any age)					

Differentials 101: Small Round Blue Cell Tumors (SRBCT) of Childhood[1]					
Diagnosis	Age/Clinical	Location	Histologic Clues	Key immu-nostains	Cytogenetics
Lymphoblastic lymphoma (LBL) (>80% are T cell)	Peaks in adolescence, rare in adults Boys>>girls #1 pediatric malignancy (together with leukemia)	Thymus (>50%), nodes, spleen, other	Dense medium-size lymphocytes, blastic ("fine lacey") chromatin, inconspicuous nucleoli No molding (cells are discohesive) Many mitoses, sometimes "starry sky" pattern (similar to Burkitt lymphoma)	CD45 variable, TdT+, CD34+ CD3+ (if T cell) frequently CD99+	Various translo-cations
Neuroblastoma	Peak age 2yrs, 90% by age 8, rare in young adults #1 solid extra-cranial malignancy and #3 overall malignancy (after leukemia/ lymphoma and CNS) in kids	Adrenal medulla, sympathetic ganglia	Fibrillar stroma (neuropil) and fibrillar (Homer Wright) rosettes Ganglion cells and schwannian stroma in better differentiated tumors No molding (cells are evenly spaced apart)	NE markers +	Poor prognosis: N-*myc* amplifica-tion, −1p, +17q Good prognosis: age <1 year, hyperdiploidy
Ewing Sarcoma (ES) /PNET[2]	Mean age 11–15 yo, but can occur at any age; very rare in ages <5 and >30 Presents as rapidly growing painful mass. Skeletal form clinically mimics osteomyelitis.	1) Skeletal: lower extremities and pelvis 2) Soft tissue: paravertebral, ex-tremities, retroperi-toneum	Monomorphic uniform cells Vesicular (open) chromatin +/– Homer Wright rosettes Cytoplasmic vacuoles (glycogen/PAS+) No neuropil outside rosettes and no ganglion cells (unlike neuroblastoma)	CD99+ NE markers +	t(11;22) EWS-FLI1– 80%
Rhabdomyosarcoma, solid alveolar variant	Peak age 9, can occur up to age 30 (older than embryonal) #1 pediatric sarcoma	Deep muscles of extremities; trunk (distinct from em-bryonal)	Look for hints of myogenic differentia-tion: pink cytoplasmic inclusions (cross-striations are rarely evident) and multinu-cleated giant cells Dense chromatin (unlike Ewing sar-coma/PNET) Cell are discohesive	Actin+, Desmin+ (can highlight cross-striations), MyoD+, Myo-genin+	t(2;13) PAX3-FKHR t(1;13) PAX7-FKHR
Wilms tumor (nephroblastoma), blastema predominant	Peak age 3.5 yo, range 3mo–6yrs; always >3mo & <16yrs of age #1 pediatric renal tumor	Kidney	May see areas with classic triphasic histology Molding present (unlike lymphoma, neuroblastoma) [8]	WT1+	11p13 (*WT1* gene) deletion/ mutation, Trisomy 12
Medulloblastoma	Peak age 7 yo; usually <20 yo (70% under age 16)	Cerebellum	High grade SRBCT Homer Wright rosettes Sometimes nodular architecture	SYN+	Isochromosome 17q
Retinoblastoma	Young children	Retina	Flexner-Wintersteiner rosettes		13q14 (*RB* gene) deletion/mutation
Hepatoblastoma, small cell variant	90% in kids under age 5	Liver	Diagnosis requires areas of better-differentiated hepatoblastoma		

1) DDx also includes Small Cell Osteosarcoma and Mesenchymal chondrosarcoma (see SRBCT of adulthood). Note that not all "blastomas" are pediatric small round cell tumors: for example, pulmonary blastoma and hemangioblastoma are tumors of adulthood that are non-SRBCT of adulthood.

2) PNET (primitive neuroectodermal tumor) and Ewing sarcoma (ES) are now regarded as morphological manifestations of one tumor type; both are char-acterized by t(11;22) translocation. In general, ES arises within the bone and PNET arises within soft tissues. In addition, there are usually more neuroendo-crine features in PNET whereas ES is thought to be a more undifferentiated tumor. However, there is a considerable overlap in clinical presentation and morphology and many experts no longer separate these entities.

Quick Morpho-logic References

There's Fungus among us! Quick Reference for Histologic Identification of Fungi

Fungi that cause deep invasive infections can be categorized as **opportunistic** (limited to immunocompromised host) versus **pathogenic** (able to infect immunocompetent host). Classic opportunistic fungi include *Aspergillus*, Zygomycetes, and *Candida*. Classic pathogenic fungi include dimorphic fungi, which exist as molds in nature and yeast in tissue: *Histoplasma*, *Blastomyces*, *Coccidioides* and *Paracoccidioides*. *Cryptococcus* and *Pneumocystis* are predominantly opportunistic. Your differential diagnosis should vary according to a patient's immune status.

Fungi are generally inconspicuous in H&E sections, and are best visualized by "pan-fungal" stains – GMS and PAS, although some larger fungi (*Blasto*, *Cocci*, Zygomycetes) as well as Crypto are visible in H&E. The size of a RBC and a lymphocyte nucleus are ~7 um; these may be used as a handy size reference. The most common histologic response to fungi is granulomatous inflammation, but some may manifest with other features, such as acute purulent inflammation (*Blasto*) or frothy intra-alveolar exudate (*Pneumocystis*).

Disease (organism)	Appearance (GMS or PAS)	Key Histologic Features	Comment
Budding Yeast in Tissue			
Histoplasmosis (*Histoplasma capsulatum*)	"tiny critters in a macrophage (MF)"	• 2–5 um • narrow-based "tear-drop" budding • surrounded by clear space/pseudocapsule (hence "*Capsulatum*") • predominantly intracellular but usually spill into surrounding tissue, where organisms tend to remain in clusters • **DDx:** other small "yeast in tissue" (particularly *Crypto*) and small intracellular protozoa (*Leishmania*)	Ohio-Mississippi river valley carrier: birds and bats ("cave fever") sites: lung, GI, disseminated old lesions typically hyalinize/calcify
Blastomycosis (*Blastomyces dermatitidis*)	"snowman"	• 8–15 um • broad-based budding • thick double walls ("double contour") • multinucleation • cell walls can be weakly positive for mucin stains	Ohio-Mississippi river valley sites: lung, skin, bone, disseminated
Paracoccidioidomycosis/ aka South American Blastomyces (*Paracoccidioides braziliensis*)	"mariner's wheel"	• 5–30 um (wide size variation is characteristic) • large spherule with multiple peripheral narrow-based buds (although diagnostic, the multiple-budding cells are usually inconspicuous)	Africa, Central and South America sites: skin, bone, mucous membranes (clinically mimics *Blasto*
Cryptococcosis (*Cryptococcus neoformans*)	"soap bubbles"	• 2–15 um • narrow-based budding • highly variable size (unlike *Histo* or *Blasto*, which are uniform) • variable shape: spherical and elongated (football-shaped) forms • polysaccharide capsule (mucicarmine+, PAS+, AB+), but some organisms are capsule-deficient; India Ink + (historic use) • cell wall contains melanin pigment (Fontana-Masson+; pigment not apparent in H&E). Note that positive melanin stain is not entirely specific for *Crypto* – *Coccidioides* and *Sporothrix* can also be positive	carrier: pigeons (droppings) sites: meningitis, lung, other deep infections
Sporotrichosis (*Sporotrix schenckii*)	"cigar bodies"	• 2–6 um • round or elongated "cigar-shaped" budding yeast, usually rare and difficult to find in tissue • "asteroid bodies" (Splendore-Hoeppli phenomenon) – crystalline structures representing antigen-antibody complexes, classic for Sporo but not specific	"rose-gardener's disease" sites: SubQ
Non-budding Spherical Fungi in Tissue			
Coccidioidomycosis (*Coccidioides immitis*)	"bag of marbles"	• thick-walled spherule (50–200 um) packed with endospores (2–5 um) • endospores frequently spill into the surrounding tissue and may resemble *Histoplasma* (but these is no budding) • **DDx:** – *Rhinosporidium*: nasal fungus, much larger than *Cocci*, also GMS+ – Myospherulosis: surgical packing material with entrapped RBCs in the nose/sinus, GMS & PAS-negative, Hemoglobin+	Southwest American deserts ("valley fever") sites: lung, skin, disseminated
Penicilliosis (*Penicillium marneffei*)	"tiny critters in a MF"	• 2–4 um • elongated cells with septae (divides by fission, not budding) • predominantly intracellular (like *Histo*) • mimics *Histo* (but *Penicillium* is non-budding and has no pseudocapsule)	Southeast Asia AIDS patients
Pneumocystosis (*Pneumocystis carinii*, recently renamed as *P. jiroveci*)	"tea cup and saucer"	• 3–5 um • clusters of non-budding organisms in a frothy background • GMS: round and crescent-shaped cysts (described as a "cup-and-saucer" or "crushed ping-pong balls") with 2 parenthesis-shaped dots • Giemsa or Diff Quik highlight up to 8 intracystic 'trophozoites'	sites: lung AIDS patients
Chromoblastomycosis	"copper pennies"	• 6–12 um • brown (melanin-containing) organisms; Fontana-Masson+ • thick-walled spheres with horizontal and vertical septae ("copper pennies", "medlar bodies", "sclerotic bodies") • overlying pseudoepitheliomatous hyperplasia is typical	sites: SubQ

There's Fungus among us! Quick Reference for Histologic Identification of Fungi – 2

Disease (organism)	Appearance (GMS or PAS)	Key Histologic Features	Comment
Hyphae in Tissue			
Aspergillosis (*Aspergillus spp*) and other **hyalohyphomycoses** (septate non-pigmented molds)	"slingshots"	• thin (2–5um thick) hyphae WITH septae ("septate hyphae") • frequent dichotomous 45-degree branching (Y-shaped) • when invasive, tends to be angioinvasive • hyphae tend to grow in a radial "sunburst"-like fashion • occasional fruiting bodies (in aerated sites) • definitive diagnosis requires cultures because in tissue *Aspergillus* is indistinguishable from other hyalohyphomycoses, including *Pseudoallescheria boydii* and *Fusarium* (both resistant to Amphotericin B).	Types of *Aspergillus*-related diseases include 1) tissue-invasive infections (sinus, lung, disseminated) in immuno-compromised host 2) allergic bronchopulmonary aspergillosis (ABPA) and allergic fungal sinusitis in atopic host 3) aspergilloma/mycetoma/fungus ball = colonization of cavities (such as sinuses or cavitary lung disease)
Zygomycosis = Mucormycosis = Phycomycosis (*Rhizopus, Absidia, Mucor*). These organisms belong to Mucorales suborder of the Zygomycetes phylum.	"wide ribbons"	• wide (6–50um thick) hyphae with INFREQUENT septae • infrequent right-angle branching • undulating, twisting (ribbon-like), "empty-looking" hyphae • angioinvasive (like *Aspergillus*) • stain weakly with GMS and PAS; organisms best visualized by H&E • definitive diagnosis requires culture because treated or degenerating *Aspergillus* may look like Zygomycetes. *Note regarding terminology: these organisms are frequently referred to collectively as "Mucor" in pathology, but in fact the right term is Zygomycetes – *Mucor* is only one of several organisms (and not even the most common) in this group.	Aggressive tissue-invasive disease (sinus, disseminated) in immuno-compromised host. This is a life-threatening emergency. Why distinguishing *Zygomycetes* vs. *Aspergillus* is important: 1) *Zygomycetes* are more aggressive 2) *Zygomycetes* are treated with Amphotericin B. They are resistant to most azoles (except the new posaconazole).
Dermatophytosis (*Microsporum spp, Epidermophyton spp, Trichophyton spp*)		• septate hyphae with rare branching that break into segments (arthroconidia) • 2–3 um thick • hyphae confined to the skin, nails, hair	superficial infections of skin and hair ("tinea" or "ringworm")
Phaeohyphomycosis (pigmented molds)		• septate branching hyphae; may resemble *Aspergillus* in tissue though are often thinner with less branching, have constrictions at their frequent septae, and vesicular swellings • contain melanin (Fontana-Masson+) • brown pigment sometimes (but not always) evident in H&E	SubQ and deep infections

Disease (organism)	Appearance (GMS or PAS)	Key Histologic Features	Comment
Yeast & Hyphae in Tissue			
Candidiasis (*Candida spp*)	"sausage-links and yeast"	• 3–5 um budding yeast • 5–10 um pseudohyphae: elongated budding yeast joined end-to-end like "sausage-links"; occasionally true hyphae (no constrictions) are present • *C. glabrata* is unique in that it does not produce any hyphae; it may mimic *Histo* and other small yeast	mucocutaneous and deep infections
Pityriasis versicolor (*Malassezia furfur*)	"spagetti & meatballs"	• 3–8 um budding yeast (meatballs) and 5–10 um fragmented hyphae (spaghetti) often arranged end-to-end • involves epidermis only, only rarely seen in tissue (skin scraping preferred method of diagnosis)	site: skin only

Disease (organism)	Appearance (GMS or PAS)	Key Histologic Features	Comment
Mold-like Branching Filamentous Bacteria			
Nocardiosis (*Nocardia asteroides*)		• delicate narrow (1 um) beaded filaments; right-angle branching • Gram+, modified AFB (Fite)+, GMS+ • DDx includes *Streptomyces* (AFB–)	deep infection in immunocompromised host
Actinomycosis (*Actinomyces israelii*)	"dust bunnies"	• delicate narrow (<1 um) branching filaments intertwined in a dense radiating meshwork • 'sulfur granules' (grossly yellow flecks; do not, in fact, contain sulfur) • Gram+, AFB–, GMS+	• normal commensal inhabitant of the oral cavity • may become pathogenic in oropharynx with local tissue damage (such as dental work), may cause draining sinus tracts • IUD-related infections

Quick Morpho-logic References

There's Fungus among us! Quick Reference for Histologic Identification of Fungi – 3

	Organism	Key Histologic Features	Comment
Yeast-like Organisms in Tissue			
Protozoa	*Leishmania spp*	• 2–4 um round to oval aflagellate amastigotes (extra-vascular form of organisms) • amastigotes are intracellular • transverse paranuclear bar-like kinetoplast • *Leishmania* is a close mimic of Histoplasma (look for kinetoplast) • organisms stain lightly in H&E • GMS–, PAS–, Giemsa+	<u>Visceral Leishmaniasis (kala-azar):</u> • Middle East, Africa, India • Sites: reticuoendothelial system (liver, spleen, bone marrow) <u>Cutaneous Leishmaniasis:</u> Old World ("oriental sore") and New World ("chicle ulcer") <u>Mucocutaneous Leishmaniasis:</u> Central and South America
	Trypanosoma Cruzi	• organisms in tissue look identical to *Leishmania spp* • *T gambiense* and *T rhodesiense* (African trypanosomiasis) are confined to blood and do not invade tissue	*T Cruzi* (Chagas' disease): • Central and South America • usual sites: heart, colon, esophagus
	Toxoplasma gondii	• 5–7 um crescent-shaped tachyzoites (non-encysted organisms in tissue) • 10–50 um pseudocysts packed with 2–3 um round bradyzoites • basophilic in H&E (unlike yeast) • GMS+, PAS+, Giemsa+	• Worldwide disease; cat vector • sites: disseminated disease (especially brain) in immunosuppressed patients
	Cryptosporidium	• 2–6 um round organisms in the brush border of small bowel mucosa • Giemsa+	Chronic diarrhea in immunosuppressed patients
	Isospora belli	• 25–30 um elliptical organisms interposed between adjacent enterocytes • Giemsa+	
	Microsporidium	• 1–3 um round organisms in the cytoplasm of enterocytes • invisible by H&E • Gram+	
Algae	*Prototheca spp*	• 2–12 um • sporulating forms are sporangia with up to 20 polygonal or wedge-shaped endospores whose cell walls mold together ("morulas") • GMS+, PAS+	• Two human infections: cutaneous (usually immunosuppresed) and olecranon bursitis (usually otherwise healthy with a history of trauma)

References: [9–11]

Quick Reference for Histological Identification of Viruses

In general, nuclear inclusions are associated with DNA viruses (HSV, CMV, Adenovirus, JC and BK viruses). One major exception is CMV in that in addition to nuclear inclusions, it also forms cytoplasmic inclusions. Some DNA viruses do not have any recognizable cytopathic effects (EBV, HHV8). Note that HPV does not manifest as inclusions, but has a unique cytopathic effect (see below).

RNA viruses as a rule do not have recognizable cytopathic changes; few that do, have cytoplasmic inclusions (RSV, negri bodies in rabies). Measles is an exception in that it is an RNA virus that forms nuclear inclusions.

Nuclear inclusions of virally infected cells fall into two morphologic categories:
1. **Cowdry type A**: eosinophilic **"owl-eye"** nuclear inclusion (as in CMV).
2. **Cowdry type B**: (aka **"smudge cells"**) nucleus with a "homogenized, ground glass" chromatin and obliterated nuclear detail.
Note that most DNA viruses (HSV, Adenovirus) can have nuclear inclusion of either Cowdry A and/or Cowdry B type even within the same lesion. Exception is CMV in that it forms exclusively type A inclusions.

Virus	Appearance	Nuclear inclusions	Cytoplasmic inclusions	Specific features	Infected cell type	Clinical
HSV	"eggs in a basket" or "pomegranate seeds"	+ (Cowdry A or B), pink, steel gray or purple	–	The 3 M's: Multinucleation, Molding, Margination of chromatin (peripheral clearing or "halo effect")	Squamous and some glandular epithelial cells (look at the periphery of an ulcer)	Gingivostomatitis and genital lesions in immunocompetent host. Opportunistic infection of any body site (pneumonia, esophagitis, neurons in encephalitis)
CMV	"owl-eye nuclear inclusion and cytoplasmic speckles"	+ (Cowdry A), blue	+ (blue speckles)	Nuclear and cytoplasmic enlargement Nuclear inclusion has a prominent halo ("owl eye"), which corresponds to marginated chromatin pushed aside by viral particles.	Stromal and endothelial cells (look at the ulcer base); rarely in epithelial cells	Opportunistic infection of any body site (lung, bowel, retina), neurons in encephalitis
Adenovirus		+ (Cowdry A or B), blue	–		Epithelial cells (bronchial cells and pneumocytes in lung)	Opportunistic infections (bladder, kidney, lung, bowel)
HPV	"koilocyte"	–	–	Clear perinuclear vacuole (Greek *koilos* = hollow), wrinkled (raisin-like) nucleus, binucleation (common), condensed keratohyaline granules typical in skin	Squamous cells	Papillary lesions (warts, condyloma, laryngeal papillomas).
JC and BK (polyoma)	"decoy cell"	+ (Cowdry B), blue	–	Nuclear enlargement Non-haloed smudgy (type B) inclusion	JC – brain BK – urothelium (mimics CIS in urine; "decoy" cells)	JC – PML BK – cystitis in immunosuppressed
Measles	"Warthin Finkeldey giant cell"	+ (Cowdry A or B), pink	+ (pink speckles)	Giant cells with multinucleation	Depends on the site: • Lung – epithelial cells, most commonly bronchial; • Lymph node – lymphoreticular cells (infected cells in lymph node are called Warthin Finkeldey giant cells), • Brain – oligodendroglia	Pneumonitis, lymphadenitis, SSPE
RSV		–	+ (large pale-pink globs)	Giant cells with multinucleation. NO nuclear inclusion (this is an RNA virus)	Epithelial cells	Bronchiolitis and pneumonia in children (rarely biopsied)

Abbreviations: ni – nuclear inclusion; ci – cytoplasmic inclusion; PML – progressive multifocal leukoencephalopathy; SSPE – subacute sclerosing panencephalitis

Quick Reference for Tumors with Viral Associations

Detection of viral molecules is a very helpful adjunct in the diagnosis of the virally induced tumors. In tissue sections, viral proteins can be detected by immunohistochemistry (e.g. EBV-LMP), or viral nucleic acids may be identified by in situ hybridization (e.g. EBER). p16 is NOT a viral protein but an endogenous cell cycle protein that is markedly overexpressed as a result of high-risk HPV infection. In cervical cytology, the specimens are tested for HPV by a DNA-based method (Hybrid capture).

Virus	Tumor associations		Detection in Tissue

EBV	**Epithelial lesions:**
	• Nasopharyngeal carcinoma (NPC), aka lymphoepithelial carcinoma (= lymphoepithelioma [LE]) and LE-like carcinomas:
	  – EBV (+): NPC and LE-like carcinomas of upper aerodigestive tract (lung, thymus, salivary gland), and stomach
	  – EBV (–): LE-like carcinoma of non-aerodigestive tract (bladder, breast, skin, cervix)
	• Oral hairy leukoplakia
	• Gastric adenocarcinoma (5%)
			1) EBER (EBV encoded early RNA). Most sensitive marker for EBV (in situ hybridization method). ID's all EBV-related tumors.
			
			2) EBV-LMP (late membrane protein). Less sensitive that EBER. ID's PTLD and AIDS-related lymphomas, variable in NPC, Hodgkin and Burkitt lymphoma, usually negative in plasmablastic lymphoma
			
			3) EBNA (EBV nuclear antigen). Least sensitive marker. ID's PTLD and AIDS-related lymphomas only.

	Lymphoid lesions:
	• Infectious mononucleosis
	• Post-transplant lymphoproliferative disease (PTLD)
	• Hodgkin lymphoma (Mixed cellularity – 70%, AIDS-related)
	• Non-Hodgkin lymphoma:
	  – Burkitt lymphoma (endemic 100%; sporadic 20%)
	  – Nasal-type NK/T cell lymphoma (>95%)
	  – Angioimmunoblastic T cell lymphoma
	  – Lymphomatoid granulomatosis (>95%)
	  – CNS lymphoma in AIDS (95%)
	  – Primary effusion lymphoma (has both EBV and HHV8)
	  – Plasmablastic lymphoma (HIV)		

	Smooth muscle tumors in immunosuppressed (AIDS, transplant)		
HPV	**Female genital tract:** • Squamous dysplasia and carcinoma of cervix, vagina, vulva. (Simplex/differentiated VIN and associated SqCC occur in the setting of lichen sclerosus and other dermatoses in older women, and are HPV-unrelated)	HSIL and associated SqCC caused by high-risk HPV (16, 18, 31, 33) LSIL is caused by • low-risk HPV (6, 11) in 20% • high-risk HPV in 80% (therefore high-risk HPV does not distinguish HSIL and LSIL)	1) In situ hybridization for HPV 2) IHC for p16 is a surrogate marker of high-risk HPV Detection of HPV/p16 may be used to identify cervix and tonsil as origin of metastatic SqCC of unknown primary. HPV-related SqCC of some (but not all) sites have basaloid morphology: • sites where HPV-related SqCC are basaloid: oropharynx, penis, vulva • sites where HPV-related SqCC are either basaloid or conventional: cervix, anus • sites where basaloid SqCC are unrelated to HPV: breast, lung, non-oropharyngeal head and neck
	• Cervical adenocarcinoma (in situ and invasive)	HPV 18>16	
	Penis: • Squamous cell carcinoma, warty and basaloid type (verrucous and papillary SqCC are HPV-unrelated)	HPV 16	
	• Bowenoid Papulosis and Erythroplasia de Queyrat	HPV 16	
	Anus: Squamous neoplasia (in situ and invasive) – analogous to cervix	HPV 16, 18	
	Head and Neck: • Squamous cell carcinoma of the oropharynx (tonsil and base of tongue)	HPV 16, 18	
	• Laryngeal papillomatosis	HPV 6, 11	
	• Focal epithelial hyperplasia (Heck's disease) of oral mucosa	HPV 13, 32	
	Mucocutaneous: • Warts (verruca)	HPV 1, 2, 4, 7	
	• Condyloma acuminatum (genital sites)	HPV 6, 11	
HHV8	Kaposi sarcoma, primary effusion lymphoma (also has EBV), Castleman's disease (multicentric)		HHV8 can be detected by IHC
HTLV1	Adult T-cell leukemia/lymphoma		
Hepatitis B	Hepatocellular carcinoma (Hep C causes HCC indirectly – virus is not present in tumor cells)		HBsAg, HBcAg – rarely used for tumor Dx
Merkel Cell Polyomavirus	50–80% Merkel cell carcinomas		Viral antigen can be detected in Merkel cell CA by IHC, (–) in small cell carcinoma

Chapter 7 Tumor Syndromes
by Justin Bishop, Ashlie Burkart, Natasha Rekhtman

Quick Summary of Tumor Syndromes
For complete list see http://AtlasGeneticsOncology.org

A general rule of thumb for inherited tumor syndromes is that virtually all inherited mutation are **inactivating** mutations in **tumor suppressor genes**. Notice in the tables below that nearly all genes involved in inherited tumor syndromes are tumor suppressors (p53, RB, APC, VHL). The second allele is inactivated somatically later in life, which serves as a trigger for tumorigenesis. This follows a famous "two-hit model of oncogenesis", for which retinoblastoma serves as a paradigm. Since only one mutant allele needs to be inherited for disease to develop, the mode of inheritance is **autosomal dominant**. A possible explanation for this principle is that if dominant mutations were manifest in utero (as would occur with recessive inheritance of two mutated tumor suppressors or with inheritance of activating mutations of oncogenes) they would be lethal.

Note an interesting contrast of inherited tumor syndromes with sporadic tumors. Sporadic tumors may be associated either with inactivation of tumor suppressors (p53) or activation of oncogene (RAS, MYC, KIT, EGFR), whereas the latter molecules are not involved in inherited tumor syndromes. A notable exception to this rule is MENII syndrome, which is caused by inheritance of activating mutations in an oncogene RET.

Other notable exceptions to the above rule of thumb for inherited tumor syndromes (autosomal dominant inheritance of mutations in tumor suppressors) are syndromes caused by inherited defects in DNA repair (Ataxia Telangiectasia, Bloom syndrome, MYH- associated polyposis, Xeroderma pigmentosa and Fanconi anemia) – these have an autosomal recessive mode of inheritance. Exception to this exception is Lynch syndrome (HNPCC) – inherited syndrome due to mutation of DNA mismatch repair genes, which has autosomal dominant transmission.

Syndrome (other names)	Inheritance	Gene [Protein]	Chromosome	Pathology and key clinical features
Multiple Endocrine Neoplasia (MEN) Syndromes				
MENI (Wermer syndrome)	AD	MEN1 [Menin]	11q13	Pituitary adenoma or hyperplasia (~2/3) Parathyroid hyperplasia (90%) Pancreatic endocrine neoplasm/islet cell tumor (~2/3), duodenal gastrin-producing carcinoids [both are a cause of hypergastrinemia/ Zollinger–Ellison syndrome]
MENIIA (Sipple syndrome)	AD	RET	10q11	Medullary thyroid carcinoma (100%) & C cell hyperplasia Parathyroid hyperplasia (50%) Pheochromocytoma (50%)
MENIIB (MEN III, Gorlin syndrome – not to be confused with Nevoid basal cell carcinoma syndrome, also bearing Gorlin's eponym)	AD	RET	10q11	Medullary thyroid carcinoma (85%) & C cell hyperplasia Pheochromocytoma (50%) Diffuse ganglioneuromatosis of the GI tract (typically colon) (100%) Marfanoid body habitus
Neurocutaneous Syndromes				
Neurofibromatosis type 1 (von Recklinghausen disease or peripheral neurofibromatosis)	AD or sporadic	Neurofibromin (p21/ras pathway)	17q11.2	Multiple **neurofibromas** (NF): plexiform NF – nearly pathognomonic for NF1; diffuse NF in 10%, MPNST in 10% **Optic nerve gliomas** (pilocytic astrocytoma) **Other tumors:** ampullary somatostatinoma, duodenal gangliocytic paraganglioma, GIST (5–25%), pheochromocytoma, juvenile xanthogranuloma, other **Non-tumor:** Cafe au lait spots, Lisch nodules (pigmented iris hamartomas), skeletal lesions (spinal deformities and bone cysts)
Neurofibromatosis type 2 (central or acoustic neurofibromatosis)	AD or sporadic	Merlin (cytoskeletal defect)	22q12	**Bilateral acoustic schwannomas**, **Meningiomas** (may be multiple), Spinal cord **ependymomas** Cafe au lait spots, no Lisch nodules
Tuberous Sclerosis (Bourneville's disease)	AD	TSC1 [Hamartin] TSC2 [Tuberin]	9p34 16p13	**PEComas** (perivascular epithelioid cell tumors): renal angiomyolipoma, pulmonary lymphangioleiomyomatosis and sugar tumor, other **CNS:** cortical tubers, subependymal giant cell astrocytoma (SEGA), white matter heterotopias **Cardiac rhabdomyoma** **Skin:** angiofibroma (aka adenoma sebaceum), periungual fibroma, connective tissue nevi (*peau chagrin* or Shagreen patches), hypopigmented (ash-leaf) patches
Sturge-Weber (fourth phacomatosis, Encephalo-trigeminal Angiomatosis)	Not familial	Unknown		**Port-wine stain / nevus flammeus** (dilated vessels) in the distribution of trigeminal nerve Angiomatosis of the ipsilateral leptomeninges **Pheochromocytoma**

N. Rekhtman, J.A. Bishop, *Quick Reference Handbook for Surgical Pathologists*, DOI:10.1007/978-3-642-20086-1_7, © Springer-Verlag Berlin Heidelberg 2011

Tumor Syndromes

Syndrome (other names)	Inheritance	Gene Protein	Chromosome	Pathology and main clinical features
Syndromes Associated with Renal Neoplasms				
Von Hippel-Lindau	AD	VHL [pVHL] (role in ubiquitination)	3p25	**RCC**, clear cell (multiple bilateral) **Cysts** of kidney, pancreas and liver **Hemangioblastomas:** cerebellum (Lindau's tumor), spinal cord, retinal (von Hippel's tumor) **Pheochromocytomas** Pancreatic endocrine neoplasm/islet cell tumor (clear cell variant) Papillary cystadenoma of epididymis and broad ligament Endolymphatic sac tumor of the ear (Heffner tumor)
Birt-Hogg-Dube	AD	BHD [Folliculin]	17p11.2	**Renal tumors:** multiple renal cell carcinomas of various types (clear cell, chromophobe, papillary); oncocytomas; hybrid oncocytic tumors (chromophobe/oncocytoma) – the latter highly specific for this syndrome **Skin:** facial fibrofolliculomas and skin tags **Lung:** cysts/spontaneous pneumothorax
Beckwith-Wiedemann	Sporadic or AD (15%)	duplication of paternal allele	11p15	**"Overgrowth** syndrome": organomegaly, macroglossia Increased childhood **neoplasia:** Wilms tumor (<5%), hepatoblastoma, pancreatoblastoma, neuroblastoma
WAGR	Not familial	Deletion of WT1 gene	11p13	Wilms tumor (>30%), aniridia, genitourinary abnormalities, mental retardation
Denys-Drash	Not familial	WT1 point mutation	11p13	Wilms tumor (>90%), gonadoblastoma, diffuse mesangial sclerosis
Hereditary papillary renal cell cancer (PRCC)	AD	MET (acts via Hepatocyte Growth Factor)	7q34	Multiple bilateral PRCC (type 1)
Hereditary leiomyoma and renal cell carcinoma (HLRCC)	AD	Fumarate hydratase	1q42-43	PRCC (type 2) and leiomyomas (cutaneous and uterine) with distinct cytologic features (see "slide-to-syndrome")
				References: [1,2]

Syndrome	Inheritance	Gene	Chromosome	Pathology and main clinical features
Syndromes Associated with Tumors of Bone				
McCune-Albright syndrome	Non-familial	mosaicism for a mutation in the GNAS1 gene	20q13	Bone: **Fibrous dysplasia** (polyostotic) Skin: Cafe au lait spots Endocrine abnormalities: precocious puberty, thyrotoxicosis, pituitary gigantism, and Cushing syndrome
Mazabraud's syndrome	Not familial	activating GNAS1 mutations	20q13	**Fibrous dysplasia** **Soft tissue myxoma**
Ollier's disease	Not familial	PTH1R mutations may be involved in some cases	3p21-22	**Multiple enchondromas (enchondromatosis)** Increased risk of chondrosarcoma
Maffucci syndrome	Not familial	PTH1R mutations may be involved in some cases	3p21-22	**Multiple enchondromas (enchondromatosis)** PLUS **Soft tissue hemangiomas** Increased risk of chondrosarcoma and angiosarcoma
				Reference: [3]

Tumor Syndromes

Syndrome (other names)	Inheritance	Gene Protein	Chromo-some	Pathology and main clinical features
				Syndromes Associated with GI Polyps and Neoplasms *by Ashlie Burkart and Natasha Rekhtman*
Familial adenomatous polyposis (FAP)	AD	APC (adenomatous polyposis coli) Normal APC degrades β-catenin (a proto-oncogene). Muta-tion/inactivation of APC causes β-catenin to accu-mulate in the nucleus resulting in activated transcription.	5q21	**Intestine**: early onset of 100s to 1000s of adenomas. Virtually 100% will develop colorectal carcinoma if not treated with total colectomy. Small intestinal adenomas (particularly of proximal duodenum and peri-ampullary); periampullary adenocarci-noma is the major cause of death following colectomy; fundic gland polyps (25–40% of fundic gland polyps have dysplasia although these polyps are biologically inert). **Soft tissue tumors (Gardner's)**: Fibromatosis (desmoid tumor), Osteomas, Nuchal fibroma and Gardner fibroma **Skin Lesions (Gardner's)**: Epidermoid cysts, pilomatrixomas **Dental abnormalities (Gardner's)**: Unerupted teeth, supernumerary teeth **Brain tumors (Turcot's)**: Medulloblastomas **Other**: Thyroid cancers (1–2% of young women with FAP) essentially pathogno-monic for FAP is the cribriform-morular variant of papillary thyroid CA; Juvenile nasopharyngeal angiofibromas (adolescent males, 25x risk) **"Attenuated FAP"**: far fewer adenomas (~ 30 adenoma) and cancer develops ~ 10 years later *In both syndromic and sporadic setting, many FAP-associated tumors (tubular adenoma, fibromatosis, JNA, fundic gland polyps) can be identified by IHC for nuclear β-catenin.*
Hereditary nonpoly-posis colorectal can-cer (HNPCC/Lynch syndrome*)	AD	hMLH1 (40%) hMSH2 (40%) hMSH6 (10%) PMS2 (5%) – genes encoding DNA mismatch repair (MMR) proteins + EPCAM (5%)#	hMLH 3p21 hMSH2 2p22 hMSH6 2p16.3 PMS2 7p22.1	**Lynch syndrome-associated tumors**: colorectum (~80% lifetime risk), endo-metrium (~60% lifetime risk), ovary (~12% lifetime risk), stomach, pancreatobil-iary, urothelial carcinoma of upper urinary tract (particularly with inverted growth), small bowel, brain, skin (sebaceous adenomas and carcinomas and keratoacan-thomas) Whereas Lynch syndrome is caused by inherited mutations in MMR genes, these genes are also inactivated in 10–15% of sporadic colorectal cancer, primarily via promoter hypermethylation of hMLH1. *Therefore by IHC – the loss of MSH2, MSH6, or PMS2 is nearly diagnostic of Lynch syndrome (germline mutation), whereas the loss of MLH1 is more commonly sporadic.* * HNPCC/Lynch terms are frequently used interchangeably BUT by strict definition HNPCC refers to patients meeting the clinical definition of inherited colorectal carcinoma ("Amsterdam criteria") vs. Lynch syndrome is reserved only for patients with confirmed germline mutation in the mismatch repair pathway. # Recent data shows that the loss of MSH2 can be caused either by inherited muta-tion in MSH2 gene OR inherited deletion of 3' end of *EPCAM* gene leading to inactivation of adjacent MSH2 gene through methylation induction of its promoter. See below (page 117) for clinicopathologic features suggesting HNPCC/Lynch syndrome. <div align="right">Reference: [4]</div>
Gardner's (FAP variant)	AD	APC	5q21	Manifestations of FAP (see FAP) with the following skin and soft tissue lesions: Fibromatosis, nuchal fibroma, osteomas, pilomatrixomas, epidermoid cysts
Turcot's (FAP variant or HNPCC variant)	AD	PMS2		CNS tumors and polyposis. Two types: 1) medulloblastoma and FAP (2/3 cases) 2) glioblastoma and HNPCC/Lynch syndrome (1/3 cases)
Muir-Torre (HNPCC variant)	AD	MSH2 and MLH1		**HNPCC/Lynch syndrome-related tumors** (see HNPCC) and **skin tumors** (sebaceous adenomas and carcinomas and keratoacanthomas)
MYH-Associated Polyposis (MAP)	AR	MYH Two mutations account for ~85%: Y165C, G382D		Phenotypically similar to attenuated FAP (~10–100 polyps and extracolonic fea-tures). MYH is a DNA repair "care-taker" gene. Its inactivation can result in accu-mulation of mutations in APC, which is why it is so phenotypically similar to FAP. Mainly affects European populations. Think of this disease if you have a patient with attenuated FAP-like disease but no evidence of AD transmission.

Syndromes Associated with GI Polyps and Neoplasms – continued				
Hereditary diffuse gastric cancer syndrome	AD	CDH1 (E-cadherin gene)		Diffuse gastric cancer, lobular breast cancer – loss of E-cadherin demonstrated by IHC (similar to sporadic tumors, where loss of expression is due to promoter hypermethylation)
Peutz-Jeghers Syndrome (PJS)	AD	STK11/LKB1	19p13	**GI polyps:** hamartomatous polyps with arborizing smooth muscle. Most occur in the small intestine although may also occur in stomach and colon. Sporadic PJ polyps are rare. **Overall risk of malignancy:** lifetime risk 93%. **GI malignancies:** colon (39%), pancreas (36%), stomach (29%), small intestine (13%) **Tumors of reproductive organs:** ovary (21%); cervix (10%); uterus (9%); testes (29%). These particular tumors are highly associated with PJS: adenoma malignum of uterine cervix, sex-cord tumor with annular tubules (SCTAT), large cell calcifying Sertoli cell tumor **Other malignancies:** breast (54%), lung (15%) **Mucocutaneous lesions:** pigmented macules (esp. lips) Reference: [5]
Juvenile Polyposis (JP)	AD	1) SMAD4/ DPC4 2) BMPR1A 3) PTEN		**GI:** multiple juvenile polyps involving colon (juvenile polyposis coli) (defined as > 3–5 polyps or > 1 polyp and family history) or juvenile polyps involving the entire GI tract (generalized juvenile polyposis syndrome). Increased risk of colorectal carcinoma.
Cronkhite-Canada	non-familial			**GI:** numerous polyps, usually of the stomach +/– small intestine and colon. The polypoid and non-polypoid mucosa are hyperplastic polyp-like in the stomach and cystically dilated and edematous in the remainder of the bowel; presents in older adults. Sometimes associated with colorectal adenocarcinoma **Ectodermal changes:** alopecia, macular hyperpigmentation of skin, nail dystrophy
Ruval-Caba-Myhre-Smith (Bannayan-Riley-Ruvalcaba)	AD	PTEN (same as Cowden)	10q23	**GI:** hamartomatous polyps (often Peutz-Jeghers-like) **Soft tissue lesions:** lipomas, hemangiomas **Other:** macrocephaly
Other syndromes with GI polyps include Cowden's and Muir-Torre (see below)				
				References: [6,7]

Syndrome (other names)	Inheritance	Gene Protein	Chromosome	Pathology and main clinical features
Syndromes Associated with Breast Cancer				
Hereditary breast and ovarian cancer	AD	BRCA1 (40–50% of hereditary breast ca)	17q21	**Breast cancer** (>70%); enriched for medullary carcinoma **Ovarian cancer** (30–60%): serous carcinoma and tubal intraepithelial carcinoma (TIC) – entire tube MUST be submitted; greater risk than BRCA2
		BRCA2 (20–30% of hereditary breast ca)	13q	**Breast cancer** (>60%) **Ovarian cancer** Other tumors: Male breast cancer, prostate cancer, pancreatic cancer
Cowden's disease (multiple hamartoma syndrome)	AD	PTEN	10q	**Multiple neoplasms and hamartomas** of endo-, ecto-, and mesodermal origin **Breast cancer:** >50% lifetime risk (often bilateral) **Skin:** facial **trichilemmomas**; café-au-lait spots, vitiligo, epidermoid cysts **GI:** polyps of any type in ~1/3 of patients (hamartomatous, hyperplastic, adenomatous, or inflammatory) **Soft tissue:** hemangiomas, lymphangiomas, lipomas, neurofibromas, leiomyoma **Other tumors:** thyroid, RCC, Merkel cell carcinoma, lymphoma, melanoma, meningioma
Increased breast cancer also seen in Ataxia-telangiectasia syndrome (11% breast cancer risk by age 50) and Li-Fraumeni syndrome.				

Syndromes Associated with Skin Tumors				
Familial atypical multiple mole melanoma syndrome (FAMMM syndrome or B-K Mole Syndrome)	AD	p16	9p21	100 + nevi, atypical (dysplastic) nevi, increased risk of melanoma Pancreatic adenocarcinoma (12–20-fold increased risk)
Gorlin's syndrome (nevoid basal cell carcinoma syndrome, NBCCS)	AD or sporadic	PTCH (patched gene)	9q22.3-q31	**Two or more basal cell carcinomas** before age 20 **Odontogenic keratocyst** of the jaw **Ovarian fibroma** (multinodular, bilateral, calcified) **Medulloblastoma** Macrocephaly and other congenital malformations Skeletal abnormalities

References: [1,3,8]

Tumor Syndromes

Syndrome (inheritance)	Inheritance	Gene Protein	Chromosome	Pathology and main clinical features
Other				
Li-Fraumeni – syndrome of multiple sarcomas and carcinomas	AD	p53	17p13	Multiple primary tumors at young age: sarcoma, carcinoma (breast, colon, pancreas, adrenal cortex), leukemia, melanoma, glioma
Inherited Defects in DNA repair **Ataxia-telangiectasia**	AR	ATM (Ataxia-telangiectasia mutated)	11q22-23	**100-fold increased risk of various malignancies:** acute lymphoblastic leukemia in children, solid tumors in adults. Progressive ataxia, ocular and cutaneous telangiectasia, thymic hypoplasia, variable immunodeficiency (IgA). Sensitivity to ionizing radiation
Bloom syndrome	AR	BLM helicase	15	Predisposition to wide range of **cancers**, esp. leukemias. Various developmental defects
Fanconi anemia	AR	Several candidate genes identified		Predisposition to **leukemias** and **solid tumors** (HCC in 10%) Hypoplasia of bone marrow (anemia), kidney, spleen, and bone (thumbs and radii)
Carney complex or **Carney syndrome**	AD	Protein kinase A	17q22-24 and 2p16	**Myxoid lesions:** cardiac myxoma, skin angiomyxoma, myxoid fibroadenoma of breast **Pigmented and calcifying lesions:** spotty skin pigmentation, epithelioid blue nevus, pigmented nodular adrenocortical hyperplasia, psammomatous melanotic schwannoma, large cell calcifying Sertoli cell tumor **Endocrine hyperactivity:** pituitary adenoma Chondroid hamartoma
Retinoblastoma	40% inherited (AD)	RB	13q14	**Bilateral retinoblastomas** **Pineoblastoma** Increased risk of **osteosarcoma** and other sarcomas
Carney triad	?	unknown	unknown	Paraganglioma Pulmonary chondroma (chondroid hamartoma) Gastric epithelioid GIST Predominantly young females
Rendu-Osler-Weber syndrome or **Hereditary Hemorrhagic Telangiectasia**	AD	1) ACVRL1 2) ENG both involved in TGFbeta pathway	1) 12q11-14 2) 9q33-34	**Aneurysmal telangiectasias** involving multiple organs, including the skin and mucosal surfaces of the oral cavity, GI tract, respiratory tract, urinary tract and visceral organs. Complicated by bleeding.

Abbreviations: AD autosomal dominant, AR autosomal recessive

"Slide to Syndrome":
Select tumors or features that should make you think of a syndrome or clinical condition (not related to an exposure)

Tumor	Syndrome(s) or Condition	% of Cases Associated with Syndrome/Condition	Comment
Genitourinary:			
Adrenal rest tumors of the testis	Congenital Adrenal Hyperplasia	100%	Mimic of Leydig cell tumor, but are bilateral/multifocal, associated with dense fibrosis, and do not have Reinke crystals
Angiomyolipoma	Tuberous Sclerosis	20%	
Hybrid chromophobe RCC-oncocytoma	Birt-Hogg-Dube	almost 100%	
Inverted TCC of renal pelvis	HNPCC/Lynch syndrome	30%	
Papillary cystadenoma of epididymis	VHL	33% of males	Like RCC, may be PAX2+ [9]
Renal medullary carcinoma	Sickle cell trait	almost 100%	
RCC, clear cell papillary	ESRD	20%	
RCC with intratumoral calcium oxalate crystals	ESRD	almost 100%	
Papillary RCC with macronucleoli surrounded by clear halo	HLRCC	Unknown (feature is not specific)	Same peculiar nuclei also seen in leiomyomas associated with HLRCC [10]
Wilms Tumor	WAGR, Danys-Drash, BWS	10–15% overall	Nephrogenic rests (intralobar) → high risk of contralateral Wilms tumor
Gynecologic:			
Adenoma malignum (minimal deviation adenocarcinoma) of cervix	PJ	5%	
Adnexal Papillary Cystadenoma of Probable Mesonephric Origin (APMO)	VHL	100% so far	Female counterpart of epididymal papillary cystadenoma
Gonadoblastoma	Dysgenetic gonad (Turner syndrome)	>90%	
Ovarian Fibroma	Meig syndrome (ascites, right hydrothorax), NBCCS	rare	
Sex cord/stromal (either sex):			
Large cell calcifying Sertoli cell tumor	Carney complex > PJ	40%	
Sex cord tumor with annular tubules (SCTAT)	PJ	30–40%	
Skin:			
Angiofibroma (adenoma sebaceum, fibrous papule)	Tuberous Sclerosis, MEN1	high if multiple	
Angiokeratoma, corporis diffusum type	Fabry and other storage diseases	>90%	
Basal cell carcinoma (multiple tumors at young age particularly children)	NBCCS, xeroderma pigmentosum	Majority are syndromic	Basal cell carcinomas at older age are usually non-syndromic
Fibrofolliculoma	Birt-Hogg-Dube	almost 100% when multiple	
Sebaceous adenoma/carcinoma	Muir-Torre (HNPCC variant)	40% above chin, 80% elsewhere	Associated with MSH2 and occasionally MLH1 mutations
Trichilemmoma, multiple facial	Cowden	almost 100%	
Thyroid:			
PTC, cribriform-morular variant	FAP	80%	Nuclear β-catenin+
Medullary carcinoma (especially with background C cell hyperplasia)	MEN2A, MEN2B; inherited endocrinopathy (isolated site)	25% overall	
Head and neck:			
Endolymphatic sac tumor	VHL	15%	Another clear cell tumor with papillae often seen in VHL
OKC, especially multiple	NBCCS	5%	

Tumor Syndromes

Tumor	Syndrome(s) or Condition	% of Cases Associated with Syndrome/Condition	Comment
Neuro:			
Hemangioblastoma	VHL	25%	
Medulloblastoma	Turcot (FAP variant), NBCCS	10%	
Neurofibroma, plexiform and diffuse types	NF1	>90% plexiform, 10% diffuse	Plexiform schwannoma is not associated with NF1
Psammomatous melanotic schwannoma	Carney complex	>50%	
Subependymal giant cell astrocytoma	Tuberous Sclerosis	>90%	
Thoracic:			
Lymphangioleiomyomatosis of the lung	Tuberous Sclerosis	15%	Part of the "PEComa" family with angiomyolipoma, etc.
Mediastinal carcinoid tumor	MEN1	25%	% syndromic is much lower for pulmonary carcinoids
Breast:			
Breast + ovarian (serous) carcinoma	BRCA1 mutation	>50% if both	
Breast carcinoma in males	BRCA2 mutation	5–40%	
Medullary carcinoma	BRCA1 mutation	10%	
Heart:			
Fibroma	NBCCS	5%	
Myxoma	Carney complex	<5%	
Rhabdomyoma	Tuberous Sclerosis	50%	
Gastrointestinal:			
Clear cell PEN and clear cell serous cystadenoma of the pancreas	VHL	Not well defined but appears high	
Colorectal adenocarcinoma (see below for histologic and clinical features suggesting HNPCC/Lynch syndrome)	HNPCC/Lynch syndrome With polyposis syndromes – FAP, PJS, JP, MYH-1	~5% syndromic (vast majority are sporadic)	
Gangliocytic paraganglioma (duodenum)	NF1	Rare	
Ganglioneuromatous polyposis	Cowden's, JP, NF1, FAP	Almost 100% if multiple (but not well defined)	Solitary polyp has no association with syndrome
Diffuse ganglioneuromatosis	MENIIb, NF1	Almost 100%	Almost invariably present in patients with MENIIb.
Neurofibroma (of the GI tract)	NF1	Almost 100%	GI neurofibromas outside the setting of NF1 are extremely rare
Peutz-Jeghers Polyp (PJP)	PJ	Almost 100%	Sporadic PJPs are rare [11]
Gastrin-secreting PEN, Gastrinoma of duodenum	MEN1	20–25%	Most are functional resulting in Zollinger-Ellison Syndrome (peptic ulcers and thickened gastric folds)
Pancreatic endocrine microadenomatosis	MEN1, rarely VHL	>95%	References: [12,13]
Somatostatinoma (duodenum)	NF1	50%	
Endocrine/neuroendocrine:			
Adrenocortical carcinoma in children	BWS, MEN1, Li-Fraumeni	50–80% overall	
Congenital adrenal cytomegaly	BWS	% not known	Marked pleomorphism but without mitoses
Pheochromocytoma	MEN 2A, MEN 2B, VHL, NF1, Sturge-Weber, isolated familial pheochromocytoma	10–25%	
Primary pigmented nodular adrenocortical disease	Carney complex	>90%	
Well-differentiated neuroendocrine neoplasms (carcinoid, pancreatic endocrine neoplasm)	MEN1 (PEN, gastrinoma), VHL (clear cell PEN), NF1 (somatostatinoma)	Site-dependent	MEN1 association highest for mediastinum followed by pancreas, and low for lung and ileum.

Abbreviations: BRCA Breast Cancer susceptibility protein, BWS Beckwith–Wiedemann syndrome, CRC colorectal carcinoma, ESRD end-stage renal disease, FAP familial adenomatous polyposis, HLRCC Hereditary leiomyomatosis and renal cell carcinoma, HNPCC Hereditary nonpolyposis colorectal cancer, JP juvenile polyposis, MEN multiple endocrine neoplasia, MSI microsatellite instability, NBCCS Nevoid basal cell carcinoma (Gorlin) syndrome, NF neurofibromatosis, OKC odontogenic keratocyst, PEN pancreatic endocrine neoplasm, PJP Peutz-Jeghers polyp, PJS Peutz–Jeghers syndrome, VHL Von Hippel–Lindau, WAGR Wilms tumor, aniridia, genitourinary abnormalities, mental retardation syndrome

HNPCC/Lynch Syndrome:
Clinicopathologic predictors and testing algorithms (in evolution)

Which patients should undergo genetic testing for Lynch Syndrome?
[testing for inherited mutations in mismatch repair (MMR) genes – MSH2, MLH1, MSH6, PMS2*]

(1) See page 34 for interpretation of IHC for MMR proteins.

(2) MSI (microsatellite instability) is tested by PCR and is reported as MSI-high (instability in ≥2 out of 5 microsatellite markers), MSI-low (instability in 1 out of 5 microsatellite markers), or microsatellite stable (MSS).

(3) Sporadic MMR deficient/MSI-high tumors frequently have BRAF V600E mutations, whereas this mutation virtually excludes Lynch syndrome. Therefore BRAF may be included in testing algorithms.

*This represents a simplified algorithm. The testing strategies are evolving and vary by institution.

Modified from [14,15]

Amsterdam ("3-2-1") Criteria (revised in 1999 to include extracolonic cancers)
≥3 relatives with CRC (or other HNPCC-related tumors*) at least 1 of which is a first-degree relative
≥2 consecutive generations affected
1 or more family member with CRC at age <50
References: [16,17]

Revised Bethesda Guidelines (2003) Only one needs to be met:
Patients diagnosed with CRC before age 50
Patients with 2 HNPCC-related cancers, including synchronous and metachronous CRC or associated extracolonic cancers*, regardless of age
Patients with CRC with MSI-high morphology** before age 60
Patients with CRC with ≥ 2 relatives also with CRC, regardless of age
Patients with CRC with ≥ 1 1st degree relative also with CRC or other HNPCC-related tumors, one of which must have been diagnosed before age 50 (or, if a colorectal adenoma, before age 40)
Reference: [14] http://prevention.cancer.gov/files/news-events/20030129-31-guidelines.pdf

Tumor Syndromes

---

* HNPCC/Lynch syndrome-associated tumors include carcinomas of colorectum, endometrium, ovary, stomach, pancreatobiliary, urinary tract (esp. inverted urothelial carcinoma of the upper tract), small bowel, brain.

** Pathologic features of CRC associated with Lynch syndrome include: tumor infiltrating lymphocytes, Crohn-like reaction^, extracellular mucin (>10%)^, signet ring cell differentiation^, medullary growth pattern^, poorly differentiated/undifferentiated, heterogeneous histology, pushing border, right-sided location. [18]

** Pathologic features of endometrial carcinoma associated with Lynch syndrome include (recent data – not part of the revised Bethesda criteria as of 2010): tumor-infiltrating lymphocytes, tumor heterogeneity including dedifferentiated/undifferentiated histology, lower uterine segment location. [19]

^ criteria for "MSI-High histology" per the revised Bethesda Guidelines

---

Note: A recent study showed that only 44% of Lynch syndrome patients were diagnosed at an age younger than 50, and only 72% met the revised Bethesda guidelines, suggesting that all newly diagnosed CRC should be tested for MMR protein abnormality. [20,21] Alternatively, other recent studies show that that probability scores based on histologic parameters have high sensitivity for identification of MMR deficient/MSI-high tumors. [18,22,23] Stay tuned for updated guidelines!!

Abbreviations: CRC colorectal carcinoma, HNPCC hereditary non-polyposis colorectal cancer, MMR mismatch repair, MSI microsatellite instability

Chapter 8 Tumor Genetics and Cytogenetics

For complete list see http://AtlasGeneticsOncology.org
Reviewer: Meera Hameed

Recurrent chromosomal translocations have traditionally been associated with leukemias/lymphomas and sarcomas. Translocations cause either formation of chimeric proteins (such as BCR-ABL) or abnormal protein expression (such as overexpression of c-Myc as a result of translocation into Ig promoter sequences in Burkitt's lymphoma). In contrast, carcinomas generally have complex karyotypes with no recurrent translocations. Instead carcinomas typically have activating mutations in oncogenes (e.g., RAS) or inactivation of tumor suppressor genes (e.g., p53). In recent years this paradigm has shifted, and an increasing number of carcinomas are being recognized as having recurrent translocations. Notable examples are pediatric renal cell carcinoma and thyroid carcinoma.

Translocations are traditionally identified by conventional cytogenetics (karyotyping/chromosomal banding analysis), although FISH and PCR-based assays are becoming increasingly utilized. In contrast, small deletions and point mutations typical of carcinomas generally cannot be visualized by cytogenetics and require nucleic acid-based methods. In some instances immunohistochemistry (IHC) can be used to identify aberrant protein expression resulting from a translocation or mutation (such as IHC for BCL2 in follicular lymphoma). Instances where IHC can be applied as a surrogate to a molecular test are of particular relevance to anatomic pathologists, and these are ***highlighted*** in the tables below.

An interesting rule of thumb is that sarcomas with characteristic translocations are morphologically UNIFORM (rather than highly pleomorphic) and lack atypical mitoses, whereas truly pleomorphic MFH-like sarcomas typically have complex cytogenetics with multiple non-recurrent changes analogous to carcinomas.

Also note a trend for some genes (EWS, FUS) to appear with multiple translocation partners in different tumors. Even more curiously, there are rare examples of an identical translocation (ETV6-NTRK3) in histogenetically disparate tumors (infantile fibrosarcoma, congenital mesoblastic nephroma, secretory breast carcinoma, and mammary analogue secretory carcinoma of salivary glands).

By convention, translocations are designated in numerical order for chromosomes [such as t(11;22)], and in 5'-3' order for chimeric gene products [EWS-WT1], which confusingly may not necessarily be in the same order [EWS gene is on chromosome 22, and WT1 on 11].

Molecular Associations at a Glance		
Gene or protein	*Chromosome*	*Tumor associations*
Igκ	2	**B cell lymphomas** (Follicular, Mantle Cell, Lymphoplasmacytic, Burkitt, myeloma)
Igλ	22	
IgH	14	
TCR α and δ	14	**T cell leukemia/lymphoma**
TCR β and γ	7q (β); 7p (γ)	
c-Myc	8	**Burkitt lymphoma**
n-Myc	2	**Neuroblastoma**
Bcl-2	18	**Follicular lymphoma; Diffuse large B-cell lymphoma**
p53	17p	Mutated in many sporadic tumors (mutation associated with overexpression) and in Li-Fraumeni syndrome
BCR-ABL (Ph chromosome)	9 (ABL) 22 (BCR)	**CML** Ph p210>p230>>p190; **B-ALL** Ph p190>>p210* *The presence of p210 in a patient with acute leukemia should prompt consideration of CML in blast crisis
WT1	11p13	Wilms tumor 11p13 mutation or deletion; **Desmoplastic small round cell tumor** t(11;22) / EWS-WT1
EWS	22	**Ewing sarcoma** t(11;22) / EWS-FLI1; **Desmoplastic small round cell tumor** t(11;22) / EWS-WT1 **Clear cell sarcoma; Angiomatoid Fibrous Histiocytoma**: identical translocation t(12;22) / EWS-ATF1 **Myxoid liposarcoma** t(12;22) / EWS-CHOP; **Extraskeletal myxoid chondrosarcoma** t(9;22) / EWS-CHN/TEC
ALK	2	**ALCL** t(2;5) / NMP-ALK (80%); t(1;2)/ TPM3-ALK (10%); **Inflammatory myofibroblastic tumor** various translocations of 2p23; **Lung adenocarcinoma** EML4-ALK
ETV6 (TEL)	12	**Precursor B-ALL** t(12;21) / ETV6-AML1 **Myeloid neoplasms with PDGFRB rearrangement (CMML with eosinophilia)** t(5;12) / ETV6-PDGFRβ **Infantile fibrosarcoma; Congenital mesoblastic nephroma; Secretory CA of the breast; Mammary analogue secretory carcinoma of salivary glands** [1]: identical translocation t(12;15) / ETV6-NTRK3
TFE3	Xp11.2	**Alveolar soft parts sarcoma; RCC with Xp11.2**: identical translocation t(X;17) / ASPL-TFE3 **PEComas**
INI1 (hSNF5/BAF47)	22q11	**Rhabdoid tumors** (renal and extra-renal rhabdoid tumors, atypical teratoid/rhabdoid tumor of the brain) Others: epithelioid sarcoma, myoepithelial carcinoma of soft tissue, medullary carcinoma of the kidney
FUS (TLS)	16p11	**Myxoid liposarcoma** t(12;16) / FUS-CHOP; **Low grade fibromyxoid sarcoma** (Evans tumor) t(7;16) / FUS-CREB3L2 **Angiomatoid Fibrous Histiocytoma** t(12;16) / FUS-ATF1
MLL	11q23	**AML (M5), AML s/p topo II therapy, B-ALL**
VHL	3p	Sporadic and hereditary **clear cell RCC, von Hippel Lindau** syndrome

	Gene or protein	Chromosome	Tumor associations	
Tyrosine Kinase (TK) Receptors	RET	10	Activating mutations: **Thyroid** (papillary CA, medullary CA), **MEN2a, MEN2b** Inactivating mutations: **Hirschsprung's disease.**	
	MET	7	Papillary RCC (hereditary and occasionally sporadic)	
	KRAS	12	Pancreas, colon, lung, ovary (mucinous)	
	BRAF	7	Papillary thyroid CA, melanoma, colorectal carcinoma	Targeted Rx under development
	ABL	9	CML, B-ALL (Ph+)	Targeted Rx with TK inhibitor Gleevec (Imatinib)
	c-kit	4	GIST, melanoma, mastocytosis	
	PDGFR	4	GIST, myeloid & lymphoid neoplasms with eosinophila and abnormalities of PDGFRA or PDGFRB	
	EGFR	7	Mutated in lung cancer	Targeted Rx with EGFR inhibitors (see below)
	HER2	17	Amplified in breast cancer	Targeted Rx with Trastuzumab (Herceptin)

N. Rekhtman, J.A. Bishop, *Quick Reference Handbook for Surgical Pathologists*, DOI:10.1007/978-3-642-20086-1_8, © Springer-Verlag Berlin Heidelberg 2011

Cytogenetic and Genetic Changes in Leukemia/Lymphoma

by Amy Duffield

Tumor type	Chromosomal abnormality	Affected Genes/Proteins	% cases w/ mutation	Prognosis	Comment
B CELL LEUKEMIA/LYMPHOMA					
Follicular lymphoma (FL)	t(14;18)(q32;q21)	IGH-BCL2	~90%		Also in some DLBCL. Not seen in pediatric FL and rare in cutaneous FL. ***BCL2 can be detected by IHC.***
Mantle cell lymphoma	t(11;14)(q13;q32)	CCND1-IGH	75%		CCNDI = cyclin D1 or Bcl-1 ***CyclinD1 can be detected by IHC***
Extranodal marginal zone lymphoma of mucosa-associated lymphoid tissue (MALT)	t(11;18)(q21;q21)	API2-MALT1			Lung & GI; resistant to antibiotic therapy
	t(14;18)(q32;q21)	IGH-MALT1			Ocular adnexae/orbit and salivary gland
	t(3;14)(p14.1;q32)	FOXP1-IGH			Thyroid, ocular adnexae/orbit and skin
	trisomy 3				Also seen in ~20% of splenic MZL
Splenic B-cell marginal zone lymphoma	loss of 7q21-32		~40%		Not seen in extranodal or nodal marginal zone lymphoma
Chronic Lymphocytic Leukemia/Small Lymphocytic Lymphoma	del 13q14.3		50%	Good	Additional prognositic factors: Good prognosis: mutated IgV$_H$; CD38–; ZAP70– Poor prognosis: unmutated IgV$_H$; CD38+; ZAP70+
	trisomy 12		20%	Fair	
	del 11q22-23		uncommon	Poor	
	del 17p		uncommon	Poor	
	del 6q		uncommon	Poor	
Burkitt lymphoma	t(8;14)(q24;q32)	MYC-IGH	85%		Concurrent BCL2 and BCL6 translocations should not be present
	t(8;22)(q24;q11)	MYC-IGL	rare		
	t(2;8)(p12;q24)	MYC-IGK	rare		
Diffuse large B cell lymphoma	t(14;18)(q32;q21)	IGH-BCL2	30%		t(14:18) may be seen, but cytogenetic changes are variable and include abnormalities of BCL6 and MYC
Precursor B-ALL	t(9;22)(q34;q11)	BCR-ABL (Ph), p190 fusion	25% adults, 2–4% peds	Poor	Ph chromosome also seen in CML (p210 fusion)
	t(4;11)(q21;q23)	MLL-AF4	most common in infants & adults	Poor	The MLL locus can also rearrange with AF9 t(9;11)(p22;q23). Blasts are often CD19+/ CD10–/CD15+/CD24–. MLL rearrangements are also seen in AML.
	t(1;19)(q23;q13)	PBX1-E2A	6% in kids	Poor	Blasts often CD19+/CD10+/CD9+/CD34–
	hypodiploidy	<46 chromosomes	1–5%	Poor	
	t(12;21)(p13;q22)	TEL(ETV6)-AML1(RUNX1)	25% in children	Good	Blasts are often CD19+/CD10+/CD34+/CD9–/CD20–
	Hyperdiploidy	>50 but <66 chromosomes	25% in children	Good	
Multiple Myeloma	t(11;14)(q13;q32)	CCND1-IGH	16%	Good	Usually shows complex karyotypes (multiple chromosome gains and losses)
T-CELL LEUKEMIA/LYMPHOMA					
Anaplastic large cell lymphoma (ALCL), ALK-positive	t(2;5)(p23;q35)	NPM-ALK	85%	Good	ALK translocations are also present in IMT. Primary cutaneous ALCL – no translocation ***ALK can be detected by IHC***
	t(2;other)	Other (most frequently TPM3) – ALK	15%		
T-ALL (various translocations involving TCR – chr 7 and chr 14)	t(1;14)(p32;q11)	ΔTAL1 or TAL1-TCRα/δ			
	t(8;14)(q24;q11)	MYC-TCRα/δ			
	t(10;14)(q24;q11)	HOX11 (TLX1)-TCRα/δ	7–30%		
	t(5;14)(q35;q11)	HOX11L2(TLX3)-TCRα/δ	10–20%		
	del(9p)	loss of CDKN2A	30%		
Hepatosplenic T-cell lymphoma	isochromosome 7q		Common		
T-cell prolymphocytic leukemia	t(14;14)(q11;q32)	TCRα/δ-TCL1A/B	10%		Associated with abnormalities of chromosome 8
	t(X;14)(q28;q11)	MTCP1-TCRα/δ	uncommon		

Tumor Genetics and Cytogenetics

Tumor type	Chromosomal abnormality	Affected Genes/Proteins	% cases	Prognosis	Comment
MYELOID LEUKEMIA AND MYELODYSPLASTIC SYNDROME					
CML	t(9;22)(q34;q11)	BCR-ABL (Philadelphia chromosome, Ph); ABL (Chr 9) is the tyrosine kinase	>90%	Very Good	p210 fusion is most common. Variant splice forms, p230 and p190, are present in a small subset of CML. p190 is also seen in B-ALL. Targeted Rx with Gleevec
	+ Ph, +8, i17q				Changes seen in blast crisis
Myeloid & lymphoid neoplasms with eosinophila and abnormalities of PDGFRB (CMML with eosinophilia)	t(5;12)(q31~33;p13)	ETV6(TEL)-PDGFRB		?	Clinical picture more is often CMML with eosinophilia, less often similar to aCML. Targeted Rx with Gleevec
Myeloid & lymphoid neoplasms with eosinophila and abnormalities of PDGFRA (Chronic eosinophilic leukemia)	cryptic del(4)(q12;q12)	FIP1L1-PDGFRA		?	Clinical picture is similar to chronic eosinophilic leukemia. Targeted Rx with Gleevec
AML (formerly FAB M2)	t(8;21)(q22;q22)	AML1(RUNX1)-ETO (RUNX1T1) (eight twenty one)	~5% of AML	Good	Granulocytic sarcoma may be present at presentation
AML: acute promyelocytic leukemia (formerly FAB M3)	t(15;17)(q22;q12) t(5;17)(q35;q12) t(11;17)(q23;q12) t(11;17)(q13;q12) t(11;17)(q11;q12)	PML-RARA NPM1-RARA ZBTB16(PLZF)-RARA NUMA1-RARA STAT5B-RARA	5–8% of AML	Very good	t(15;17) responds to all-trans retinoic acid (ATRA); some variant translocations are ATRA sensitive (NPM1) but some (ZBTB16, STAT5B) are unresponsive to ATRA
AML (formerly FAB M4 Eo)	inv(16)(p13.1q22) t(16;16)(p13.1;q22)	CBFB-MYH11a	5–8% of AML	Good	Associated with increased abnormal eosinophils and granulocytic sarcoma
AML (formerly FAB M4, M5)	11q23 rearrangements Commonly: t(9;11)(p22;q23)	MLL rearrangements MLLT3-MLL		Poor	Over 80 different translocations with over 50 partner genes. Also seen in AML s/p topo II inhibitors (t-AML) and infants with precursor B-ALL
AML (formerly FAB M7)	t(1;22)(p13;q13)	RBM15-MKL1	<1%	Fair	Most commonly seen in infants and children; not associated with Down syndrome
AML, various FAB classifications	t(6;9)(p23;q34)	DEK-NUP214	1–2%	Poor	Associated with monocytic features, basophilia and multilineage dysplasia
	inv(3)(q21q26.2) or t(3;3)(q21;q26.2)	RPN1-EVI1	1–2%	Very poor	Normal or elevated platelet counts and atypical megakaryocytes
AML, various types (M2, M3, M5, M6)	none	FLT3 internal tandem duplications or point mutations		Poor	Adverse prognosis in cytogenetically normal AML; trials with targeted therapy are in progress
Treatment related AML — Alkalating agents (cyclophosphamide) and radiation therapy	Same as MDS: −7, del(7q), −5, del(5q)		70–80%	Poor	5–10 year lag, presents with treatment-related MDS (marrow failure and cytopenias)
Treatment related AML — Topoisomerase II inhibitors (doxorubicin)	11q23 translocations	MLL	20–30%	Poor	1–5 year lag, presents as overt acute leukemia with no MDS phase
MDS	Isolated del(5q) ("5q- syndrome")	bands q31-q33 are invariably deleted (? loss of EGR1, CTNNA1, RPS14)		Good	Middle-aged women, severe macrocytic anemia, increased platelets, monolobated micromegakaryocytes
	Isolated del (20q)			Good	Involvement of erythroid and megakaryocytic lines
	−7, del(7q), −5, del(5q) *Often seen as part of a complex karyotype			Poor	The gene(s) deleted in del(5q) are thought to be distinct from gene(s) deleted in "isolated 5q- syndrome".
	del(17p)			Poor	MDS and AML with pseudo Pelger-Huet cells and small vacuolated PMNs; associated with therapy related MDS
Chronic myeloproliferative diseases	None	JAK2 V617F or variant mutations including abnormalities of exon 12 of JAK2	Varies		Invariably seen in polycythemia vera May be seen in primary myelofibrosis (50%) and essential thrombocytosis (40–50%), rarely in chronic eosinophilic leukemia
	del(13)(q12-22) OR der(6)t(1;6)(q21-23;p21.3)				Highly suggestive of primary myelofibrosis (previously called chronic idiopathic myelofibrosis)
	None	KIT point mutations (often D816V)			Mastocytosis D816V is resistant to imatinib
	Recurrent non-specific alterations: +8, +9, del (13q), del(20q), del(9p)				

Hematopathology Abbreviations: ALCL anaplastic large cell lymphoma, ALL acute lymphoid leukemia, AML acute myeloid leukemia, CML chronic myelogenous leukemia, CMML chronic myelomonocytic leukemia, FAB French-American-British, MDS myelodysplastic syndrome, MZL marginal zone lymphoma

Cytogenetic and Genetic Changes in Solid Tumors

by Justin Bishop, Ashlie Burkhart, Natasha Rekhtman

SELECT SOLID TUMORS WITH RECURRENT GENETIC ALTERATIONS				
Tumor type	Chromosomal abnormality	Genes/Proteins	% cases w/ mutation	Comment
Alveolar Soft Parts Sarcoma	t(X;17)(p11;q25) = derX	ASPL-TFE3 Xp11.2 = site of TFE3	>90%	Same translocation present in translocation carcinomas of the kidney. **TFE (+) by IHC.**
Angiomatoid Fibrous Histiocytoma	t(12;16)(q13:p11) t(12;22)(q13;q12) t(2;22)(q33;q12)	FUS/TLS-ATF1 EWS-ATF1 EWS-CREB1	most	FUS/TLS – ATF1 thought to be specific for this tumor.
Clear Cell Sarcoma of Tendon Sheath (Melanoma of Soft Parts)	t(12;22)(q13;q12) t(2;22)(q34;q12)	EWS-ATF1 EWS-CREB1	>90%	
Congenital mesoblastic nephroma, cellular type	see infantile fibrosarcoma			
Dermatofibrosarcoma protuberans (DFSP)	t(17;22)(q22;q13) ring chromosome 17	COL1A (collagen gene)-PDGFβ	>90% >75%	Same translocation present in giant cell fibroblastoma (regarded as a pediatric variant of DFSP).
Endometrial stromal sarcoma	t(7;17)(p15;q21)	JAZF1-JJAZ1	60%	
Extraskeletal Myxoid Chondrosarcoma	t(9;22)(q22;q12) t(9;17)(q11;q11)	EWS-CHN (TEC) RBP56-CHN (TEC)	75%	
Ewing sarcoma/PNET	t(11;22)(q24;q12) t(21;22)(q22;q12) t(7;22)(p22;q12) t(17;22)(q12;q12)	EWS-FLI1 EWS-ERG EWS-ETV1 EWS-E1AF	90% 5% rare rare	FLI1 (or ERG) and EWS have variant translocation breakpoints. Most common breakpoint (type 1) is associated with a favorable prognosis. **FLI1 detected by IHC but is not specific.**
Gastrointestinal stromal tumor (GIST)	n/a (mutations are not detectable via cytogenetic analyses)	c-kit mutation PDGFRA mutation	~80% ~5–7%	**95% c-kit (+) by IHC.** c-kit (–) GISTs are often epithelioid and may have PDGFRA mutations. Different mutations confer different responses to Gleevec; see targeted therapies section.
Inflammatory Myofibroblastic Tumor (IMT)	translocations of 2p23	ALK1 fusions	50%	ALK gene also rearranged in ALCL via t(2;5). **ALK (+) by IHC in 30% of cases.**
Infantile Fibrosarcoma	t(12;15)(p13;q25)	ETV6(TEL)-NTRK3	90%	Same translocation in Congenital mesoblastic nephroma and Secretory CA of the breast
Intraabdominal Desmoplastic Small Round Cell Tumor	t(11;22)(p13;q12)	EWS-WT1	99%	**WT1 (+) by IHC.**
Liposarcoma, myxoid and round cell	t(12;16)(q13;p11) t(12;22)(q13;q12)	FUS/TLS-CHOP EWS-CHOP	>90% rare	
Liposarcoma, well differentiated	ring chromosome 12	HMGA2, MDM2 amplification	80%	**MDM2 (+) by IHC (lipoma is MDM2-negative)**
Low grade fibromyxoid sarcoma (Evans tumor)	t(7;16)(q34;p11) t(11;16) (p11;p11)	FUS-CREB3L2 FUS-FUS-CREB3L1	~100%	Same translocation found in hyalinizing spindle cell tumor with giant rosettes; now considered a variant of the same entity. [2]
Neuroblastoma	–1p or deletion 1p32-36	gene unknown	30%	bad prognosis
	Double minutes	N-myc amplification	30%	bad prognosis
	+17q		50%	bad prognosis
	Hyperdiploidy		40%	good prognosis
PEComa	TFE3 rearrangements or amplification	TFE3	17%	**TFE3 (+) by IHC** (though positivity is not specific for a gene alteration)[3]
Rhabdomyosarcoma, alveolar	t(2;13)(q35;q14) t(1;13)(p36;q14)	PAX3-FKHR PAX7-FKHR	70% rare	unfavorable prognosis favorable prognosis
Rhabdomyosarcoma, embryonal	loss of 11p15 no recurrent translocations			11p15 also mutated in Beckwith-Wiedeman syndrome; Recent studies suggest that "fusion-negative" ARMS are clinically/molecularly indistinguishable from ERMS [4]
Rhabdoid tumor of the kidney and extra-renal sites	22q11.2 deletion or mutation	INI1(HSNF5)	>70%	Same gene mutated in AT/RT. **Loss of INI1 expression by IHC.**
Seminoma and other germ cell tumors	Isochromosome (12p)(p10)		~100%	
Synovial Sarcoma (SS)	t(X;18)(p11;q11) t(X;18)(p11;q11)	SYT-SSX1 SYT-SSX2	80% 35%	Monophasic or biphasic SS Monophasic SS; better prognosis in localized tumors.
Wilms tumor	11p13 deletion/mutation	WT1	15%	Same mutation present in syndromic Wilms tumors (WAGR; Denys-Drash)
	11p15 mutation	"WT2" locus (? gene)	3%	Mutation present in Wilms tumors associated with Beckwith-Wiedeman syndrome.
	Trisomy 12		25%	

BRAIN AND MENINGES				
Medulloblastoma	Isochromosome 17q	unknown	50%	
Oligodendroglioma	1p/19q deletion (loss of heterozygocity)	unknown	80%	LOH can be used to distinguish oligo from astrocytoma.
Atypical teratoid/rhabdoid tumor (AT/RT)	22q11.2 deletion or mutation	INI1(hSNF5)	75%	Same gene mutated in renal/extra-renal rhabdoid tumors. 75% have detectable deletion or mutations, almost all show loss of INI1 expression. ***Loss of INI1 expression by IHC.***
Retinoblastoma	13q14 deletion/mutation	RB inactivation	100%	
Meningioma	Monosomy 22			
Pilocytic astrocytoma	7q34 duplication	BRAF-KIAA1549 fusion → BRAF activation	80% of juvenile	Specific for juvenile pilocytic astrocytomas [5]

RECURRENT GENETIC ALTERATIONS IN SELECT CARCINOMAS – SPORADIC				
(see Tumor Syndromes section for genetic alterations in inherited tumor syndromes)				
Tumor type	*Chromosomal abnormality*	*Genes/ Proteins*	*% cases with mutation/ genetic alteration*	*Comment*
Colorectal carcinoma (CRC)	n/a	APC (adenomatous polyposis coli)	• 80% of sporadic CRC	• Germline mutation in APC → Familial adenomatous polyposis (FAP) syndrome (see page 111) • APC inhibits oncogene β-catenin. Mutation of APC → ***nuclear shift of β-catenin (detected by IHC)***
	n/a	hMLH1 >95% hMSH2, hMSH6, PMS2 rare [DNA mismatch repair (MMR) genes]	• 10–15% of sporadic CRC	• Germline mutation in MMR genes → HNPCC/Lynch syndrome (see page 111) vs promoter hypermethylation (primarily of hMLH1) → sporadic tumors • ***Loss of MMR proteins is detected by IHC***: the loss of hMLH1 is more commonly sporadic, whereas the loss of hMSH2, hMSH6 and PMS2 is nearly diagnostic of Lynch syndrome. • Tumors with defective MMR proteins have distinctive pathologic and clinical features (see pages 34 and 117).
	n/a	KRAS	35%	Mutation testing is used to select which patients (KRAS-mutant) will not respond to EGFR-targeted antibody therapy (Cetuximab). See Targeted Therapies section for details.
Breast cancer	n/a	HER2 (ErbB 2) amplification	~25%	• ***IHC and/or FISH are used to select pts for targeted rx with*** Trastuzumab (Herceptin).
Breast, secretory carcinoma	See under infantile fibrosarcoma			
Lung cancer	n/a	EGFR (HER1)	15%	• Clinicopathologic associations: woman, Asian, non-smoker, adeno with BAC component most common (but adeno with any histology may have a mutation and should be tested) • EGFR mutations (not expression by IHC) predict response to EGFR-targeted agents – Gefitinib (Iressa®) and Erlotinib (Tarceva®). • ***Antibodies specific to mutant EGFR are being developed for IHC – stay tuned.***
	n/a	KRAS	30%	• Strongest predictor for lack of response to EGFR inhibitors (better negative predictor than EGFR mutation is a positive predictor) • Clinicopatologic associations: smoker, mucinous histology
	Inv(2)	EML4-ALK	5%	• Optimal method of detection (FISH vs. IHC) under investigation. • Clinicopathologic associations: young, non-smoker, higher stage, solid histology with signet-ring cells and mucin. • Targeted therapy with Crizotinib (PF02341066®)
Thyroid, papillary carcinoma	10q11.2 translocation or inversion	RET fusion to PTC1, PTC3, or several other genes (RET/PTC)	20% (highest in children and post-radiation)	• Screening for these mutations has been suggested as an ancillary tool in FNA of thyroid nodules. • Only BRAF mutations seem to be entirely specific for carcinoma (RAS mutations are the least specific)
	1q21 translocations	NTRK1 fusions	5–10%	
	n/a	BRAF V600E mutations	30–50% (highest in tall cell variant)	
	n/a	RAS mutations	10%	

(For Lung cancer EGFR, KRAS, and EML4-ALK rows: "mutually exclusive mutations")

Tumor Genetics and Cytogenetics

Thyroid, follicular carcinoma	t(2;3)(q13;p25)	PAX8-PPARγ1	30–40%	• Translocation is not specific for follicular carcinoma (has been seen in follicular adenomas and occasionally follicular variants of PTC)
	n/a	RAS	40–50%	
Thyroid, medullary carcinoma	n/a	RET activating mutations		Mutation present in syndromic (MEN2) and sporadic CA. There are no ret/PTC rearrangements typical of PTC.
Thyroid, anaplastic carcinoma	n/a	TP53 mutations	70%	• *Strong immunoreactivity for p53 supports the diagnosis of anaplastic carcinoma vs. mimickers* (e.g., squamous metaplasia in PTC)
	n/a	Beta-catenin mutations	60%	• BRAF mutations are specific for anaplastic carcinomas that arose from BRAF mutant PTC
	n/a	RAS mutations	50%	
	n/a	V600E BRAF mutations	20%	
Kidney, clear cell RCC	3p deletion	VHL gene – encodes ubiquitin ligase	70% of sporadic CC-RCC	• Germline mutations in VHL → Von Hippel-Lindau syndrome • ↑CAIX is a consequence of VHL gene incactivation. *Diffuse reactivity for CAIX is a hallmark of CC-RCC* (see diagram in Targeted therapies section)
Kidney, papillary RCC	Trisomy 7 and 17 Deletion Y	MET (chr. 7) activating mutations		Mutations of MET are present in both inherited and some sporadic (~15%) forms of PRCC (type 1 histology).
Kidney, translocation carcinomas	t(X;17)(p11.2;q25)	ASPL-TFE3		*TFE3 (+) by IHC.* Distinct features: young age, papillary architecture, clear cells, psammoma bodies. Identical translocation (ASPL-TFE3) also seen in alveolar soft parts sarcoma.
	t(X;1)(p11.2;q21)	PRCC-TFE3		
	t(X;1)(p11.2;q34)	PSF-TFE3		
	t(6;11)(p21;q12)	Alpha-TFEB		*TFEB (+) by IHC.* [6] Distinct features: young age, clear and eosinophilic cells in nests and tubules
Melanoma, skin	n/a	BRAF — mutually exclusive mutations	40–50%	Potential target of directed therapy. Mutation not seen in mucosal melanomas.
	n/a	c-KIT	5–20%	• More common in acral and mucosal sites. [7] • Unlike GIST, most are deletions or insertions.
Myoepithelial carcinoma of soft tissue	t(19;22)(q13;q12) t(16;22)(p11;q12) t(1;22)(q23;q12)	EWS-ZNF444 EWS-POUF1 EWS-PBX1	45% have EWS rearrangements [8]	Often seen in children. These molecular alterations are not seen in myoepithelial tumors of the salivary glands. Can display loss of INI1. [9,10]
NUT Midline carcinoma	t(15;19)(q14;p13.1)	BRD4-NUT	67%	Invariably lethal midline CA arising adjacent to respiratory tract in children and young adults. *NUT IHC is very sensitive and specific,* [11] *but not yet commercially available*
	t(9;15)(q34;q14)	BRD3-NUT	33%	
Prostate cancer	21q22.2-3 deletion	TMPRSS2-ERG	50%	Specific for prostate cancer. Associated with low Gleason scores [12] *Translocation-specific antibody to ERG recently developed – stay tuned!* [13]
Salivary gland, mucoepidermoid carcinoma	t(11;19)(q21;p13)	MECT1-MAML2	66%	Translocation activates NOTCH signalling. Associated with lower grade histology and favorable prognosis [14] Appears to be specific among salivary tumors [15,16]
Salivary gland, pleomorphic adenoma	8q12 rearrangements	PLAG1	70%	Reference: [17]
Salivary gland, mammary analogue secretory carcinoma	See under infantile fibrosarcoma			Reference: [1]
Granulosa cell tumor, adult type	n/a	FOXL2 mutation	Almost 100%	This mutation appears to be specific for granulosa cell tumor. [18]

Abbreviations: ARMS alveolar rhabdomyosarcoma, ERMS embryonal rhabdomyosarcoma,

n/a – non-applicable (indicates that a mutation or deletion is too small to be detected by karyotypic analysis)

Chapter 9 Quick Clinical References for Pathologists
by Justin Bishop and Natasha Rekhtman

Metastasis "To and From": a Quick Reference
General principles

Carcinomas generally metastasize via lymphatics (i.e. initial spread is to lymph nodes). Notable exceptions are renal cell carcinoma and follicular carcinoma of thyroid, which disseminate hematogenously. In contrast to carcinomas, **sarcomas** generally metastasize hematogenously to organs such as liver and lung, bypassing the lymph nodes. Lymph node metastases are rare or in some cases (such as Ewing sarcoma) never occur. Exceptions are clear cell sarcoma/melanoma of soft parts, epithelioid sarcoma, alveolar rhabdomyosarcoma, synovial sarcoma, malignant fibrous histiocytoma, angiosarcoma – these sarcomas are an exception in that they frequently metastasize to lymph nodes.

Some metastases follow a predictable route of dissemination based on the circulatory map. As such, tumors in organs drained by portal circulation (bowel, pancreas) metastasize to the liver first. In contrast, tumors in organs drained by the inferior vena cava (such as kidney, rectum) metastasize first to the lung. However, usual circulatory flow can be disrupted due to obstruction by the tumor or as a result of surgery and/or radiation; therefore tumor spread not conforming to normal circulatory map is not unusual. In addition, certain tumors show proclivity for metastasis to unusual sites not based on vascular drainage. Notable examples are lobular breast carcinoma and renal cell carcinoma, which tend to metastasize to unusual sites, such as GI tract. In addition, certain sites such as bone (not a particularly vascular organ) appear to be the preferential target of metastasis.

Tumors known to have late metastases (may present as metastases many years after primary diagnosis):
- Renal cell carcinoma
- Salivary gland carcinomas (particularly adenoid cystic carcinoma)
- Breast cancer
- Carcinoid tumors
- Melanoma
- Granulosa cell tumor of the ovary
- Sarcomas (endometrial stromal sarcoma, alveolar soft part sarcoma, extraskeletal myxoid chondrosarcoma, synovial sarcoma)

Organs where metastasis are more common than primary tumors:
- Liver
- Lung, pleura (except for solitary nodules)
- Heart
- Bone (in adult)
- Brain
- Adrenal (most "incidentalomas" are adrenocortical adenomas, whereas majority of malignant tumors are metastasis rather than primary)

Most common sites of distant metastases:
- lung, liver, bone, brain

Metastasis in children:
- Clear cell sarcoma of kidney (in infants)
- Rhabdoid tumor
- Wilms tumor
- Neuroblastoma

Carcinoma of unknown primary (CUP) = carcinoma initially presenting with metastasis, where the primary site is occult (inapparent clinicoradiologically). The site of origin may be identified by morphology/IHC, or may be found only at autopsy. Most common sites (if discovered) are
- Pancreaticobiliary
- Lung
- Gastric

Patterns of lung metastasis and differentials: Lung is THE most common site of distant metastases because 1) entire systemic circulation from right heart goes through lung; 2) lung is the first capillary bed encountered by lymphatic drainage (thoracic duct → subclavian → right heart → lung); and 3) lung has densest capillary bed in the body.

Pattern of mets in the lung	Classic Primary	Clinical DDx	Comment
Multiple nodules	any	granulomas, abscesses, infarcts	Most common pattern of metastasis
Solitary nodule	sarcoma, melanoma, germ cell tumor, colorectal	granuloma (usually PET+), lung primary	
Lymphangitic	breast, stomach, pancreas, lung, prostate	pulmonary edema, infectious, interstitial lung disease (ILD)	Interstitial (reticular) pattern on CT + thickened septae and bronchovascular structures. Ominous clinically.
Bronchioloalveolar/"airway"	pancreaticobiliary	Bronchioloalveolar CA, ILD	
Pleural seeding	lung, breast, ovary, thymoma	mesothelioma	
Miliary	thyroid, RCC	TB, carcinoid tumorlets, minute meningotheliod nodules	usually associated with highly vascular neoplasms

References: [1,2]

N. Rekhtman, J.A. Bishop, *Quick Reference Handbook for Surgical Pathologists*,
DOI:10.1007/978-3-642-20086-1_9, © Springer-Verlag Berlin Heidelberg 2011

Metastasis "To and From": a Quick Reference

Metastasis FROM	TO – Lymph Nodes (LN)	TO – Distant Sites
Adrenocortical	Regional LNs (aortic, retroperitoneal)	Liver, lung, peritoneal and pleural surfaces, bone
Anus	Above the dentate line: inferior mesenteric LNs Below the dentate line: superficial inguinal LNs	Liver, lung
Bladder	Regional LNs (hypogastric, obturator, iliac, perivesical pelvic, sacral, presacral)	Retroperitoneal lymph nodes, lung, bone, and liver
Breast	Axillary, internal mammary, supraclavicular LNs	Ductal carcinoma: lungs, bone, liver, brain, adrenal Lobular carcinoma: tendency to metastasize to unusual sites (GI tract, GYN tract, bone marrow, endocrine organs, meninges, mesothelial surfaces/produces effusions)
Colon	Regional LNs	Liver, peritoneum, lung, ovaries
Carcinoid tumor of the GI tract	Regional LNs	Mets to liver first (typical presentation of ileal carcinoid is massive liver metastasis in otherwise healthy patient with unknown primary; an unlikely scenario for carcinoma). Can also metastasize to bone, skin, or almost any organ.
Carcinoid tumor of the lung	Regional LNs (hilar)	Bone – common site of extra-thoracic mets Late mets possible (need 10+ yr follow-up)
GYN tract Uterus	Pelvic and periaortic LNs	Lung, vagina, peritoneal surfaces and omentum for serous and clear cell carcinoma
Cervix	Pelvic, inguinal LNs	Lung
Ovaries	Regional LNs (iliac, obturator, para-aortic, inguinal, pelvic, retroperitoneal)	Intra-peritoneal spread typical. Mets to lung, pleura
Liver, HCC	Regional LNs (hilar, hepatoduodenal ligament, inferior phrenic, caval)	Lung, bone, adrenal
Liver, cholangiocarcinoma	Regional LNs (porta hepatis)	Lung, bone, adrenal, peritoneal surfaces
Lung, non-small cell carcinoma	Regional LNs (hilar), supra-clavicular	Adrenal (lung is the most common origin of adrenal metastasis), bone, brain
Lung, small cell carcinoma	Regional LNs (hilar), supra-clavicular. Classic presentation – massive hilar adenopathy (with or without obvious lung primary)	Extra-thoracic metastasis at presentation in majority of pts. Brain mets in >50% (therefore prophylactic cranial radiation recommended). Other common sites – liver, adrenal, bone, bone marrow.
Melanoma	Regional LNs depending on primary site	Any site is possible. Common source of unknown primary. Common sites include soft tissue, skin, liver, brain, bone, GI tract. May form solitary metastasis in the lung (DDx primary non-small cell carcinoma).
Pancreas	Regional LNs surrounding the pancreas	Liver, peritoneal cavity, lung (metastases may colonize alveolar walls, mimicking mucinous bronchioloalveolar CA)
Parathyroid	Regional LNs (cervical or mediastinal)	Lung, liver, bone
Pheochromocytoma	Regional LNs	Predilection for bone mets (always need bone scan), liver
Prostate	Regional: true pelvis (LNs below the bifurcation of the common iliac arteries: pelvic, NOS, hypogastric, obturator, internal and external iliac, sacral) Distant (staged as M1): paraaortic, common iliac, inguinal, cervical/supra-clavicular	Hematogenous spread (via spinal cord venous plexus) to AXIAL skeleton – spine, femur, pelvis, ribs Non-bony distant metastases are uncommon (particularly in the absence of skeletal metastasis). Common sites include lung, liver, and adrenal gland.
Renal cell carcinoma	LN mets are rare (mets usually hematogenous)	Hematogenous mets to lung, bone, liver, brain, adrenal, other Proclivity for mets to unusual sites (small bowel, thyroid, soft tissue, scapula) and late mets (10+yrs)
Salivary gland	Regional LNs in an orderly fashion, first nodes within/adjacent to the gland, then to cervical nodes	Lung. Adenoid cystic CA – late metastasis characteristic
Stomach	Regional LNs (perigastric greater curvature, lesser curvature, and pancreatic/splenic areas).	Liver, peritoneal surfaces and distant lymph nodes. Classic sites include supraclavicular node (Virchow), periumbilical (Sister Mary Joseph nodule), ovary (Krukenberg tumor)
Testis	Lymphatic to retroperitoneal (para-aortic) LNs, later mediastinal and left supraclavicular (not inguinal)	Lung (most common), liver, brain, bone Note: Lymphatic route is typical of seminoma vs. hematogenous route is typical of non-seminoma germ cell tumors (particularly choriocarcinoma).
Thyroid	Papillary: Mets via lymphatics (to regional LNs, especially central neck level VI). Surprisingly, lymph node mets are of limited prognostic significance	Follicular: Hematogenous mets to distant sites (lung and bone)
Thyroid, medullary	Spread similar to papillary thyroid carcinoma, though much more prognostically significant	Distant mets common (miliary pattern of metastasis typical in the lung)

Metastasis "To and From": a Quick Reference

Pediatric Tumors:		
Neuroblastoma	Lymphatic spread to LNs	Common sites: liver, bone, lymph nodes, ovary Rare sites: lung Blue-gray skin mets ("blueberry muffin" babies)
Wilms tumor	Mets to lymph nodes, liver, lung ("the three L's"). Mets to bone or brain – rare	
Clear cell sarcoma of kidney		Proclivity for bone mets (i.e., "bone metastasizing renal tumor of childhood"); also mets to usual sites (e.g. brain, soft tissue) – Wilms tumor almost never mets to these sites
Sarcomas:		
Alveolar soft parts sarcoma		Lung, brain, bone
Ewing sarcoma	NEVER mets to LNs	Lung, bone
PNET (bone)	Regional LN mets rare	Lungs and pleura, other bones, CNS
Myxoid liposarcoma		Mets to other soft tissue sites (and lung)

Metastasis TO	FROM
Adrenal	Lung, breast, kidney, stomach, pancreas (adrenocortical adenoma "CT-incidentaloma" is much more common than mets)
Bone	Most common mets to large bones are from Breast, Lung, Thyroid, Kidney, Prostate (mnemonic = "BLT and Kosher Pickle") *Osteolytic:* Lung, Thyroid, Kidney *Osteoblastic:* Prostate *Either:* Breast Children: primary bone tumors > metastasis vs. Adults: metastasis > primary bone tumors
Brain	Lung, breast, melanoma, RCC, colon, thyroid
Heart	Lung, melanoma, breast, RCC
Liver	Overall 90% mets, 10% primary In non-cirrhotic liver: 98% mets In cirrhotic liver: 75% mets, 25% primary (HCC) Mets in adult: colorectum, pancreas, stomach, breast, lung, kidney, melanoma (prostate unusual) Mets in children: neuroblastoma, Wilms tumor, rhabdomyosarcoma, germ cell tumor
Lung	Most common destination of metastasis. Overall mets>primary tumors. Sites of origin: any carcinoma (frequency reflects population incidence – breast, colon, etc), melanoma, sarcoma, germ cell tumors
Lymph nodes:	
Submental (cervical level IA)	Anterior floor of mouth, anterior tongue, anterior mandibular ridge, lower lip
Submandibular (level IB)	Oral cavity, anterior nasal cavity, midfacial soft tissue, submandibular gland
Upper jugular (level II)	Oral cavity, Waldeyer's ring, nasal cavity, supraglottis, glottis, floor of mouth
Midjugular (level III)	Hypopharynx, oropharynx, nasopharynx, larynx, oral cavity
Lower jugular (level IV)	Hypopharynx, base of tongue, thyroid, cervical esophagus, larynx
Posterior triangle (level V)	Nasophayrnx, oropharynx, thyroid, skin of posterior scalp and neck
Central neck (level VI)	Papillary thyroid CA, larynx, cervical esophagus, lung
Intraparotid	SqCC, melanoma, and Merkel cell (all of the overlying facial skin), primary salivary gland
Supraclavicular (Virchow node)	<50% from head and neck sites (left = right) >50% from visceral organs (left>>right) Virchow node = supraclavicular node with metastasis from visceral organs, classically left-sided
Axillary	Breast, lung, melanoma
Intra-thoracic	Adult – lung, breast Pediatric – germ cell tumor, Ewing sarcoma/PNET, lymphoma
Intra-abdominal	Adult – GI tract, GYN, pancreato-biliary, lymphoma Pediatric – Wilms tumor, germ cell tumor, neuroblastoma, lymphoma
Superficial inguinal	Lower extremity, vulvar/penile
Deep inguinal	Anorectal, GYN, genitourinary, melanoma
Iliac	Prostate
Para-umbilical (Sister Mary Joseph)	Visceral organs (stomach is classic site)
Meninges	Melanoma, breast, leukemia in pediatric
Pleura	Mets >> primary Most common lung, breast; mets from any organ are possible
Skin	Adult – lung, breast, colon, melanoma, oral cavity Pediatric – leukemia, rhabdomyosarcoma, neuroblastoma
Soft tissue	Lung, breast, RCC, aerodigestive tract, melanoma

References: [3–5]

Malignant effusions	Most common sites of origin
Pleural	Lung, breast (in female), lymphoma
Peritoneal	Female: GYN tract (ovary, endometrium, cervix) > GI Male: GI (colon, rectum, stomach)

Quick Clinical References

Serologic Tumor Markers:
Common Associations

Serum Marker	Main Association(s)	Comment
α-FP	HCC, yolk sac tumor	diagnosis of HCC unlikely in the setting of normal α-FP (except fibrolamellar variant)
βHCG	Choriocarcinoma, trophoblastic tumors, various tumors with admixed syncytiotrophoblasts	
CA125	Ovary	non-specific, used for monitoring (e.g. following treatment)
CA19.9	Pancreas	non-specific
CA27.29	Breast	non-specific
Calcitonin	Medullary thyroid carcinoma	
Catecholamines (serum and urine)	Pheochromocytoma, neuroblastoma	most sensitive for pheochromocytoma is plasma metanephrines/normetanephrines; most sensitive for neuroblastoma is urinary vanillylmandelic acid/homovanillic acid
CEA	Colon, pancreas, medullary thyroid carcinoma	non-specific
Chromogranin A	NE neoplasms, NE differentiation in prostate cancer after androgen-deprivation Rx (unresponsive to hormone Rx)	
Hypercalcemia	Lung SqCC (PTH-like hormone secretion), ovarian small cell carcinoma hypercalcemic type, ATLL	
Lipase	Acinar cell carcinoma	widespread subcutaneous fat necrosis, polyarthritis, and eosinophilia ("Schmid's triad")
Hormones		
Insulin	PEN, SFT	symptoms of hypoglycemia (anxiety, tremor)
Glucagon	PEN	necrotizing migratory erythema, diabetes
Gastrin	PEN	gastric ulcers
Somatostatin	PEN	diabetes, $\downarrow H^+$, steatorrhea
Pancreatic polypeptide (PP)	PEN	asymptomatic
Vasoactive intestinal peptide (VIP)	PEN	watery diarrhea, $\downarrow H^+$, $\downarrow K^+$
Serotonin	Small bowel carcinoid (uncommon for NE tumors of lung, thymus, pancreas)	carcinoid syndrome (flushing, diarrhea). Usually develops with mid-gut carcinoid metastatic to liver (presumably due to overwhelmed clearance)
ACTH, cortisol	ACTH due to pituitary adenoma Ectopic ACTH due to SmCC, thymic carcinoid Cortisol due to adrenocortical tumors Unrelated to tumor (exogenous steroids)	Cushing syndrome (central obesity, glucose intolerance, hypertension, striae, hirsutism)
Prolactin	Pituitary adenoma	galactorrhea, hypogonadism, infertility
Growth hormone	Pituitary adenoma	acromegaly
TSH	Pituitary adenoma	asymptomatic or hyperthyroidism
LH, FSH	Pituitary adenoma	asymptomatic
ADH (vasopressin)	Pulmonary SmCC, intracranial tumors	symptoms of siADH/$\downarrow Na^+$ – fluid overload, neurologic
Estrogen	Granulosa cell tumor, thecoma	precocious puberty, endometrial hyperplasia/bleeding
Androgens in women	Sertoli-Leydig and steroid cell tumors ($\uparrow$testosterone, nl or low 5DHEA) Adrenocortical tumors ($\uparrow$5DHEA)	virilization
PSA	Prostate cancer, BPH	normal <4, equivocal= 4–10, high= 10 (though normal levels increase with age, obesity, etc.). May be negative in some high-grade carcinomas, equivocal in BPH
PSA ratio	Prostate cancer >> BPH	more specific for carcinoma than PSA
PSA, percent free	Prostate cancer << BPH	The lower the value, the higher the risk. Most useful in patients with PSA from 4–10.
Thyroglobulin	Thyroid cancer	Used to monitor recurrence (requires total thyroidectomy or I* ablation). 15–20% have anti-thyroglobulin antibodies, which interfere with test

Abbreviations: α-FP alpha fetoprotein, βHCG beta human chorionic gonadotropin, ACTH adrenocorticotropic hormone, ADH antidiuretic hormone, ATLL adult T cell leukemia/lymphoma, BPH benign prostatic hyperplasia, CEA carcinoembryonic antigen, DHEA dehydroepiandrosterone, FSH follicle stimulating hormone, H^+ hydrogen, K^+ potassium, LH luteinizing hormone, Na^+ sodium, PEN pancreatic endocrine neoplasm, PSA prostate specific antigen, PTH parathyroid hormone, SFT solitary fibrous tumor, siADH syndrome of inappropriate antidiuretic hormone, TSH thyroid stimulating hormone

Reference: [6]

Targeted Therapies and Predictive Markers – Welcome to the Future!
Examples of therapies targeted to specific mutations or aberrant protein expression with emphasis on predictive marker testing on pathologic specimens (established or in development).

Reviewer: Peter Illei

Tumor type	Altered gene or expression (frequency)	Drug	*Predictive Marker Testing and Other Comments*
Solid Tumors			
Many cancers	RAS/RAF/MEK/ERK pathway	Multiple inhibitors in development	This oncogenic pathway is activated at various points in many cancers.
Many cancers	PI3K/AKT/mTOR/S6K1 pathway (inhibited by PTEN)	Multiple inhibitors in development, particularly mTOR inhibitors – rapamycin analogs, such as Temsirolimus (Torisel®)	Pathway deregulated in multiple cancers most prominently in glioma, melanoma, prostate CA, endometrioid CA, and RCC. Predictive testing of this pathway by IHC is under intense investigation (including loss of PTEN, and activation of AKT/mTOR/S6K1).
Many cancers	VEGF	Bevacizumab (Avastin®)	Risk of life-threatening hemorrhage in pulmonary SqCC, therefore use is restricted to adenocarcinoma.
Lung Adenocarcinoma	EGFR (15–30%)	Tyrosine kinase inhibitors (TKIs): Gefitinib (Iressa®), Erlotinib (Tarceva®)	*EGFR* mutation is best predictor of response, not IHC or in situ hybridization. IHC antibodies specific to exon 19 & 21 mutant EGFR recently developed, and likely to be used in the future for predictive testing. Clinical associations: woman, Asian, non-smoker. Histologic associations: adenoCA with bronchioloalveolar component most common, but every adenoCA should be tested
	KRAS (30%)	none	Strongest predictor for lack of response to TKI's (better negative predictor than *EGFR* mutation is a positive predictor) Clinical associations: smoker
	EML4-ALK rearrangements (4%)	Crizotinib (PF02341066 or 1066®)	FISH is needed, since IHC with standard ALK antibody does not correlate with presence of translocation (however novel highly sensitive and specific ALK antibody recently developed) [7] Clinical associations: young, non-smoker, higher stage. Histologic associations: solid with signet-ring cells and mucin. Reference: [8]
Colon	EGFR overexpression	Cetuximab (Erbitux®), Panitumumab (Vectibix®)	*KRAS* mutation best negative predictor for response to anti-EGFR Rx. EGFR IHC is no longer recommended.
	BRAF (10%)	none	Mutation is a negative predictor to response to anti-EGFR Rx.
	KRAS (40%)	none	Mutations in codons 12 and 13 are resistant to anti-EGFR Rx. [9,10]. Emerging evidence that mutations in codons 61 and 146 also resistant. [10]
	UGT1A1 polymorphism	Irinotecan (Camptosar®)	Certain genotypes have increased risk for drug-induced toxicity to Irinotecan. This is not a targeted agent, but in this case testing is predictive of inability to metabolize the drug.
Melanoma	BRAF (40–50%)	BRAF or MEK inhibitors	Efficacy of these therapies not yet clear, but promising results reported with PLX4032 (Plexxikon), a BRAF inhibitor in metastatic melanoma Reference: [11]
	c-kit (5–20%)	Imatinib (Gleevec®)	More common in acral and mucosal sites Mutually exclusive with BRAF mutations. Unlike GIST, most are deletions or insertions Reference: [12]
Gastrointestinal stromal tumor	c-kit (~ 80%) PDGFRA (~5–7%) Wild type (~10–15%)	Imatinib (Gleevec®), Sunitinib (Sutent®)	Mutation testing (not IHC) predicts response to TKIs for non-surgically resectable disease. Typically molecular testing is only used for patients with advanced disease refractory to treatment. Response to Imatinib is based on type of mutation: (*by Ashlie Burkart*) Tumors with KIT mutations: Exon 11 mutations (67%): best response. [13] Exon 9 (10%): poor response. Responds better to higher doses. Exon 13 and 17 (rare): partial response. Tumors with PDGFRA mutations: Exon 18 with D842V mutation: resistant to Imatinib. Exon 18 without D842V: variable response. Exon 12 (rare): respond well. Wild type: respond better than exon 9 tumors, but not as well as exon 11. Sunitinib is a newer drug often used for patients whose tumors are resistant to Imatinib.

Quick Clinical References

Kidney, CC-RCC	VHL	Small molecule inhibitors of VDGF and PDGF (Sunitinib, Sorafenib), and mTOR inhibitor (Temsirolimus)	VHL normally causes degradation of Hypoxia Inducible Factor (HIF), which in turn regulates expression of CAIX, VEGF and PDGF (proliferative and pro-angiogenic factors, accounting for high vascularity of clear cell RCC). VHL mutation in clear cell RCC (or hypoxia in any tumor) leads to activation of HIF and its downstream targets. In a separate pathway, mTOR controls the synthesis of HIF. See diagram below for summary of this pathway and targeted agents. *This pathway explains high expression of CAIX in clear cell RCC and focal CAIX in any tumor with necrosis (related to hypoxia). CAIX is also a target of G250 – monoclonal antibody to CAIX which is used in molecular imaging for clear cell RCC (investigational).
Breast*	ER, PR expression (60–75%)	Tamoxifen (Soltamox®)	Preferred method is immunohistochemistry using formalin fixed paraffin embedded tissue sections
	HER2 amplification/ overexpression (~15%)	Trastuzumab (Herceptin®), Lapatinib (Tykerb®)	Tykerb given in combination with Xeloda (Capecitabine), a conventional chemotherapeutic agent
Gastric or Gastro-esophageal adenoCA	HER2 amplification/ overexpression (20–30%)	Trastuzumab (Herceptin®)	Herceptin given in combination with traditional chemotherapy improves survival. Amplification more common with intestinal histology. Reference: [14]
Thyroid, papillary CA	BRAF (30–50%)	BRAF inhibitors and tyrosine kinase inhibitors	Promising early results for patients with advanced BRAF-mutated papillary CA Reference: [15]

* Onco*type* DX® is something (created by Genomic Health) that you have probably heard about and is worth mentioning. It looks at expression of 21 genes by RT-PCR (including ER, PR, and HER2 but also less-obvious genes like Survivin, Cyclin B1, Stromelysin 3, etc.) to come up with a "recurrence score." It is used in women with early stage, node-negative, ER+ invasive cancer to see what benefit they would get from adjuvant chemotherapy. (www.oncotypedx.com)

Abbreviation: HIF hypoxia inducible factor, TKI tyrosine kinase inhibitor

Selected Hematopoietic Tumors		
Tumor type	Altered gene or expression	Drug
Chronic Myelogenous Leukemia	BCR-ABL translocation	Targeted Rx with tyrosine kinase inhibitor Gleevec (Imatinib)
Precursor B Acute Lymphoid Leukemia		
Chronic myelo-monocytic leukemia with eosinophilia	ETV6(TEL)-PDGFRB translocation	
Chronic eosinophilic leukemia	FIP1L1-PDGFRA translocation	
Acute promyelocytic leukemia	RAR translocations (such as PML-RAR)	Targeted Rx with all-trans retinoic acid (ATRA). The most common t(15;17) responds to all-trans retinoic acid (ATRA); some variant translocations are ATRA sensitive (NPM1) but some (ZBTB16, STAT5B) are not
B cell lymphomas	CD20 expression	Retuximab (Retuxan) is an antibody to CD20. Note that B cell lymphoma may become CD20-negative after therapy, and require alternative marker such as CD79a to confirm the diagnosis
Acute myeloid leukemia	FLT3 mutation	FLT3 mutations are associated with a worse prognosis in AML. Trials with FLT3 TK inhibitors are in progress. [16]

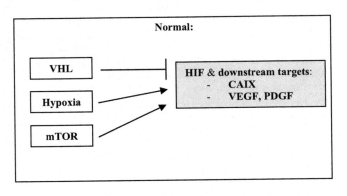

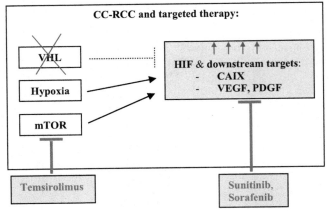

Abbreviations: CAIX carbonic anhydrase IX, CC-RCC clear cell renal cell carcinoma, HIF hypoxia inducible factor, mTOR mammalian target of Rapamycin, PDGF platelet derived growth factor, TKI tyrosine kinase inhibitor, VEGF vascular endothelial growth factor

Chapter 10 Pathology Web Resources

by *Terina Chen*
(updated September 2010)
Also see references: [1,2]

Source/Site	URL	Features
General		
Pathology Outlines	http://www.pathologyoutlines.com/	Ever expanding resource. AP and CP topics. Outlines pathologic processes, organized by organ/topic. Links to images & primary references. Info on jobs & fellowships.
Robbins and Cotran Pathologic Basis of Disease, 8th edition (on MD Consult)	http://www.mdconsult.com/php/198002462-2/homepage	Go to "Books" tab → Pathology. Full text. May require subscription.
Henry's Clinical Diagnosis and Management by Laboratory Methods, 21st edition (on MD Consult)	http://www.mdconsult.com/php/198002462-2/homepage	Go to "Books" tab → Pathology. Full text. May require subscription.
WebPath: Internet Pathology Laboratory – University of Utah/Mercer University School of Medicine	http://library.med.utah.edu/WebPath/webpath.html	Gross & microscopic images, variety of tutorials and quizzes. Includes Forensic Pathology.
The Virtual Slidebox – University of Iowa	http://www.path.uiowa.edu/virtualslidebox/	Virtual microscopy, including normal histology and histopathology.
PathWeb Virtual Pathology Museum – University of Connecticut	http://pathweb.uchc.edu/	Gross and microscopic images of disease processes organized by organ system. Includes outlines.
Pathology Education Instructional Resource (PEIR) Digital Library – University of Alabama	http://peir2.path.uab.edu/pdl/dbra.cgi?uid=default&view_search=1 http://peir2.path.uab.edu/reslinks/	Gross and microscopic image database with search capability.
Pathmax	http://www.pathmax.com/main.html	Links to multiple pathology-related websites.
Surgical Pathology		
United States & Canadian Academy of Pathology (USCAP) Specialty Conference Cases	http://www.uscap.org/newindex.htm?92nd/specialtyh.htm	Cases from USCAP annual meetings.
Surgical Pathology Unknowns Conference – Johns Hopkins Hospital	http://pathology2.jhu.edu/sp/	Multiple choice quiz format. Includes discussion/didactic on each case. Searchable.
Case of the Month – University of Pittsburgh	http://path.upmc.edu/casemonth/ap-casemonth.html	Includes radiology, gross, ancillary tests.
PathCONSULT	http://www.pathconsultddx.com/pathCon/home	Outline format. Can compare diagnoses side by side.
California Tumor Tissue Registry (CTTR)	http://www.cttr.org/	Offers online case of the month. Digital or glass slide sets available for purchase.
Webpathology.com	http://webpathology.com/atlas_map.asp?section=4	Gross and microscopic pathology images. Currently limited to GU, Breast, Lymph nodes/Spleen, Mediastinum.
Cytopathology		
Cytopathology Interesting Case Conference (ICC) – Johns Hopkins Hospital	http://pathology2.jhu.edu/cytopath/welcome.cfm	Quiz format.
NCI Bethesda System Web Atlas	http://www.cytopathology.org/NIH/	Online Bethesda book on cervical cytology. Self-test available.

N. Rekhtman, J.A. Bishop, *Quick Reference Handbook for Surgical Pathologists*,
DOI:10.1007/978-3-642-20086-1_10, © Springer-Verlag Berlin Heidelberg 2011

Gynecologic/Placental Pathology		
Tumors of the Female Reproductive Organs	http://www.bioscience.org/atlases/tumpath/freprod/freprod.htm	Gross and microscopic images.
Endometrium.org – Brigham & Women's Hospital	http://www.endometrium.org/	EIN (alternative to hyperplasia system). Didactics, cases, quiz.
Placental Pathology Index – WebPath (see above)	http://medlib.med.utah.edu/WebPath/PLACHTML/PLACIDX.html	
Gastrointestinal & Liver Pathology		
GI & Liver Pathology Case Conference – Johns Hopkins Hospital	http://pathology2.jhu.edu/gicases/	Multiple choice quizzes with didactic explanations.
PanIN and Cystic lesions of the Pancreas – Johns Hopkins Hospital	http://pathology.jhu.edu/pancreas/professionals/DuctLesions.php	Didactic on PanIN with images. Didactic on evaluation of pancreatic cystic lesions.
Grading Dysplasia in Barrett's esophagus – Johns Hopkins Hospital	http://pathology2.jhu.edu/beweb/study_images.cfm	Images with consensus diagnoses and discussion.
Endoatlas (Atlas of Gastrointestinal Endoscopy) – Atlanta, GA	http://www.endoatlas.com/index.html	Endoscopy images.
Genitourinary Pathology		
Prostate Cancer Gleason Grading Tutorial & Testing – Johns Hopkins Hospital	http://162.129.103.34/prostate/	Needle biopsies with a consensus Gleason grade. Pre and post-tutorial assessments.
The WHO/ISUP Consensus Classification of Urothelial Neoplasms Tutorial – Johns Hopkins Hospital	http://pathology.jhu.edu/bladder/	Urothelial lesions with teaching on tumor classification system.
Renal Pathology & Transplant Pathology		
American Journal of Kidney Diseases (AJKD) Renal Pathology Atlas – Vanderbilt University	http://www2.us.elsevierhealth.com/ajkd/atlas/	Medical renal disease atlas, includes IF & EM, micro descriptions.
Transplant Pathology Internet Services (TPIS) – University of Pittsburgh	http://tpis.upmc.com/TPIShome/	Multiple organs. Tutorials, classification system summaries, biopsy templates. Case conference with forum discussion. Transplant links.
Transfusion Medicine		
Blood Bank Guy	http://www.bbguy.org/	Fun site with blood bank FAQs, Osler course notes and quizzes.
American Association of Blood Banks (AABB)	http://www.aabb.org/Pages/Homepage.aspx	Professional Development section contains variety of presentations/ didactics. May require an account.
TM Resources links	http://www.patletendre.com/tm-education.html	Links to transfusion medicine-related sites.
Microbiology		
Dr. Fungus	http://www.doctorfungus.com/	Extensive site with didactic materials.
Morphology of Medically Important Fungi – UCSF	http://labmed.ucsf.edu/education/residency/fung_morph/launchpage.html	Great pictures (including plates) with brief didactics.
CDC DPDx Parasitology	http://www.dpd.cdc.gov/dpdx/Default.htm	Includes many great pictures, information on life cycles, etc.
Microbiology & Immunology Online – University of South Carolina	http://pathmicro.med.sc.edu/book/welcome.htm	Medical school level didactics with great pictures.

Immunohistochemistry		
Immunoquery	https://immunoquery.pathiq.com/PathIQ/Login.do	Information on antibodies, what tumors stain for what, etc. Side by side comparisons. Requires registration.
Immunohistochemistry (IHC) World	http://www.ihcworld.com	Includes methods/protocols, extensive list of links.
Nordic Immunohistochemistry Quality Control (NordiQC)	http://www.nordiqc.org (go to "epitopes")	Information on epitopes, pitfalls, background, references, etc.
Propathlab	http://www.propathlab.com (go to "newsletters" and "immunohistochemistry")	Collection of newsletters pertaining to various IHC topics.
Phenopath	http://www.phenopath.com (go to "site map" and "case studies")	Case studies and other handy references.
Dakocytomation	http://www.dakocytomation.dk (go to "products" and "antibody algorithm")	Panels and algorithms with hyperlinks for common differentials.
Immunohistochemistry vade mecum	http://e-immunohistochemistry.info	Notes on IHC and histology with primary literature references; lots of links.
Electron Microscopy		
Society for Ultrastructural Pathology	http://www.ultrapath.org/	Board review slide lectures.
Molecular Pathology & Genetics		
Genetics Home Reference – National Library of Medicine	http://ghr.nlm.nih.gov/	General reference on genetic disorders. For a lay audience but includes key facts and additional links.
Atlas of Genetics and Cytogenetics in Oncology and Hematology	http://atlasgeneticsoncology.org/	Genetics of tumors and genetic disorders with increased risk of tumors.
NCBI Gene Tests	http://www.genetests.org/	Educational materials, genetics glossary, lab testing, directories.
Organizations		
College of American Pathologists (CAP)	http://www.cap.org/apps/cap.portal	Includes educational programs, tumor reporting checklists, etc.
United States and Canadian Academy of Pathology (USCAP)	http://www.uscap.org/	Includes educational materials from annual meetings.
American Society for Clinical Pathology (ASCP)	http://www.ascp.org/	
American Society of Cytopathology (ASC)	http://www.cytopathology.org/	
National Association of Medical Examiners	http://www.thename.org/	Includes cause of death tutorial.
Association for Pathology Informatics	http://www.pathologyinformatics.org/index.htm	
Miscellaneous		
PathMD Board Review Letter	http://www.pathmd.com/	Board review questions with online images.
StatSoft Electronic Statistics Textbook	http://www.statsoft.com/textbook/	Online statistics didactics.
Learningradiology.com	http://www.learningradiology.com/	Images, didactic presentations and quizzes.
Chest Radiology tutorial	http://www.med-ed.virginia.edu/courses/rad/cxr/index.html	Great basic chest imaging tutorial.
Mammography and Breast Imaging – University of Washington	http://www.rad.washington.edu/breast/	Cases in mammography. Links to other breast imaging sites.
Medicalstudent.com	http://www.medicalstudent.com/	Any medicine topic under the sun linked here. Includes online textbooks.

Pathology Web Resources

Chapter 11 CPT (Current Procedural Terminology) Coding Quick Reference

by Diana Molavi

The following codes are for the gross and microscopic examination of anatomic specimens. All codes begin with 8830-; the last digit ranges from 2 to 9, and is listed below by specimen.

Abdominal	8830x		Ditzels cont'd	8830x
Adrenal gland	7		Cyst, skin/soft tissue	4
Hernia sac	2		Debridement	4
Omentum	5		Diverticulum	4
Peritoneal biopsy	5		Finger or toe amputation, disease	5
Bone and joint			Finger or toe amputation, trauma	2
Bone biopsy or path fracture	7		Fistula	4
Bone fragments, no fracture	4		Foreskin, newborn	2
Bone, exostosis or bunion	5		Foreskin, not newborn	4
Bone, path. fracture	7		Gross only, any*	0
Bone resection	9		Hemorrhoids	4
Bursa	4		Hernia sac	2
Disc, intervertebral	4		Sympathetic ganglion	2
Femoral head, fracture	5		**Gastrointestinal**	
Femoral head, no fracture	4		Appendix, incidental	2
Ganglion	4		Appendix, other	4
Joint, biopsy or resection	5		Colon, partial, non tumor	7
Joint, loose body	4		Colon, total, non tumor	9
Meniscus	4		Colon, tumor	9
Muscle biopsy	5		Donuts, for tumor resection	5
Shavings	4		Esophagus biopsy	5
Synovium, biopsy	5		Esophagus resection	9
Tendon	4		Gallbladder, any	4
Breast			Liver biopsy	7
Biopsy, core or excisional, no margins	5		Liver resection	7
Mass (lumpectomy, excision) with margins	7		Pancreas biopsy	7
Mastectomy, simple, no nodes*	7		Pancreas resection (including Whipple)	9
Mastectomy, with nodes*	9		Small bowel biopsy or polyp	5
Reduction mammoplasty	5		Small bowel resection, non tumor	7
Sentinel node	7		Small bowel resection, tumor	9
Cardiovascular			Stoma	4
Aneurysm or plaque	4		Stomach biopsy	5
Artery, biopsy	5		Stomach resection, tumor	9
Heart valve	5		Stomach resection, non tumor	7
Hematoma, thrombus	4		**Genitourinary**	
Myocardium	7		Bladder biopsy	5
Pericardium, biopsy	5		Bladder resection	9
Vein, varicose	4		Bladder TURBT	7
Central nervous system			Kidney biopsy	5
Brain biopsy	7		Kidney resection	7
Brain or meninges, tumor	7		Prostate biopsy	5
Brain or meninges resection, not for tumor	5		Prostate resection w/ seminal vesicles and vas	9
Meninges, biopsy	5		Prostate TURP	5
Pituitary, tumor	5		Spermatocele, varicocele	4
Ditzels			Testicular appendage	4
Abscess	4		Testis biopsy	7
Arm/leg amputation, disease	7		Testis resection, non tumor	5
Arm/leg amputation, for tumor	9		Testis resection, tumor	9
Arm/leg amputation, trauma	5		Ureter resection	7
Cholesteatoma	4		Ureter/urethra biopsy	5
			Vas deferens, other	4
			Vas deferens, sterilization	2

N. Rekhtman, J.A. Bishop, *Quick Reference Handbook for Surgical Pathologists*,
DOI:10.1007/978-3-642-20086-1_11, © Springer-Verlag Berlin Heidelberg 2011

CPT

Gynecologic	8830x
Cervix biopsy/ECC	5
Cervix LEEP or cone	7
Ectopic pregnancy	5
Endometrium, biopsy	5
Fallopian tubes, biopsy	5
Fallopian tubes, sterilization	2
Fetus, with dissection	9
Myomectomy	5
Omentum	5
Ovary, biopsy or wedge	5
Ovary and/or fallopian tube, non tumor	5
Ovary and/or fallopian tube, tumor	7
Placenta, 1–2nd trimester	5
Placenta, 3rd trimester	7
Products of conception, induced	4
Products of conception, spontaneous/missed	5
Uterus, leiomyomas	7
Uterus, prolapse	5
Uterus, tumor*	9
Vagina, biopsy	5
Vulva biopsy	5
Vulva resection	9
Head and neck	
Conjunctiva, any	4
Cornea or lens	4
Eye, enucleation	7
Eyelid, plastics	2
Eyelid biopsy	5
Larynx biopsy	5
Larynx resection, no nodes	7
Larynx resection, nodes	9
Lip biopsy	5
Nasal mucosa, biopsy	5
Nasal polyp	4
Odontogenic cyst	5
Odontogenic tumor	7
Oropharynx, biopsy	5
Parathyroid	5
Salivary gland biopsy	5
Salivary gland resection	7
Salivary mucocele	4
Sinus, biopsy	5
Thyroid	7
Tongue biopsy	5
Tongue resection, tumor	9
Tonsil biopsy	5

Tonsil, adenoids, uvula, non tumor	4
Tonsil, tumor	9
Hematopathology	
Bone marrow biopsy or clot section	5
Lymph node dissection*	7
Lymph node, biopsy/excision	5
Sentinel node for tumor	7
Spleen	5
Thymus, tumor	7
Peripheral blood smear	85060
Marrow aspirate smear	85097
Lungs and mediastinum	
Branchial cleft cyst	5
Bronchus biopsy	5
Lung biopsy	5
Lung total/lobe resection	9
Lung wedge	7
Mediastinal mass, resection	7
Pleura biopsy	5
Pleural peel	4
Thymus, incidental	2
Thymus, tumor	7
Thyroglossal duct cyst	5
Trachea biopsy	5
Skin	
Biopsy	5
Plastics repair	2
Sentinel node	7
Skin cyst	4
Skin tag	4
Wide excision, with margins	5
Soft tissue	
Biopsy of tumor	7
Debridement	4
Lipoma	4
Mass, extensive resection	9
Mass, simple excision	7
Nerve biopsy	5
Nerve, incidental	2
Neuroma	4
Other	
Consult or outside slide review	88321

* Bundling rules:
- Many organs are considered bundled with adjacent parts. For example, a mastectomy with a separate axillary dissection is billed as a radical mastectomy (88309) and not a mastectomy + axilla (88307x2). The same applies to laryngectomies.
- The uterus is also bundled, with adnexa rather than nodes. A hysterectomy for any reason includes the tubes and ovaries, which may not be billed separately, even if received in different containers. The exception to this rule is if there is a separate pathologic process or tumor involving a tube or ovary, in which case it can be billed as its own specimen. A uterus removed as part of an ovarian tumor resection is an 88307 by itself, or 88309 if there is a concurrent uterine malignancy.
- The gross only code, when used with other AP codes, requires a –59 modifier. For example, a gallbladder plus a separately received biliary stent would be 88304 + 88300-59.
- Extra organs in a single specimen can be billed individually, other than the exceptions above. For example, a distal pancreas and spleen may be coded as 88309 +88305.

Ancillary studies

Intraoperative		Stains and processing	
Gross evaluation	88329	Bug stains (AFB, GMS, PAS)	88312
1st frozen, each part	88331	Copper stain	88318
Additional frozens, each block within a part	88332	Decalcification, each part	88311
Touch prep, no frozen	88333	Histochemical (special) stains	88313
Touch prep, additional parts	88334	Immunohistochemistry, each antibody	88342
Touch prep w/ frozen	No $	In situ hybridization, tissue, qualitative	88365
Dissection for molecular studies	88388	In situ hybridization, tissue, quantitative	88368
Oil red O	88314	Packaging for sendout of fresh tissue	99001
Fetus, dissection for cytogenetics	99001	Quantitative IHC (ER, PR, Ki67, etc)	88360
		Quantitative IHC, computer-assisted	88361
		No tissue in container	No $
		TID/did not survive processing	88300

Special rules:

Decalcification is charged per part. For example, a three-part bone case can charge 88311 x 3 for decalcification. Individual ancillary studies are charged per stain, per block. A sentinel node with S-100 and HMB45 staining on three different slides is charged 88342 x 6. However, you cannot charge for a repeat or duplicate stain on the same block.

Cytology

For a single service, you may select <u>one</u> of the following codes for each procedure and part. You may not add these codes together unless they represent distinct specimens, in which case you need to clarify that with a –59 modifier on the end of the lesser code. Use the highest appropriate code: if you do a thin-prep on an FNA case, you may only bill for the FNA code (88173). Cell blocks and stains are the exception and can be added to other codes.

Cervicovaginal smear (see note)	
Pathologist interpretation, excluding QA review	88141
Fluids, washings, brushings (except cerv-vag): Bronchial brushings/washing/BAL, biliary brushings, CSF, urine, ascitic fluid, breast cyst aspirates, etc.	
Smear only	88104
Cytospin, such as for CSF	88108
Thin prep or similar liquid prep	88112
Direct smears examination that is NOT a washing or brushing: i.e. sputum, skin scraping, Tzanck prep, or nipple discharge:	
Screening and interpretation	88160
Smear preparation, screening, and interpretation	88161
FNA of any site, as long as it is not a breast cyst aspirate:	
Screening and interpretation	88173
Immediate evaluation of adequacy, each pass (up to 3 passes allowed, more than that require the –59 modifier)	88172
Immediate evaluation of adequacy, each additional pass, on the same site	88177
Additional services codes that can be added to the above:	
Cell block preparation	88305
Special stains and IHC codes as performed	
Performing the FNA on the patient	10021
Performing the FNA with imaging guidance	10022
Note: Billing for cervico-vaginal smears is complex, and as most smears are handled at the cytotechnologist level, will not be explored in detail here. The code for physician review does not change by method, and should be added to the appropriate code for the screening of the slide.	

Reference: [1]

Chapter 12 It Looks Like WHAT?
An Illustrated Glossary of Histopathologic Descriptors.

by Natasha Rekhtman and Kathryn Villa

Illustrations (in the definitions column) by Terry Helms.
Also see Chapter 2 in "The Practice of Surgical Pathology: A Beginner's Guide to the Diagnostic Process" by Diana Molavi.
Thanks to Diana Molavi for sharing some of the entries and many helpful discussion for this section.

Descriptors of Architectural Patterns		
Term	*Definition*	*Example(s)*
Alveolar	resembling lung alveoli. A pattern seen in some tumors in which nests of cells are centrally discohesive (fall apart) and paucicellular thereby appearing like empty spaces in the lung alveoli.	alveolar soft part sarcoma (shown), alveolar rhabdomyosarcoma
Basaloid	resembling basal cell carcinoma (BCC) in that tumor cells are small, tightly packed, and grow as islands with peripheral palisading, similar to BCC. Basaloid morphology is typical of squamous cell cancers of head and neck.	basaloid squamous cell carcinoma
Chicken wire	branching ("crow feet"-like) and anastomosing network of vessels, typically seen in liposarcoma and oligodendroglioma. Calcifications in chondroblastoma are also described as chicken wire-like.	vessels in myxoid liposarcoma
Cribriform	perforated like a sieve; having "Swiss cheese"-like spaces. Etymology: Latin *cribrum*, sieve.	adenoid cystic carcinoma (shown), cribriform DCIS
Discohesive (dyshesive)	falling apart into single cells. In a setting of a poorly differentiated neoplasm, discohesion suggests a lymphoma.	lymphoma (shown), LCIS

N. Rekhtman, J.A. Bishop, *Quick Reference Handbook for Surgical Pathologists*,
DOI:10.1007/978-3-642-20086-1_12, © Springer-Verlag Berlin Heidelberg 2011

Fascicular	fascicle = bundle of cells (as in muscle fascicle). Generally used to describe a bundle of spindle cells streaming in unison (like the school of fish). Fascicles may intersect perpendicularly, as in smooth muscle tumors, or at acute angles, as in fibrosarcoma (see "herringbone" pattern).	 leiomyosarcoma
Festoon-like Garland-like	undulating appearance, as in a festoon or a garland (an ornament suspended between two points). "*Festoon pattern*" is used to describe the projection of dermal papillae into blister cavity in some bullous skin diseases, as well as undulating cell ribbons in carcinoid tumors and granulosa cell tumors. "*Garland necrosis*", where undulating collars of tumor project into necrotic center, is typical of colon cancer and epithelioid sarcoma.	 pemphigus vulgaris (shown)
Filigree-like	complex intertwining threads (from Latin filum, *thread*), as in filigree style of jewelry. The term is most commonly used to describe complex intertwining papillae in micropapillary serous carcinoma of the ovary (aka the "medusa-head pattern"). In addition, the term has been applied to a pattern of infiltration, wherein the tumor cells are invading as complex cords (such as filigree pattern in Ewing sarcoma).	 micropapillary serous carcinoma
Glandular	forming glands (easy!). This is a defining feature of adenocarcinoma. Sometimes "tubular" and "ductal" are used synonymously with glandular to describe an adenocarcinoma.	 adenocarcinoma of the colon
Geographic	(as in geographic necrosis): large confluent areas of necrosis with an irregular outline resembling outlines of a continent on a map (where water would = viable tumor)	 Wegener's granulomatosis (shown), small cell carcinoma
Glomeruloid	resembling a glomerulus: tufts or tangles of vascular or epithelial structures protruding into a clear space. Glomeruloid epithelial structures are diagnostic of prostate cancer, and glomeruloid vascular proliferation is a hallmark feature GBM.	 glomeruloid structure in prostate cancer

Glossary

Gyriform, watered silk, 'moiré' pattern	ribbons or cords of cells that undulate and/or form loops, resembling a topographic map (courtesy of Diana Molavi). From the Greek *gyros,* a circle.	carcinoid tumor (shown), granulosa cell tumor
Herringbone pattern	a pattern resembling the spine of a herring; characterized by alternating cellular fascicles intersecting at acute angles. Prototype is fibrosarcoma, but this pattern may be seen in other neoplasms (e.g. MPNST, synovial sarcoma).	fibrosarcoma
Hobnail	resembling a large-headed nail (like the ones used to protect the soles of shoes). Describes cells, which project into a lumen of a vessel or a gland.	angiosarcoma (shown), clear cell carcinoma of the female genital tract
Indian-file (= single file)	cells arranged in linear rows as if one following in the footstep of the other. The term refers to the "notion of Amerindian people's way of walking along a trail" [1]	lobular breast carcinoma
Insular	literally, resembling an "island" (insula = island); basically a term for large nests.	carcinoid with an insular growth pattern
Lepidic	scale-like (from Greek "lepis" scale). Term used to describe the superficial (scale-like) growth pattern of lung bronchioloalveolar carcinoma (metastatic carcinomas to the lung, particularly pancreas can assume this growth pattern!)	Bronchioloalveolar carcinoma

Lobular	referring to an anatomic unit (as in breast lobule). When describing a lesion, the term implies that the lesion has a smooth (non-infiltrative) contour, conforming to or resembling normal anatomic structures. Sometimes used synonymously with nodular. Lobular breast carcinoma relates to the anatomic origin rather than the growth pattern.	 lobular capillary hemangioma
Microcystic	tightly packed small cysts, honeycomb-like	 serous cystadenoma of the pancreas, microcystic
Micropapillary	papillary-shaped epithelial projections **without** a true fibrovascular core (cells surround avascular cores) 	 micropapillary DCIS
Nested	packets or groups of cells separated by stroma	 pheochromocytoma
Neuroendocrine (NE)	**NE pattern** is defined by two components: architecture and cytology. **NE architecture** refers to formation of nests, ribbons/trabeculae and rosettes (this is vaguely reminiscent of ribbons and nests formed by normal neuroendocrine structures, such as the Islets of Langerhans). **NE cytology** refers to cells being monotonous/uniform (not overtly pleomorphic like most carcinomas). Cells have finely stippled "salt and pepper" chromatin with NO prominent nucleoli (see below under "salt and pepper").	 carcinoid (trabecular/ribbon-like pattern)

Glossary

Nodular	refers to a discrete collection of cells with a smooth rounded border. Generally nodules refer to larger cell aggregates than nests.	 nodular sclerosis Hodgkin lymphoma (shown), multinodular thyroid hyperplasia
Organoid	cells showing some features of organization (into nests, glands, papillae, etc) rather than growing as sheets – i.e. epithelial organ-like. In an unknown malignancy, presence of organoid structures argues against a lymphoma. DDx includes carcinoma (most common), few types of sarcoma (most notably alveolar soft parts sarcoma), and also melanoma. In practice, the term is used almost exclusively to describe cells aggregating into nests in neuroendocrine neoplasms (pheochromocytoma, carcinoid). The reason for this selective use is completely unclear to us. More intuitively, the term is also used to describe structures resembling various normal organs in a teratoma.	 pheochromocytoma
Pagetoid	resembling Paget's disease of the nipple in that the large malignant cells ascend singly or in nests in the epidermis in a buckshot-like fashion. True Paget's disease must be differentiated from other lesions with a "pagetoid growth": Bowen's disease (squamous cell carcinoma in situ) and melanoma in situ.	 Paget's disease of the nipple
Palisading	cells lining up in parallel arrays; resembling a picket fence. Peripheral palisading is a defining feature of basal cell carcinoma. Palisading in a spindle cell neoplasm is classic for schwannoma (but few other tumors, such as smooth muscle neoplasms, can palisade). Also histiocytes may palisade in so-called "palisading granulomas" (as in a rheumatoid nodule). Etymology: French *palissade,* a fence of stakes. 	 basal cell carcinoma
Papillary	fronds of finger-like projections containing fibrovascular cores (stroma with blood vessels) that support the overlying epithelium. If papillary structures grow endophytically, the process is called "inverted" (as in inverted papilloma of the bladder or sinuses) Etymology: papilla = *nipple* (Latin), or nipple-like protrusion. FV core = Stroma + Vessels	 papillary thyroid carcinoma

Peritheliomatous	an older term for "perivascular". The term "peritheliomatous growth" relays that the tumor cells are viable around vessel, but are necrotic away from vessels. May be a feature of melanoma, small cell carcinoma, or any other very high grade neoplasm that outgrows its blood supply.	 melanoma
Plexiform	resembling or forming a plexus (like the brachial plexus); interwoven network; said to resemble a "bag of worms". Generally a macroscopic term. Etymology: From Latin *plexus*, braid. 	 plexiform neurofibroma
Reticular or **Retiform**	resembling a complex lattice, network or spider web. May resemble a honeycomb with cells of variable size and shape. The term is applied to connective tissue (reticular framework in liver, nodes, etc.) as well as to describe a pattern in neoplasms (classically a feature of yolk sac tumors). Etymology: From Latin *rete*, net.	 yolk sac tumor, reticular pattern
Rosette (also see table below)	Etymology: Rosette = structure with a circular arrangement of parts radiating out from the center resembling the petals of a rose. In pathology, "rosette" is a term used to describe structures with cells arranged radially around a central point. Different from a gland in that basally-located cell are not supported by a basement membrane (but merge with the rest of tumor cells). See table below for details on rosettes and pseudorosettes. Window Rosette in a Cathedral (based on photo by Enrique Villa)	 ependymoma (perivascular pseudorosette)
Sarcomatoid	term generally applied to spindle cell growth in a carcinoma	 sarcomatoid renal cell carcinoma

Serpiginous or **serpentine**	snake-like: undulating, wavy	wavy spaces in usual duct hyperplasia of the breast, wavy nuclei of neurofibroma
Sheet-like or solid pattern	a sea of back to back cells with no particular architecture	any poorly differentiated malignancy (lymphoma [shown], carcinoma, melanoma, sarcoma)
Staghorn (hemangio-pericytoma-like) **vessels**	branching thin-walled vessels that have staghorn or antler-like shapes. Prototype is hemangiopericytoma (HPC).	solitary fibrous tumor
Storiform	short fascicles of spindle cells that intersect or intertwine at various angles thereby resembling the weaving of a **doormat** OR **cartwheel**, **pinwheel**, or **starburst.** *Storea* is Latin for woven straw mat [2] The storiform pattern is also said to resemble a **cartwheel**, **pinwheel**, or **starburst** in that intersecting spindle cells have radial orientation emanating from a common point.	prototype is DFSP (shown): both the doormat-like and cartwheel-like arrangement of cells can be discerned (with some imagination)
Syncytial	having indistinct cell borders	lymphoepithelioma-like carcinoma (shown), medullary carcinoma of the breast

Tissue culture-like growth pattern	pattern resembling the growth of cultured fibroblasts in a tissue culture plate: spindle cells are loosely arranged and are randomly oriented; cells have plump nuclei and dendrite-like extension of cytoplasmic processes. Cultured fibroblasts growing in a Petri dish	 inflammatory myofibroblastic tumor (shown), nodular fasciitis
Trabecular	Etymology: Latin *trabes,* beam-like. [3] The term is used to describe the "beam-like" arrangement of cells in rows, cords, ribbons, or strands; cells may form parallel arrays or tram-tracks (as in trabecular pattern in carcinoid tumors). In addition, the term describes the beam-like strands of connective tissue (as in splenic trabeculae) or macroscopic beam-like structures (as in trabecular bone). trabecular bone	 carcinoid, trabecular pattern
Verrucous Verrucoid Verruciform Warty	resembling a verruca (clinical wart) – a lesion with pointed church spire-like epithelium covered by hyperkeratosis (abundant keratin). **"Verrucous carcinoma"** and **"warty carcinoma"** are specific entities of mucosal surfaces, which have additional defining features (e.g. broad pushing border in the former). Note that warts are HPV-related lesions, containing koilocytes (cells with crinkly nuclei, perinuclear halos) +/– chunky keratohyaline granules. Some lesions with "verrucous" architecture are also HPV-related, even if koilocytes are not prominent (e.g. some verrucous carcinomas), whereas other verrucous lesions are HPV-unrelated (e.g. verrucoid keratosis of the skin, verruciform xanthoma, verrucous dysplasia of the mucosa).	 verrucous carcinoma
Villous	having finger-like projections. In essence same as papillary, except that, by convention, when referring to intestinal epithelium – the process is called villous.	 villous adenoma of the colon
Whorled	swirled arrangement of cells. Prototypical tumor with true 360-degree whorls is meningioma.	 meningioma
Zellballen	German for "cellular ball". Basically another term for nested. The term is usually applied to pheochromocytoma and paraganglioma, where nests are surrounded by supportive (sustentacular) cells and vascular stroma.	see pheochromocytoma under "nested"

Rosettes at a Glance

Rosettes are structures with radial arrangement of cells around a central point (like rose petals). In general, presence of rosettes in an unknown neoplasm is a clue to its **neuroglial differentiation** (neuroblastic, neuroendocrine or ependymal). In addition, rosette-like structure may be present in several non-neuroglial neoplasms: thymoma, ovarian granulosa cell tumor (Call-Exner bodies), other.

The terminology of "pseudo" versus "true" rosettes is inconsistently applied. In general, the term "pseudo" is applied to perivascular rosettes to distinguish them from "true" rosettes, which do not surround a central vessel.

Homer Wright Rosettes (aka **"fibrillary** or **neuroblastic"** rosettes) have a <u>central tangle of fibrillar processes</u> (neuropil). There is no central vessel or lumen. DDx: fibrillar rosettes are **pathognomonic for neuroblastic tumors** (tumors with primitive neuron differentiation) – neuroblastoma, medulloblastoma, PNET, pineoblastoma, retinoblastoma. (Named after one person, James Homer Wright, which is why there is no hyphen between the names.)	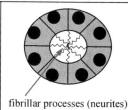 fibrillar processes (neurites)	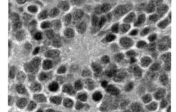 neuroblastoma
Perivascular Pseudorosettes: as above, but fibrillar processes are projecting toward a <u>central blood vessel</u>, resembling "spokes around the hub of wheel". Prototype is ependymoma. DDx: **ependymoma** (prominent in nearly all cases), central neurocytoma, rarely neuroblastic tumors (neuroblastoma, medulloblastoma, PNET).	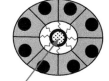 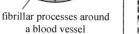 fibrillar processes around a blood vessel	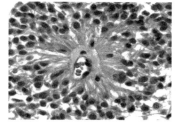 ependymoma
Luminal Rosettes: cells polarized around a <u>central lumen</u>. Lumen is formed by apical cell borders. These are different from a gland in that the cells are not surrounded by a basement membrane. DDx: **Ependymoma:** "True Ependymal Rosettes" (recapitulate embryonic ependymal canal). These are less numerous than perivascular pseudo-rosettes. **Retinoblastoma:** "Flexner-Wintersteiner Rosettes" (photoreceptor-like differentiation). Lumen has hypereosinophilic border. **Neuroendocrine neoplasms** (e.g. carcinoid, pancreatic neuroendocrine tumor/islet cell tumor). Rosettes are commonly present.	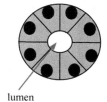 lumen	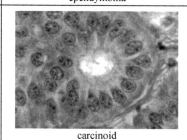 carcinoid

148

12 It Looks Like WHAT? An Illustrated Glossary of Histopathologic Descriptors.

Cytologic Descriptors		
Term	*Definition/Appearance*	*Example*
Amphophilic (cytoplasm)	color that is a mixture of blue and pink due to affinity for both hematoxylin (blue dye) and eosin (pink dye), resulting in an intermediate purplish color	pheochromocytoma
Cerebriform (nucleus)	convoluted outline like in cerebral cortex; flower-like; classic descriptor nuclei in peripheral T cell lymphomas	Sezary cells in Mycosis Fungoides (appearance in peripheral smears)
Coffee bean-like (nucleus)	containing a longitudinal groove or fold (based on photo by Enrique Villa)	papillary thyroid cancer (shown), granulosa cell tumor
Fried egg-like cell	cells with a perfectly round nucleus, surrounded by either a clear halo (as in oligodendroglioma) or by pale cytoplasm (chondroblastoma). Remember the poultry-theme in both of these tumors: chicken-wire vasculature in the former and chicken-wire calcifications in the latter.	oligodendroglioma
Grooved (nucleus)	containing an indentation or a cleft; synonymous with reniform, grooved, or cleaved (see coffee-bean-like)	urothelial cells, papillary thyroid cancer (longitudinal groove), granulosa cell tumor (shown), "buttock lymphocytes" in follicular lymphoma
Ground glass	glass that has been ground or etched to create a roughened nontransparent surface; "frosted glass", as seen in glass bottle stoppers. In pathology, the term is classically used to describe optical clearing of nuclei (washed out look with loss of chromatin detail) in papillary thyroid cancer and homogenized cytoplasmic inclusions of Hepatitis B virus-infected hepatocytes. In radiology, the term is used to describe hazy opacities characteristic of interstitial pneumonias, BAC (buzzword is "GGO" = ground glass opacity) or fibrous dysplasia of bone.	papillary thyroid cancer: note the optically cleared ("ground glass") nuclei

Leukocytoclastic	fragmentation of neutrophils; looks like blue cell dust	leukocytoclastic vasculitis
Oncocytic cell, Hürthle cell, Oxyphil cell	having abundant pink granular cytoplasm (due to lots of mitochondria) and bland small round nuclei. Oncocytic neoplasms are grossly mahogany brown (e.g. oncocytic neoplasms of the kidney or salivary gland). Oncocytic cells are called Hürthle or Askanazy cells in the thyroid and Oxyphil cells in the pituitary and parathyroid (all terms are basically synonymous, but different names are inconveniently applied in different organs). Etymology: Oncocyte is Greek for "swollen cells"	oncocytoma (salivary)
Orphan Annie eyes-like	Little Orphan Annie is a character in a comic strip from 1924, who has "vacant circles for eyes". The term is used interchangeably with "ground glass" to describe optical clearing of nuclei in papillary thyroid cancer. Reproduced with permission by Tribune Media Services, Inc. ("TMS")	papillary thyroid cancer (see under "ground glass" above)
Physaliphorous	foamy (cytoplasm). Etymology: Greek *physalis* – bubbles or vacuoles; *phoros* – bearing	chordoma
Plasmacytoid	resembling plasma cell in that the nucleus is eccentrically-placed and is round (unlike signet-ring cell, in which the nucleus is eccentric but is indented due to cytoplasmic mucin)	plasmacytoid variant of urothelial carcinoma (shown), neuroendocrine neoplasms

Polygonal	relatively vague descriptor typically denoting tumor cells with sharp "squared" cell membranes (fitting together like boulders). Classic examples are squamous cell carcinoma and seminoma. 	 seminoma
Reniform (nucleus)	kidney-shaped, indented, containing a groove	 histiocytes in Langerhans cell histiocytosis
Rhabdoid	cells with bright pink globular cytoplasmic inclusions resembling primitive skeletal muscle cells (rhabdomyoblasts). Usually accompanied by vesicular nuclei with prominent nucleoli. Prototypes are rhabdoid tumors of kidney and brain (inclusions are aggregates of intermediate filaments); both have chr. 22 rearrangements. There are many tumors that have rhabdoid appearance, where it is usually a sign of poor differentiation. Melanoma can look rhabdoid and must be ruled out!	 rhabdoid tumor of the kidney
Salt and pepper chromatin (=neuroendocrine chromatin)	granular finely speckled chromatin, which is evenly distributed throughout the nucleus; consists of intermixed finer and larger particles (like salt 'n pepper!) Is a defining feature of neuroendocrine neoplasms. salt pepper salt 'n pepper Diagram based on Atkinson, Atlas of Diagnostic Cytopathology.	 carcinoid
Serous	"Serous fluid" refers to clear watery fluid, which resembles *serum*. "Serous cells" are those cells that secrete serous fluid (as opposed to mucinous secretions and cells). There are 4 types of serous cells/lesions: 1) serous cells of the salivary gland (have zymogen granules), 2) serous tumors of the ovary, 3) serous cysts of various organs (e.g. serous cystadenoma of the pancreas), 4) serous cells lining body cavities/serosal surfaces (pleura, peritoneum, pericardium); these are referred to as mesothelial cells. Note that the above cells and lesions are histologically dissimilar, and they bear the same designation ("serous") only by virtue of their ability to elaborate clear secretions, NOT because of histologic relatedness.	 serous cystadenoma of the pancreas
Signet-ring	cytoplasmic vacuole (usually containing mucin) that compresses the nucleus. Signet = bookmark or seal; signet ring = portable version of a signet. [4] 	 gastric carcinoma, signet-ring type

Stellate cell	star-shaped, with several pointed cytoplasmic tails; typical morphology of fibroblasts and myofibroblasts	 chondromyxoid fibroma
Strap cell	Strap-shaped (elongated like a strap of a shoulder bag; tad-pole-like). Describes the shape of rhabdomyoblasts in rhabdomyosarcoma. With rare luck, cross-striations may be visible. 	 rhabdomyosarcoma
Vesicular (chromatin)	chromatin that appears porous or bubbly. This occurs due to clumping of the chromatin, which leaves behind cleared-out spaces resembling vesicles. Nuclei appear light, almost transparent. Frequently vesicular appearance correlates with a higher degree of dysplasia (e.g. higher grades of ductal carcinoma in situ are vesicular). 	 high grade intraductal carcinoma (shown), embryonal carcinoma

	General Descriptors of Cell Shape (used to define 3 broad groups of tumor differentials)	
Epithelioid	resembling epithelial cells in that the cells have plump round to oval nuclei (as opposed to spindle or small cells), abundant cytoplasm, and well-defined cell borders. The term also usually implies that the cells are cohesive (as epithelioid histiocytes in a granuloma). In a setting of a poorly differentiated neoplasm, the term "epithelioid" implies that a neoplasm looks like carcinoma, but could also be epithelioid melanoma, sarcoma or even lymphoma.	 DDx: carcinoma, epithelioid melanoma (shown), epithelioid sarcoma, large cell lymphoma
Spindle (fusiform)	cells that are elongated and have tapered (pointed) ends. Usually both the nucleus and cytoplasm are elongated, but the term still applies for cells with spindle-shaped cytoplasmic outline but rounded (or only slightly oval) nucleus. In a setting of malignant neoplasm, the differential diagnosis includes sarcoma (e.g. muscle, neural, vascular) AND spindle-cell variants of carcinoma (sarcomatoid carcinoma) and melanoma! "Fusiform" is derived from the Latin "fusus" meaning "spindle" 	 DDx: sarcoma (shown leiomyosarcoma), sarcomatoid carcinoma, melanoma
Small round blue cell	sheets of small round blue cells. Cells are blue because they have very little cytoplasm. Subtle morphologic clues may be present (as in rosettes in neuroblastoma and PNET) but generally diagnosis requires immunostains +/– molecular studies+/– cytogenetics. DDx is age-dependent (see "Potpourri of Differentials" section).	 DDx (for pediatric SRBCT): neuroblastoma (shown), PNET, alveolar rhabdomyosarcoma, Wilms, lymphoblastic lymphoma, other

12 It Looks Like WHAT? An Illustrated Glossary of Histopathologic Descriptors.

153

Descriptors of Giant cells (For more images and differentials see http://www.granuloma.homestead.com/)		
Langhans type giant cells	peripheral semi-circular nuclei (horseshoe-like); characteristic of TB

Named after Theodor Langhans, who was not the same person as Paul Langerhans of the Langerhans cell and islets of Langerhans eponyms | |
| Foreign-body type giant cells | haphazardly arranged nuclei often aggregating towards the center of the cell; characteristic of reaction to a foreign body | |
| Touton giant cells | a full ring of nuclei with eosinophilic cytoplasm centrally and foamy cytoplasm at the periphery. Seen in lesions with high lipid content such as xanthoma, juvenile xanthogranuloma, and fat necrosis; also common in dermatofibroma.

Named after Karl Touton – a German dermatologist | |
Floret cell	wreath of hyperchromatic peripheral nuclei. Hallmark of pleomorphic lipoma, but these cells may rarely be present in liposarcoma as well.	
Osteoclast-like giant cell	multiple **bland** central nuclei, ruffled cell membrane (feature well seen in smears but not in H&E sections). Seen in giant cell-rich tumors of bone and soft tissue (e.g. giant cell tumor) and admixed in various high-grade carcinomas (e.g. pancreatic undifferentiated carcinoma with osteoclast-like giant cells). In the latter case, these cells are non-neoplastic (as may be confirmed by negative CKs and positive CD68 by IHC)	
Tumor giant cells	pleomorphic (scary-looking) cytology; featured in anaplastic carcinomas and high grade sarcomas	
Viral infections	HSV, respiratory syncitial virus (RSV), Measles	

Glossary

Descriptors of Granulomas and Differential Diagnoses		
Term	*Definition/Appearance*	*Differential Diagnosis*
Granuloma NOS	Granuloma = rounded aggregate of histiocytes. Histiocytes in a granuloma have abundant cytoplasm (are "epithelioid") and indistinct cell borders such that they seem to merge into a syncytium. Giant cells are usually but not always present. If syncytial aggregates of histiocytes/giant cells are in sheets (rather than in a discreet nodule) the preferred term is "granulomatous inflammation" rather than granuloma.	• Foreign body or particles (suture, beryllium) • Sarcoidosis • Infection (usually but not always granulomas are necrotizing) • Autoimmune (Crohn's, hypersensitivity pneumonitis, primary biliary cirrhosis) • Drug reactions • Chronic granulomatous disease (rare)
Necrotizing (caseating) granuloma	Caseating: cheese (specifically, cottage-cheese or curd-cheese) -like appearance (strictly speaking a macroscopic term) Necrotizing: microscopic counterpart to "caseating"	• Infection (TB, fungus) • Sarcoidosis (minimal necrosis is allowed) • also see necrobiotic granulomas
Suppurative granuloma	Granulomas with central collections of neutrophils. Coalescent abscesses in granulomas have been termed "stellate microabscesses".	Classic differential: • Cat scratch disease (*Bartonella henselae*) • Lymphogranuloma venereum *(Chlamydia trachomatis)* • Tularemia • *Yersinia* Also rule out Mycobacteria, Fungi
Necrobiotic granuloma	See below for definition of "necrobiosis"	• Granuloma annulare (central mucin) • Rheumatoid nodule • Necrobiosis lipoidica diabeticorum (shins; cake-like horizontal layers) • Wegener's ("blue" necrobiosis) • Post-transurethral resection (TUR) granuloma (prostate, bladder)
"Special" granulomas	Either frank misnomers (pyogenic granuloma) or lesions where histiocytes are present but are not prominent (plasma cell granuloma). This is because the term is loosely applied (usually by non-pathologists) to refer to a nodule (as in a clinical term "suture granuloma").	• Plasma cell granuloma (lung) = Inflammatory myofibroblastic tumor • Eosinophilic granuloma (lung) = Langerhans cell histiocytosis • Pulmonary hyalinizing granuloma = sclerosing lesion analogous to sclerosing mediastinitis • Pyogenic granuloma = Lobular capillary hemangioma • Lethal midline granuloma = NK/T lymphoma nasal type

Descriptors of Stroma		
Term	Definition/Appearance	Example
Hyaline	Etymology: from Latin *hyalinus,* transparent or nearly so and homogeneous. [5] The term is etiologically non-specific. There is no one molecule that corresponds to "hyaline" material. Instead, "hyaline" is a descriptive term, which refers to any material that looks homogeneous (non-fibrillar, non-granular), glassy, almost refractile (like hyaline cartilage) and usually bright pink in H&E. The term is used to describe a variety of processes, including • *hyalinized collagen* (as in hyalinized fibroadenoma): the term refers to collagen which has lost its fibrillar quality and appears homogenized and glassy; the molecular basis for this change is unknown; usually a feature of a long-standing benign process • *hyalinized vessels* (as in schwannoma or nephrosclerosis): the term refers to deposition of glassy pink material in vessel walls; here hyaline material consists of extravasated plasma proteins and basement membrane matrix • other: *hyaline membranes* in the lung (fibrin), *Russell bodies* in plasma cells (immunoglobulins), *Mallory hyaline* in the liver (cytokeratins), *hyaline globules* in various tumors, etc.	 hyalinizing trabecular adenoma of the thyroid
Desmoplastic	host response to a neoplasm manifesting as fibroblast proliferation and deposition of collagen	 desmoplastic small round cell tumor
Fibrotic, Fibrosis	having an abundant collagen deposition. Sometimes sclerotic is used synonymously with fibrotic (see below).	 scar
Mucinous (colloid)	slimy viscous material (a component of mucus) that looks purplish and stringy on H&E. Carcinomas may produce abundant mucin (e.g. mucinous or colloid carcinomas, mucoepidermoid carcinoma)	 intraductal papillary mucinous neoplasm of the pancreas
Myxoid	gelatinous material produced by soft tissue cells. Resembles epithelial mucin, but is not as thick (looks like watered-down mucin – it is not as blue or stringy). By convention, mucoid material produced by soft tissues is called "myxoid" rather than mucinous material. These substances are biochemically distinct: stromal mucin contains hyaluronic acid, whereas epithelial mucin does not (see section on Special Stains for details). **Chondromyxoid** material is bluish and refractile, like cartilage.	 myxoid liposarcoma

(see table)

| **Necrobiotic** | In surgical pathology, the term "necrobiosis" or "bionecrosis" is generally used to describe the blue-red granular necrosis ("granular soup") characteristic of Wegener's granulomatosis. The granularity represents karyorrhectic debris (nuclear dust) from degenerated neutrophils superimposed on degenerated collagen.
In the dermpath literature, necrobiosis is used to indicate "collagenolysis" or degeneration of collagen, wherein collagen takes on an amorphous bluish appearance (nuclear dust may not be prominent). When surrounded by epithelioid histiocytes, the process is called "necrobiotic granuloma" (as seen in necrobiosis lipoidica diabeticorum and granuloma annulare). [6,7] | Wegener's granulomatosis (shown), necrobiosis lipoidica diabeticorum, granuloma annulare |
| **Sclerotic (sclerosis)** | etiologically non-specific term describing "thickening or hardening". may be used to describe microscopic fibrosis/collagen deposition (as in sclerosing adenosis of the breast, sclerotic glomeruli, systemic sclerosis), formation of macroscopically firm plaques (as in multiple sclerosis) or vessel hardening (arteriosclerosis). | sclerosing adenosis |

12 It Looks Like WHAT? An Illustrated Glossary of Histopathologic Descriptors.

157

Descriptors of Collagen		
Term	*Definition/Appearance*	*Example*
Keloidal collagen	thick ropey bundles of eosinophilic hyalinized (bright pink and glassy) collagen. Prototype is a keloid. This type of collagen is typical of fibromatosis, solitary fibrous tumor and spindle cell lipoma.	 keloid (shown)
Amianthoid collagen	resembling amianth: earth-flax or mountain flax; composed of delicate filaments resembling threads of silk. [8] The term is used to describe collagen nodules with fibrillar "frayed" border (as in palisaded myofibroblastoma).	 palisaded myofibroblastoma
Carrot shavings-like collagen	long wavy, curly, wiry strands of collagen. A classic feature of neurofibroma and malignant peripheral nerve sheath tumor (MPNST).	 neurofibroma (shown), MPNST
Skeinoid fibers	collagen fibers "so-named after their peculiar appearance by electron microscopy simulating skeins of yarn". [9] By light microscopy, these are rounded collagen globules or short fibers. Present in ~15% of gastrointestinal stromal tumors (GIST).	 GIST

	Descriptors of Necrosis	
Term	Definition/Appearance	Example
Coagulative necrosis	dead cells are seen as cell shadows or ghosts but the overall architecture is preserved (as if mummified)	 ischemia (except brain, where ischemia causes liquefaction)
Liquefactive necrosis	dead cells are completely digested away and normal architecture is obliterated. Usually caused by infection and is associated with inflammatory cells.	 abscess
Caseating (caseous) necrosis	Central necrosis within a granuloma. Named after the "cheesy" macroscopic appearance.	 TB
Fibrinoid necrosis	fibrin-like. The term "fibrinoid necrosis" is mainly applied to necrotic vessels with deposition of pink hyaline material (as in leukocytoclastic vasculitis). It consists of plasma proteins, including fibrin.	 fibrinoid necrosis in vasculitis

Common Dermatopathologic Descriptors		
Term	Definition/Appearance	Example
Acanthosis	increased thickness of the epidermis	Psoriasis
Acantholysis	the loss of cohesion between keratinocytes	Acantholytic squamous cell carcinoma, Pemphigus vulgaris
Dyskeratosis	premature keratinization of individual keratinocytes before they have reached the surface layer. Dyskeratotic cells have a dense pink cytoplasm and they usually become rounded.	Squamous Dysplasia, Erythema Multiforme, Graft vs. Host Disease
Grenz zone	a narrow area of uninvolved dermis between the upper edge of a dermal lesion (neoplastic or inflammatory) and the epidermis. "Grenz" is German for "border".	Dermatofibroma (Grenz zone present) versus dermatofibrosarcoma protuberans (Grenz zone absent)
Hyperkeratosis	increased thickness of the stratum corneum (clinically a scale)	Actinic Keratosis
Lentiginous	junctional (dermo-epidermal) growth; used in reference to melanocytes	Lentigo Maligna
Lichenoid dermatitis (synonymous with "interface dermatitis")	junctional (dermal-epidermal or DE) inflammatory process, manifesting as band-like lymphocytic infiltrate ("lichenoid infiltrate") and basal cell damage. Basal cell damage leads to formation of vesicles at DE junction ("basilar vacuolopathy" or "liquefaction degeneration").	Lichen Planus (prototype)
Orthokeratosis	normal "basket-weave" pattern of the stratum corneum (no nuclear retention as in parakeratosis)	Normal skin
Parakeratosis	retention of nuclei in the stratum corneum. Reflects a hyperproliferative state. Normal on mucous membranes.	Psoriasis
Papillomatosis	upward displacement of the dermal papillae, giving skin surface a finger-like or "church-spire"-like appearance	Verruca Vulgaris (clinical wart)
Spongiosis	intercellular edema in the epidermis seen as an increase in intercellular spaces	Allergic contact dermatitis

References

Chapter 1 Immunostains: Introduction

1. Moll R, Franke WW, Schiller DL, Geiger B, Krepler R. The catalog of human cytokeratins: patterns of expression in normal epithelia, tumors and cultured cells. Cell 1982;31:11–24.
2. Moll R, Divo M, Langbein L. The human keratins: biology and pathology. Histochem. Cell Biol. 2008;129:705–733.
3. Chu PG, Weiss LM. Keratin expression in human tissues and neoplasms. Histopathology 2002;40:403–439.
4. Cooper D, Schermer A, Sun TT. Classification of human epithelia and their neoplasms using monoclonal antibodies to keratins: strategies, applications, and limitations. Lab. Invest. 1985;52:243–256.
5. Dabbs DJ. Diagnostic Immunohistochemistry: Theranostic and Genomic Applications. 3rd ed. New York: Saunders; 2010.
6. Taylor CR, Cote RJ. Immunomicroscopy: A Diagnostic Tool for the Surgical Pathologist. 3rd ed. Philadelphia: Saunders; 2006.
7. True L. Atlas of Diagnostic Immunohistopathology. Philadelphia: Lippincott Williams & Wilkins; 1990.
8. Zhang PJ, Shah M, Spiegel GW, Brooks JJ. Cytokeratin 7 immunoreactivity in rectal adenocarcinomas. Appl. Immunohistochem. Mol. Morphol. 2003;11:306–310.
9. Carpentieri DF, Nichols K, Chou PM, Matthews M, Pawel B, Huff D. The expression of WT1 in the differentiation of rhabdomyosarcoma from other pediatric small round blue cell tumors. Mod. Pathol. 2002;15:1080–1086.
10. Montgomery E, Lee JH, Abraham SC, Wu TT. Superficial fibromatoses are genetically distinct from deep fibromatoses. Mod. Pathol. 2001;14:695–701.
11. Aleixo PB, Hartmann AA, Menezes IC, Meurer RT, Oliveira AM. Can MDM2 and CDK4 make the diagnosis of well differentiated/dedifferentiated liposarcoma? An immunohistochemical study on 129 soft tissue tumours. J. Clin. Pathol. 2009;62:1127–1135.
12. Hammond ME, Hayes DF, Dowsett M, Allred DC, Hagerty KL, Badve S, et al. American Society of Clinical Oncology/College of American Pathologists guideline recommendations for immunohistochemical testing of estrogen and progesterone receptors in breast cancer. Arch. Pathol. Lab. Med. 2010;134:907–922.
13. Wolff AC, Hammond ME, Schwartz JN, Hagerty KL, Allred DC, Cote RJ, et al. American Society of Clinical Oncology/College of American Pathologists guideline recommendations for human epidermal growth factor receptor 2 testing in breast cancer. Arch. Pathol. Lab. Med. 2007;131:18–43.
14. DAKO HercepTest™. A Manual for Interpretation, http://pri.dako.com/28630_herceptest_interpretation_manual.pdf.
15. Dako EGFR pharmDx™ Interpretation Manual, http://pri.dako.com/08052_egfr_pharmdx_interpretation_manual.pdf.

Chapter 2 Immunostains: Organ Systems

1. Werling RW, Hwang H, Yaziji H, Gown AM. Immunohistochemical distinction of invasive from noninvasive breast lesions: a comparative study of p63 versus calponin and smooth muscle myosin heavy chain. Am. J. Surg. Pathol. 2003;27:82–90.
2. Bratthauer GL, Moinfar F, Stamatakos MD, Mezzetti TP, Shekitka KM, Man YG, et al. Combined E-cadherin and high molecular weight cytokeratin immunoprofile differentiates lobular, ductal, and hybrid mammary intraepithelial neoplasias. Hum. Pathol. 2002;33:620–627.
3. Grin A, O'Malley FP, Mulligan AM. Cytokeratin and estrogen receptor immunohistochemistry as a useful adjunct in identifying atypical papillary lesions on breast needle core biopsy. Am. J. Surg. Pathol. 2009;33:1615–1623.
4. Tse GM, Tan PH, Moriya T. The role of immunohistochemistry in the differential diagnosis of papillary lesions of the breast. J. Clin. Pathol. 2009;62:407–413.
5. Collins LC, Schnitt SJ. Papillary lesions of the breast: selected diagnostic and management issues. Histopathology 2008;52:20–29.
6. Lacroix-Triki M, Geyer FC, Lambros MB, Savage K, Ellis IO, Lee AH, et al. beta-catenin/Wnt signalling pathway in fibromatosis, metaplastic carcinomas and phyllodes tumours of the breast. Mod. Pathol. 2010;23:1438–1448.
7. Tse GM, Tan PH, Lui PC, Putti TC. Spindle cell lesions of the breast – the pathologic differential diagnosis. Breast Cancer Res. Treat. 2008;109:199–207.
8. Rosai J. Rosai and Ackerman's Surgical Pathology. 9th ed. St. Louis: Mosby; 2004.
9. Sheridan T, Herawi M, Epstein JI, Illei PB. The role of P501S and PSA in the diagnosis of metastatic adenocarcinoma of the prostate. Am. J. Surg. Pathol. 2007;31:1351–1355.
10. Epstein JI, Netto GJ. Biopsy Interpretation of the Prostate. 4th ed. Philadelphia: Lippincott Williams & Wilkins; 2008.
11. Coleman JF, Hansel DE. Utility of diagnostic and prognostic markers in urothelial carcinoma of the bladder. Adv. Anat. Pathol. 2009;16:67–78.
12. McKenney JK, Desai S, Cohen C, Amin MB. Discriminatory immunohistochemical staining of urothelial carcinoma in situ and non-neoplastic urothelium: an analysis of cytokeratin 20, p53, and CD44 antigens. Am. J. Surg. Pathol. 2001;25:1074–1078.
13. Paner GP, Brown JG, Lapetino S, Nese N, Gupta R, Shen SS, et al. Diagnostic use of antibody to smoothelin in the recognition of muscularis propria in transurethral resection of urinary bladder tumor (TURBT) specimens. Am. J. Surg. Pathol. 2010;34:792–799.
14. Council L, Hameed O. Differential expression of immunohistochemical markers in bladder smooth muscle and myofibroblasts, and the potential utility of desmin, smoothelin, and vimentin in staging of bladder carcinoma. Mod. Pathol. 2009;22:639–650.
15. Raspollini MR, Nesi G, Baroni G, Girardi LR, Taddei GL. Immunohistochemistry in the differential diagnosis between primary and secondary intestinal adenocarcinoma of the urinary bladder. Appl. Immunohistochem. Mol. Morphol. 2005;13:358–362.
16. Wang HL, Lu DW, Yerian LM, Alsikafi N, Steinberg G, Hart J, et al. Immunohistochemical distinction between primary adenocarcinoma of the bladder and secondary colorectal adenocarcinoma. Am. J. Surg. Pathol. 2001;25:1380–1387.
17. Herawi M, Drew PA, Pan CC, Epstein JI. Clear cell adenocarcinoma of the bladder and urethra: cases diffusely mimicking nephrogenic adenoma. Hum. Pathol. 2010;41:594–601.
18. Sun K, Huan Y, Unger PD. Clear cell adenocarcinoma of urinary bladder and urethra: another urinary tract lesion immunoreactive for P504S. Arch. Pathol. Lab. Med. 2008;132:1417–1422.
19. Tong GX, Weeden EM, Hamele-Bena D, Huan Y, Unger P, Memeo L, et al. Expression of PAX8 in nephrogenic adenoma and clear cell adenocarcinoma of the lower urinary tract: evidence of related histogenesis? Am. J. Surg. Pathol. 2008;32:1380–1387.
20. Chuang AY, DeMarzo AM, Veltri RW, Sharma RB, Bieberich CJ, Epstein JI. Immunohistochemical differentiation of high-grade prostate carcinoma from urothelial carcinoma. Am. J. Surg. Pathol. 2007;31:1246–1255.

N. Rekhtman, J.A. Bishop, *Quick Reference Handbook for Surgical Pathologists*,
DOI:10.1007/978-3-642-20086-1, © Springer-Verlag Berlin Heidelberg 2011

21. Dabbs DJ. Diagnostic Immunohistochemistry: Theranostic and Genomic Applications. 3rd ed. New York: Saunders; 2010.

22. Wang HY, Mills SE. KIT and RCC are useful in distinguishing chromophobe renal cell carcinoma from the granular variant of clear cell renal cell carcinoma. Am. J. Surg. Pathol. 2005;29:640–646.

23. Argani P, Aulmann S, Illei PB, Netto GJ, Ro J, Cho HY, et al. A distinctive subset of PEComas harbors TFE3 gene fusions. Am. J. Surg. Pathol. 2010;34:1395–1406.

24. Ross H, Argani P. Xp11 translocation renal cell carcinoma. Pathology 2010;42:369–373.

25. Martignoni G, Pea M, Gobbo S, Brunelli M, Bonetti F, Segala D, et al. Cathepsin-K immunoreactivity distinguishes MiTF/TFE family renal translocation carcinomas from other renal carcinomas. Mod. Pathol. 2009;22:1016–1022.

26. Went P, Dirnhofer S, Salvisberg T, Amin MB, Lim SD, Diener PA, et al. Expression of epithelial cell adhesion molecule (EpCam) in renal epithelial tumors. Am. J. Surg. Pathol. 2005;29:83–88.

27. Tong GX, Yu WM, Beaubier NT, Weeden EM, Hamele-Bena D, Mansukhani MM, et al. Expression of PAX8 in normal and neoplastic renal tissues: an immunohistochemical study. Mod. Pathol. 2009;22:1218–1227.

28. Tickoo SK, Gopalan A. Pathologic features of renal cortical tumors. Urol. Clin. North Am. 2008;35:551–61; v.

29. Olgac S, Hutchinson B, Tickoo SK, Reuter VE. Alpha-methylacyl-CoA racemase as a marker in the differential diagnosis of metanephric adenoma. Mod. Pathol. 2006;19:218–224.

30. Gobbo S, Eble JN, Grignon DJ, Martignoni G, MacLennan GT, Shah RB, et al. Clear cell papillary renal cell carcinoma: a distinct histopathologic and molecular genetic entity. Am. J. Surg. Pathol. 2008;32:1239–1245.

31. Truong LD, Shen SS. Immunohistochemical diagnosis of renal neoplasms. Arch. Pathol. Lab. Med. 2011;135:92–109.

32. Reuter VE, Tickoo SK. Differential diagnosis of renal tumours with clear cell histology. Pathology 2010;42:374–383.

33. Browning L, Bailey D, Parker A. D2-40 is a sensitive and specific marker in differentiating primary adrenal cortical tumours from both metastatic clear cell renal cell carcinoma and phaeochromocytoma. J. Clin. Pathol. 2008;61:293–296.

34. Jones TD, Ulbright TM, Eble JN, Baldridge LA, Cheng L. OCT4 staining in testicular tumors: a sensitive and specific marker for seminoma and embryonal carcinoma. Am. J. Surg. Pathol. 2004;28:935–940.

35. Cao D, Li J, Guo CC, Allan RW, Humphrey PA. SALL4 is a novel diagnostic marker for testicular germ cell tumors. Am. J. Surg. Pathol. 2009;33:1065–1077.

36. Lau SK, Weiss LM, Chu PG. D2-40 immunohistochemistry in the differential diagnosis of seminoma and embryonal carcinoma: a comparative immunohistochemical study with KIT (CD117) and CD30. Mod. Pathol. 2007;20:320–325.

37. Leroy X, Augusto D, Leteurtre E, Gosselin B. CD30 and CD117 (c-kit) used in combination are useful for distinguishing embryonal carcinoma from seminoma. J. Histochem. Cytochem. 2002;50:283–285.

38. Hammerich KH, Ayala GE, Wheeler TM. Application of immunohistochemistry to the genitourinary system (prostate, urinary bladder, testis, and kidney). Arch. Pathol. Lab. Med. 2008;132:432–440.

39. Rosai J, Carcangiu ML, DeLellis RA. Undifferentiated (Anaplastic) Carcinoma. Tumors of the Thyroid GlandWashington, D.C.: ARP Press; 1992, p.135–159.

40. Mendelsohn G, Wells SA,Jr, Baylin SB. Relationship of tissue carcinoembryonic antigen and calcitonin to tumor virulence in medullary thyroid carcinoma. An immunohistochemical study in early, localized, and virulent disseminated stages of disease. Cancer 1984;54:657–662.

41. Nonaka D, Tang Y, Chiriboga L, Rivera M, Ghossein R. Diagnostic utility of thyroid transcription factors Pax8 and TTF-2 (FoxE1) in thyroid epithelial neoplasms. Mod. Pathol. 2008;21:192–200.

42. Bishop JA, Sharma R, Westra WH. PAX8 immunostaining of anaplastic thyroid carcinoma: A reliable means of discerning thyroid origin for undifferentiated tumors of the head and neck. Human pathology In Press.

43. Gill AJ, Clarkson A, Gimm O, Keil J, Dralle H, Howell VM, et al. Loss of nuclear expression of parafibromin distinguishes parathyroid carcinomas and hyperparathyroidism-jaw tumor (HPT-JT) syndrome-related adenomas from sporadic parathyroid adenomas and hyperplasias. Am. J. Surg. Pathol. 2006;30:1140–1149.

44. Wenig BM, Dulguerov P, Kapadia SB, Prasad ML, Fanburg-Smith JC, Thompson LDR. Neuroectodermal tumours. In: Barnes L, Eveson JW, Reichart P, Sidranksy D, editors. World Health Organization Classification of Tumours. Pathology and Genetics of Head and Neck Tumors.Lyon, France: IARC Press; 2005, p.65–75.

45. Maxwell JH, Kumar B, Feng FY, McHugh JB, Cordell JB, Eisbruch A, et al. HPV-positive/p16-positive/EBV-negative nasopharyngeal carcinoma in white North Americans. Head Neck. 2010;32:562–567.

46. Lo EJ, Bell D, Woo J, Li G, Hanna EY, El-Naggar AK, Strugis EM. Human papillomavirus and WHO type I nasopharyngeal carcinoma. Laryngoscope. 2010;120:1990–1997.

47. Shingi AD, Califano J, Westra WH. High-risk human papillomavirus in nasopharyngeal carcinoma. Head Neck; In Press.

48. Gillison ML, Koch WM, Capone RB, Spafford M, Westra WH, Wu L, et al. Evidence for a causal association between human papillomavirus and a subset of head and neck cancers. J. Natl. Cancer Inst. 2000;92:709–720.

49. Haack H, Johnson LA, Fry CJ, Crosby K, Polakiewicz RD, Stelow EB, et al. Diagnosis of NUT midline carcinoma using a NUT-specific monoclonal antibody. Am. J. Surg. Pathol. 2009;33:984–991.

50. Wenig BM. Undifferentiated malignant neoplasms of the sinonasal tract. Arch. Pathol. Lab. Med. 2009;133:699–712.

51. Begum S, Westra WH. Basaloid squamous cell carcinoma of the head and neck is a mixed variant that can be further resolved by HPV status. Am. J. Surg. Pathol. 2008;32:1044–1050.

52. Serrano MF, El-Mofty SK, Gnepp DR, Lewis JS, Jr. Utility of high molecular weight cytokeratins, but not p63, in the differential diagnosis of neuroendocrine and basaloid carcinomas of the head and neck. Hum. Pathol. 2008;39:591–598.

53. Emanuel P, Wang B, Wu M, Burstein DE. p63 Immunohistochemistry in the distinction of adenoid cystic carcinoma from basaloid squamous cell carcinoma. Mod. Pathol. 2005;18:645–650.

54. Bishop JA, Sciubba J, Westra WH. Squamous cell carcinoma of the oral cavity and oropharynx. Surg. Pathol. Clin.; In Press.

55. Wenig BM. Atlas of Head and Neck Pathology. 2nd ed. Philadelphia: Saunders Elsevier; 2008.

56. Ellis GL, Auclair PL. Tumors of the Salivary Glands. Washington, D.C.: ARP Press; 2008.

57. Ji H, Isacson C, Seidman JD, Kurman RJ, Ronnett BM. Cytokeratins 7 and 20, Dpc4, and MUC5AC in the distinction of metastatic mucinous carcinomas in the ovary from primary ovarian mucinous tumors: Dpc4 assists in identifying metastatic pancreatic carcinomas. Int. J. Gynecol. Pathol. 2002;21:391–400.

58. Parwani AV, Geradts J, Caspers E, Offerhaus GJ, Yeo CJ, Cameron JL, et al. Immunohistochemical and genetic analysis of non-small cell and small cell gallbladder carcinoma and their precursor lesions. Mod. Pathol. 2003;16:299–308.

59. Adsay NV, Merati K, Andea A, Sarkar F, Hruban RH, Wilentz RE, et al. The dichotomy in the preinvasive neoplasia to invasive carcinoma sequence in the pancreas: differential expression of MUC1 and MUC2 supports the existence of two separate pathways of carcinogenesis. Mod. Pathol. 2002;15:1087–1095.

60. Moniaux N, Andrianifahanana M, Brand RE, Batra SK. Multiple roles of mucins in pancreatic cancer, a lethal and challenging malignancy. Br. J. Cancer 2004;91:1633–1638.

61. Hruban RH, Bishop Pitman M, Klimstra DS. Tumors of the Pancreas. Washington, D.C.: ARP Press; 2007.

62. Marsh WL, Colonna J, Yearsley M, Bloomston M, Frankel WL. Calponin is expressed in serous cystadenomas of the pancreas but not in adeno-carcinomas or endocrine tumors. Appl. Immunohistochem. Mol. Morphol. 2009;17:216–219.

63. Kloppel G, Detlefsen S, Chari ST, Longnecker DS, Zamboni G. Autoimmune pancreatitis: the clinicopathological characteristics of the subtype with granulocytic epithelial lesions. J. Gastroenterol. 2010;.

64. Dhall D, Suriawinata AA, Tang LH, Shia J, Klimstra DS. Use of immunohistochemistry for IgG4 in the distinction of autoimmune pancreatitis from peritumoral pancreatitis. Hum. Pathol. 2010;41:643–652.

65. Klimstra DS, Pitman MB, Hruban RH. An algorithmic approach to the diagnosis of pancreatic neoplasms. Arch. Pathol. Lab. Med. 2009;133:454–464.

66. Ormsby AH, Goldblum JR, Rice TW, Richter JE, Falk GW, Vaezi MF, et al. Cytokeratin subsets can reliably distinguish Barrett's esophagus from intestinal metaplasia of the stomach. Hum. Pathol. 1999;30:288–294.

67. Das KM, Prasad I, Garla S, Amenta PS. Detection of a shared colon epithelial epitope on Barrett epithelium by a novel monoclonal antibody. Ann. Intern. Med. 1994;120:753–756.

68. Glickman JN, Shahsafaei A, Odze RD. Mucin core peptide expression can help differentiate Barrett's esophagus from intestinal metaplasia of the stomach. Am. J. Surg. Pathol. 2003;27:1357–1365.

69. Walsh SV, Loda M, Torres CM, Antonioli D, Odze RD. P53 and beta catenin expression in chronic ulcerative colitis – associated polypoid dysplasia and sporadic adenomas: an immunohistochemical study. Am. J. Surg. Pathol. 1999;23:963–969.

70. Kane MF, Loda M, Gaida GM, Lipman J, Mishra R, Goldman H, et al. Methylation of the hMLH1 promoter correlates with lack of expression of hMLH1 in sporadic colon tumors and mismatch repair-defective human tumor cell lines. Cancer Res. 1997;57:808–811.

71. Hampel H, Frankel WL, Martin E, Arnold M, Khanduja K, Kuebler P, et al. Feasibility of screening for Lynch syndrome among patients with colorectal cancer. J. Clin. Oncol. 2008;26:5783–5788.

72. Hatch SB, Lightfoot HM, Jr, Garwacki CP, Moore DT, Calvo BF, Woosley JT, et al. Microsatellite instability testing in colorectal carcinoma: choice of markers affects sensitivity of detection of mismatch repair-deficient tumors. Clin. Cancer Res. 2005;11:2180–2187.

73. Watanabe T, Wu TT, Catalano PJ, Ueki T, Satriano R, Haller DG, et al. Molecular predictors of survival after adjuvant chemotherapy for colon cancer. N. Engl. J. Med. 2001;344:1196–1206.

74. Ribic CM, Sargent DJ, Moore MJ, Thibodeau SN, French AJ, Goldberg RM, et al. Tumor microsatellite-instability status as a predictor of bene-fit from fluorouracil-based adjuvant chemotherapy for colon cancer. N. Engl. J. Med. 2003;349:247–257.

75. Pino MS, Mino-Kenudson M, Wildemore BM, Ganguly A, Batten J, Sperduti I, et al. Deficient DNA mismatch repair is common in Lynch syndrome-associated colorectal adenomas. J. Mol. Diagn. 2009;11:238–247.

76. Muller CI, Schulmann K, Reinacher-Schick A, Andre N, Arnold D, Tannapfel A, et al. Predictive and prognostic value of microsatellite instabil-ity in patients with advanced colorectal cancer treated with a fluoropyrimidine and oxaliplatin containing first-line chemotherapy. A report of the AIO Colorectal Study Group. Int. J. Colorectal Dis. 2008;23:1033–1039.

77. De Jong AE, Morreau H, Van Puijenbroek M, Eilers PH, Wijnen J, Nagengast FM, et al. The role of mismatch repair gene defects in the devel-opment of adenomas in patients with HNPCC. Gastroenterology 2004;126:42–48.

78. Iino H, Simms L, Young J, Arnold J, Winship IM, Webb SI, et al. DNA microsatellite instability and mismatch repair protein loss in adenomas presenting in hereditary non-polyposis colorectal cancer. Gut 2000;47:37–42.

79. Yan BC, Gong C, Song J, Krausz T, Tretiakova M, Hyjek E, et al. Arginase-1: a new immunohistochemical marker of hepatocytes and hepato-cellular neoplasms. Am. J. Surg. Pathol. 2010;34:1147–1154.

80. Wang FH, Yip YC, Zhang M, Vong HT, Chan KI, Wai KC, et al. Diagnostic utility of glypican-3 for hepatocellular carcinoma on liver needle biopsy. J. Clin. Pathol. 2010;63:599–603.

81. Lau SK, Prakash S, Geller SA, Alsabeh R. Comparative immunohistochemical profile of hepatocellular carcinoma, cholangiocarcinoma, and metastatic adenocarcinoma. Hum. Pathol. 2002;33:1175–1181.

82. Ojanguren I, Ariza A, Castella EM, Fernandez-Vasalo A, Mate JL, Navas-Palacios JJ. P53 Immunoreactivity in Hepatocellular Adenoma, Focal Nodular Hyperplasia, Cirrhosis and Hepatocellular Carcinoma. Histopathology 1995;26:63–68.

83. Coston WM, Loera S, Lau SK, Ishizawa S, Jiang Z, Wu CL, et al. Distinction of hepatocellular carcinoma from benign hepatic mimickers using Glypican-3 and CD34 immunohistochemistry. Am. J. Surg. Pathol. 2008;32:433–444.

84. Libbrecht L, Severi T, Cassiman D, Vander Borght S, Pirenne J, Nevens F, et al. Glypican-3 expression distinguishes small hepatocellular carcinomas from cirrhosis, dysplastic nodules, and focal nodular hyperplasia-like nodules. Am. J. Surg. Pathol. 2006;30:1405–1411.

85. Wang HL, Anatelli F, Zhai QJ, Adley B, Chuang ST, Yang XJ. Glypican-3 as a useful diagnostic marker that distinguishes hepatocellular carci-noma from benign hepatocellular mass lesions. Arch. Pathol. Lab. Med. 2008;132:1723–1728.

86. Bishop JA, Benjamin H, Cholakh H, Chajut A, Clark DP, Westra WH. Accurate classification of non-small cell lung carcinoma using a novel microRNA-based approach. Clin. Cancer Res. 2010;16:610–619.

87. Rekhtman N, Ang DC, Sima CS, Travis WD, Moreira AL. Immunohistochemical algorithm for differentiation of lung adenocarcinoma and squamous cell carcinoma based on large series of whole tissue sections with validation in small specimens. Mod. Pathol. 2011 In press.

88. Rekhtman N. Neuroendocrine tumors of the lung: an update. Arch. Pathol. Lab. Med. 2010;134:1628–1638.

89. Gaffey MJ, Mills SE, Askin FB. Minute pulmonary meningothelial-like nodules. A clinicopathologic study of so-called minute pulmonary chemodectoma. Am. J. Surg. Pathol. 1988;12:167–175.

90. Hishima T, Fukayama M, Hayashi Y, Fujii T, Ooba T, Funata N, et al. CD70 expression in thymic carcinoma. Am. J. Surg. Pathol. 2000;24:742–746.

91. Kojika M, Ishii G, Yoshida J, Nishimura M, Hishida T, Ota SJ, et al. Immunohistochemical differential diagnosis between thymic carcinoma and type B3 thymoma: diagnostic utility of hypoxic marker, GLUT-1, in thymic epithelial neoplasms. Mod. Pathol. 2009;22:1341–1350.

92. Nakagawa K, Matsuno Y, Kunitoh H, Maeshima A, Asamura H, Tsuchiya R. Immunohistochemical KIT (CD117) expression in thymic epithelial tumors. Chest 2005;128:140–144.
93. Dorfman DM, Shahsafaei A, Chan JK. Thymic carcinomas, but not thymomas and carcinomas of other sites, show CD5 immunoreactivity. Am. J. Surg. Pathol. 1997;21:936–940.
94. Ordonez NG. The immunohistochemical diagnosis of mesothelioma: a comparative study of epithelioid mesothelioma and lung adenocarcinoma. Am. J. Surg. Pathol. 2003;27:1031–1051.
95. Carella R, Deleonardi G, D'Errico A, Salerno A, Egarter-Vigl E, Seebacher C, et al. Immunohistochemical panels for differentiating epithelial malignant mesothelioma from lung adenocarcinoma: a study with logistic regression analysis. Am. J. Surg. Pathol. 2001;25:43–50.
96. Sato A, Torii I, Okamura Y, Yamamoto T, Nishigami T, Kataoka TR, et al. Immunocytochemistry of CD146 is useful to discriminate between malignant pleural mesothelioma and reactive mesothelium. Mod. Pathol. 2010;.
97. Kato Y, Tsuta K, Seki K, Maeshima AM, Watanabe S, Suzuki K, et al. Immunohistochemical detection of GLUT-1 can discriminate between reactive mesothelium and malignant mesothelioma. Mod. Pathol. 2007;20:215–220.
98. Attanoos RL, Griffin A, Gibbs AR. The use of immunohistochemistry in distinguishing reactive from neoplastic mesothelium. A novel use for desmin and comparative evaluation with epithelial membrane antigen, p53, platelet-derived growth factor-receptor, P-glycoprotein and Bcl-2. Histopathology 2003;43:231–238.
99. Hornick JL, Dal Cin P, Fletcher CD. Loss of INI1 expression is characteristic of both conventional and proximal-type epithelioid sarcoma. Am. J. Surg. Pathol. 2009;33:542–550.
100. Jagdis A, Rubin BP, Tubbs RR, Pacheco M, Nielsen TO. Prospective evaluation of TLE1 as a diagnostic immunohistochemical marker in synovial sarcoma. Am. J. Surg. Pathol. 2009;33:1743–1751.
101. Kosemehmetoglu K, Vrana JA, Folpe AL. TLE1 expression is not specific for synovial sarcoma: a whole section study of 163 soft tissue and bone neoplasms. Mod. Pathol. 2009;22:872–878.
102. Louis DN, Ohgaki H, Wiestler OD, Cavenee WK. WHO Classification of Tumours of the Central Nervous System. 4th ed. Lyon, France: IARC Press; 2007.
103. Burger PC, Minn AY, Smith JS, Borell TJ, Jedlicka AE, Huntley BK, et al. Losses of chromosomal arms 1p and 19q in the diagnosis of oligodendroglioma. A study of paraffin-embedded sections. Mod. Pathol. 2001;14:842–853.
104. Takei H, Powell SZ. Novel immunohistochemical markers in the diagnosis of nonglial tumors of nervous system. Adv. Anat. Pathol. 2010;17:150–153.
105. Hoang MP, Amirkhan RH. Inhibin alpha distinguishes hemangioblastoma from clear cell renal cell carcinoma. Am. J. Surg. Pathol. 2003;27:1152–1156.
106. Jung SM, Kuo TT. Immunoreactivity of CD10 and inhibin alpha in differentiating hemangioblastoma of central nervous system from metastatic clear cell renal cell carcinoma. Mod. Pathol. 2005;18:788–794.
107. Weinbreck N, Marie B, Bressenot A, Montagne K, Joud A, Baumann C, et al. Immunohistochemical markers to distinguish between hemangioblastoma and metastatic clear-cell renal cell carcinoma in the brain: utility of aquaporin1 combined with cytokeratin AE1/AE3 immunostaining. Am. J. Surg. Pathol. 2008;32:1051–1059.
108. Rivera AL, Takei H, Zhai J, Shen SS, Ro JY, Powell SZ. Useful immunohistochemical markers in differentiating hemangioblastoma versus metastatic renal cell carcinoma. Neuropathology 2010;.
109. Cho HY, Lee M, Takei H, Dancer J, Ro JY, Zhai QJ. Immunohistochemical comparison of chordoma with chondrosarcoma, myxopapillary ependymoma, and chordoid meningioma. Appl. Immunohistochem. Mol. Morphol. 2009;17:131–138.
110. Huse JT, Pasha TL, Zhang PJ. D2-40 functions as an effective chondroid marker distinguishing true chondroid tumors from chordoma. Acta Neuropathol. 2007;113:87–94.
111. Sangoi AR, Dulai MS, Beck AH, Brat DJ, Vogel H. Distinguishing chordoid meningiomas from their histologic mimics: an immunohistochemical evaluation. Am. J. Surg. Pathol. 2009;33:669–681.
112. Kong CS, Beck AH, Longacre TA. A panel of 3 markers including p16, ProExC, or HPV ISH is optimal for distinguishing between primary endometrial and endocervical adenocarcinomas. Am. J. Surg. Pathol. 2010;34:915–926.
113. Sanati S, Huettner P, Ylagan LR. Role of ProExC: a novel immunoperoxidase marker in the evaluation of dysplastic squamous and glandular lesions in cervical specimens. Int. J. Gynecol. Pathol. 2010;29:79–87.
114. Walts AE, Bose S. p16, Ki-67, and BD ProExC immunostaining: a practical approach for diagnosis of cervical intraepithelial neoplasia. Hum. Pathol. 2009;40:957–964.
115. Comin CE, Saieva C, Messerini L. h-caldesmon, calretinin, estrogen receptor, and Ber-EP4: a useful combination of immunohistochemical markers for differentiating epithelioid peritoneal mesothelioma from serous papillary carcinoma of the ovary. Am. J. Surg. Pathol. 2007;31:1139–1148.
116. Nofech-Mozes S, Khalifa MA, Ismiil N, Saad RS, Hanna WM, Covens A, et al. Immunophenotyping of serous carcinoma of the female genital tract. Mod. Pathol. 2008;21:1147–1155.
117. Ordonez NG. Value of immunohistochemistry in distinguishing peritoneal mesothelioma from serous carcinoma of the ovary and peritoneum: a review and update. Adv.Anat.Pathol. 2006;13:16–25.
118. Zhao C, Barner R, Vinh TN, McManus K, Dabbs D, Vang R. SF-1 is a diagnostically useful immunohistochemical marker and comparable to other sex cord-stromal tumor markers for the differential diagnosis of ovarian sertoli cell tumor. Int. J. Gynecol. Pathol. 2008;27:507–514.
119. McCluggage WG, Young RH. Immunohistochemistry as a diagnostic aid in the evaluation of ovarian tumors. Semin.Diagn.Pathol. 2005;22:3–32.
120. Baker PM, Oliva E. Immunohistochemistry as a tool in the differential diagnosis of ovarian tumors: an update. Int. J. Gynecol. Pathol. 2005;24:39–55.
121. Yemelyanova A, Ji H, Shih I, Wang TL, Wu LS, Ronnett BM. Utility of p16 expression for distinction of uterine serous carcinomas from endometrial endometrioid and endocervical adenocarcinomas: immunohistochemical analysis of 201 cases. Am. J. Surg. Pathol. 2009;33:1504–1514.
122. Reid-Nicholson M, Iyengar P, Hummer AJ, Linkov I, Asher M, Soslow RA. Immunophenotypic diversity of endometrial adenocarcinomas: implications for differential diagnosis. Mod. Pathol. 2006;19:1091–1100.
123. Lax SF, Pizer ES, Ronnett BM, Kurman RJ. Clear cell carcinoma of the endometrium is characterized by a distinctive profile of p53, Ki-67, estrogen, and progesterone receptor expression. Hum. Pathol. 1998;29:551–558.
124. Kobel M, Kalloger SE, Carrick J, Huntsman D, Asad H, Oliva E, et al. A limited panel of immunomarkers can reliably distinguish between clear cell and high-grade serous carcinoma of the ovary. Am. J. Surg. Pathol. 2009;33:14–21.

125. Oliva E, Young RH, Amin MB, Clement PB. An immunohistochemical analysis of endometrial stromal and smooth muscle tumors of the uterus: a study of 54 cases emphasizing the importance of using a panel because of overlap in immunoreactivity for individual antibodies. Am. J. Surg. Pathol. 2002;26:403–412.

126. Irving JA, Carinelli S, Prat J. Uterine tumors resembling ovarian sex cord tumors are polyphenotypic neoplasms with true sex cord differentiation. Mod. Pathol. 2006;19:17–24.

127. Czernobilsky B. Uterine tumors resembling ovarian sex cord tumors: an update. Int. J. Gynecol. Pathol. 2008;27:229–235.

128. Carlson JW, Jarboe EA, Kindelberger D, Nucci MR, Hirsch MS, Crum CP. Serous tubal intraepithelial carcinoma: diagnostic reproducibility and its implications. Int. J. Gynecol. Pathol. 2010;29:310–314.

129. Zhao C, Vinh TN, McManus K, Dabbs D, Barner R, Vang R. Identification of the most sensitive and robust immunohistochemical markers in different categories of ovarian sex cord-stromal tumors. Am. J. Surg. Pathol. 2009;33:354–366.

130. Shih I. Trophogram, an immunohistochemistry-based algorithmic approach, in the differential diagnosis of trophoblastic tumors and tumorlike lesions. Ann. Diagn. Pathol. 2007;11:228–234.

131. Castrillon DH, Sun D, Weremowicz S, Fisher RA, Crum CP, Genest DR. Discrimination of complete hydatidiform mole from its mimics by immunohistochemistry of the paternally imprinted gene product p57KIP2. Am. J. Surg. Pathol. 2001;25:1225–1230.

132. Kipp BR, Ketterling RP, Oberg TN, Cousin MA, Plagge AM, Wiktor AE, et al. Comparison of fluorescence in situ hybridization, p57 immunostaining, flow cytometry, and digital image analysis for diagnosing molar and nonmolar products of conception. Am. J. Clin. Pathol. 2010;133:196–204.

133. Busam KJ, Chen YT, Old LJ, Stockert E, Iversen K, Coplan KA, et al. Expression of melan-A (MART1) in benign melanocytic nevi and primary cutaneous malignant melanoma. Am. J. Surg. Pathol. 1998;22:976–982.

134. Nonaka D, Chiriboga L, Rubin BP. Sox10: a pan-schwannian and melanocytic marker. Am. J. Surg. Pathol. 2008;32:1291–1298.

135. Ramos-Herberth FI, Karamchandani J, Kim J, Dadras SS. SOX10 immunostaining distinguishes desmoplastic melanoma from excision scar. J. Cutan. Pathol. 2010;37:944–952.

136. Prieto VG, Shea CR. Use of immunohistochemistry in melanocytic lesions. J. Cutan. Pathol. 2008;35 Suppl 2:1–10.

137. Mahmood MN, Lee MW, Linden MD, Nathanson SD, Hornyak TJ, Zarbo RJ. Diagnostic value of HMB-45 and anti-Melan A staining of sentinel lymph nodes with isolated positive cells. Mod. Pathol. 2002;15:1288–1293.

138. Thurber SE, Zhang B, Kim YH, Schrijver I, Zehnder J, Kohler S. T-cell clonality analysis in biopsy specimens from two different skin sites shows high specificity in the diagnosis of patients with suggested mycosis fungoides. J. Am. Acad. Dermatol. 2007;57:782–790.

139. Bandarchi B, Ma L, Marginean C, Hafezi S, Zubovits J, Rasty G. D2-40, a novel immunohistochemical marker in differentiating dermatofibroma from dermatofibrosarcoma protuberans. Mod. Pathol. 2010;23:434–438.

140. Busam KJ, Jungbluth AA, Rekthman N, Coit D, Pulitzer M, Bini J, et al. Merkel cell polyomavirus expression in merkel cell carcinomas and its absence in combined tumors and pulmonary neuroendocrine carcinomas. Am. J. Surg. Pathol. 2009;33:1378–1385.

141. Gleason BC, Calder KB, Cibull TL, Thomas AB, Billings SD, Morgan MB, et al. Utility of p63 in the differential diagnosis of atypical fibroxanthoma and spindle cell squamous cell carcinoma. J. Cutan. Pathol. 2009;36:543–547.

142. Hall JM, Saenger JS, Fadare O. Diagnostic utility of P63 and CD10 in distinguishing cutaneous spindle cell/sarcomatoid squamous cell carcinomas and atypical fibroxanthomas. Int. J. Clin. Exp. Pathol. 2008;1:524–530.

143. Hultgren TL, DiMaio DJ. Immunohistochemical staining of CD10 in atypical fibroxanthomas. J. Cutan. Pathol. 2007;34:415–419.

144. Goldblum JR, Hart WR. Perianal Paget's disease: a histologic and immunohistochemical study of 11 cases with and without associated rectal adenocarcinoma. Am. J. Surg. Pathol. 1998;22:170–179.

145. Swerdlow SH, Campo E, Harris NL, Jaffe ES, Pileri SA, Stein H, et al. WHO Classification of Tumours of Haematopoietic and Lymphoid Tissues. 4th ed. Lyon, France: IARC Press; 2008.

146. Jaffe E, Harris NL, Stein H, Campo E, Pileri SA, Swerdlow SH. Introduction and Overview of the Classification of the Lymphoid Neoplasms. In: Swerdlow SH, Campo E, Harris NL, Jaffe ES, Pileri SA, Stein H, et al, editors. WHO Classification of Tumours of Haematopoetic and Lymphoid Organs. 4th ed. Lyon, France: IARC Press; 2008, p.157–168.

147. Ioachim HL, Medirus LJ. The Normal Lymph Node. In: Ioachim HL, Medirus LJ, editors. Ioachim's Lymph Node Pathology. Philedelphia: Lippioncott Williams & Wilkins; 2009, p.2–15.

148. Bell A, Sallah S, Diggs LW. Hematopoiesis. In: Bell A, Sallah S, Diggs LW, editors. Morphology of Human Blood Cells. 7th ed.: Abbott Laboratories; 2005, p.1–12.

149. Sagaert X, Sprangers B, De Wolf-Peeters C. The dynamics of the B follicle: understanding the normal counterpart of B-cell-derived malignancies. Leukemia 2007;21:1378–1386.

150. Hans CP, Weisenburger DD, Greiner TC, Gascoyne RD, Delabie J, Ott G, et al. Confirmation of the molecular classification of diffuse large B-cell lymphoma by immunohistochemistry using a tissue microarray. Blood 2004;103:275–282.

151. Berglund M, Thunberg U, Amini RM, Book M, Roos G, Erlanson M, et al. Evaluation of immunophenotype in diffuse large B-cell lymphoma and its impact on prognosis. Mod. Pathol. 2005;18:1113–1120.

152. Choi WW, Weisenburger DD, Greiner TC, Piris MA, Banham AH, Delabie J, et al. A new immunostain algorithm classifies diffuse large B-cell lymphoma into molecular subtypes with high accuracy. Clin. Cancer Res. 2009;15:5494–5502.

153. Jaffe R, Pileri SA, Facchetti F, Jones DM, Jaffe ES. Histiocytic and Dendritic cell neoplasms, introduction. In: Swerdlow SH, Campo E, Harris NL, Jaffe ES, Pileri SA, Stein H, et al, editors. WHO Classification of Tumours of Haematopoetic and Lymphoid Organs. 4th ed. Lyon, France: IARC Press; 2008, p.354–357.

Chapter 3 Immunostains: Antibody Index

1. Yan BC, Gong C, Song J, Krausz T, Tretiakova M, Hyjek E, et al. Arginase-1: a new immunohistochemical marker of hepatocytes and hepatocellular neoplasms. Am. J. Surg. Pathol. 2010;34:1147–1154.

2. Simon RA, di Sant'Agnese PA, Huang LS, Xu H, Yao JL, Yang Q, et al. CD44 expression is a feature of prostatic small cell carcinoma and distinguishes it from its mimickers. Hum. Pathol. 2009;40:252–258.

3. Wu JM, Borowitz MJ, Weir EG. The usefulness of CD71 expression by flow cytometry for differentiating indolent from aggressive CD10+ B-cell lymphomas. Am. J. Clin. Pathol. 2006;126:39–46.

4. Bing Z, Pasha T, Tomaszewski JE, Zhang P. CDX2 expression in yolk sac component of testicular germ cell tumors. Int. J. Surg. Pathol. 2009;17:373–377.
5. Kalof AN, Cooper K. D2-40 immunohistochemistry – so far! Adv. Anat. Pathol. 2009;16:62–64.
6. Ordonez NG. Podoplanin: a novel diagnostic immunohistochemical marker. Adv.Anat.Pathol. 2006;13:83–88.
7. Lau SK, Weiss LM, Chu PG. D2-40 immunohistochemistry in the differential diagnosis of seminoma and embryonal carcinoma: a comparative immunohistochemical study with KIT (CD117) and CD30. Mod. Pathol. 2007;20:320–325.
8. Miettinen M, Wang ZF, Lasota J. DOG1 antibody in the differential diagnosis of gastrointestinal stromal tumors: a study of 1840 cases. Am. J. Surg. Pathol. 2009;33:1401–1408.
9. Kandil DH, Cooper K. Glypican-3: a novel diagnostic marker for hepatocellular carcinoma and more. Adv. Anat. Pathol. 2009;16:125–129.
10. Hornick JL, Dal Cin P, Fletcher CD. Loss of INI1 expression is characteristic of both conventional and proximal-type epithelioid sarcoma. Am. J. Surg. Pathol. 2009;33:542–550.
11. Lau SK, Chu PG, Weiss LM. Immunohistochemical expression of Langerin in Langerhans cell histiocytosis and non-Langerhans cell histiocytic disorders. Am. J. Surg. Pathol. 2008;32:615–619.
12. Zafrakas M, Petschke B, Donner A, Fritzsche F, Kristiansen G, Knuchel R, et al. Expression analysis of mammaglobin A (SCGB2A2) and lipophilin B (SCGB1D2) in more than 300 human tumors and matching normal tissues reveals their co-expression in gynecologic malignancies. BMC Cancer 2006;6:88.
13. Bhargava R, Beriwal S, Dabbs DJ. Mammaglobin vs GCDFP-15: an immunohistologic validation survey for sensitivity and specificity. Am. J. Clin. Pathol. 2007;127:103–113.
14. Gill AJ, Clarkson A, Gimm O, Keil J, Dralle H, Howell VM, et al. Loss of nuclear expression of parafibromin distinguishes parathyroid carcinomas and hyperparathyroidism-jaw tumor (HPT-JT) syndrome-related adenomas from sporadic parathyroid adenomas and hyperplasias. Am. J. Surg. Pathol. 2006;30:1140–1149.
15. Zhai QJ, Ozcan A, Hamilton C, Shen SS, Coffey D, Krishnan B, et al. PAX-2 expression in non-neoplastic, primary neoplastic, and metastatic neoplastic tissue: A comprehensive immunohistochemical study. Appl. Immunohistochem. Mol. Morphol. 2010;18:323–332.
16. Mazal PR, Stichenwirth M, Koller A, Blach S, Haitel A, Susani M. Expression of aquaporins and PAX-2 compared to CD10 and cytokeratin 7 in renal neoplasms: a tissue microarray study. Mod. Pathol. 2005;18:535–540.
17. Nonaka D, Tang Y, Chiriboga L, Rivera M, Ghossein R. Diagnostic utility of thyroid transcription factors Pax8 and TTF-2 (FoxE1) in thyroid epithelial neoplasms. Mod. Pathol. 2008;21:192–200.
18. Bishop JA, Sharma R, Westra WH. PAX8 immunostaining of anaplastic thyroid carcinoma: A reliable means of discerning thyroid origin for undifferentiated tumors of the head and neck. Hum. Pathol; In Press.
19. Sheridan T, Herawi M, Epstein JI, Illei PB. The role of P501S and PSA in the diagnosis of metastatic adenocarcinoma of the prostate. Am. J. Surg. Pathol. 2007;31:1351–1355.
20. Epstein JI, Netto GJ. Biopsy Interpretation of the Prostate. 4th ed. Philadelphia: Lippincott Williams & Wilkins; 2008.
21. Gopalan A, Dhall D, Olgac S, Fine SW, Korkola JE, Houldsworth J, et al. Testicular mixed germ cell tumors: a morphological and immunohistochemical study using stem cell markers, OCT3/4, SOX2 and GDF3, with emphasis on morphologically difficult-to-classify areas. Mod. Pathol. 2009;22:1066–1074.
22. Nonaka D, Chiriboga L, Rubin BP. Sox10: a pan-schwannian and melanocytic marker. Am. J. Surg. Pathol. 2008;32:1291–1298.
23. Argani P, Aulmann S, Illei PB, Netto GJ, Ro J, Cho HY, et al. A distinctive subset of PEComas harbors TFE3 gene fusions. Am. J. Surg. Pathol. 2010;34:1395–1406.
24. Ordonez NG. Value of thyroid transcription factor-1 immunostaining in distinguishing small cell lung carcinomas from other small cell carcinomas. Am. J. Surg. Pathol. 2000;24:1217–1223.
25. Srodon M, Westra WH. Immunohistochemical staining for thyroid transcription factor-1: a helpful aid in discerning primary site of tumor origin in patients with brain metastases. Hum. Pathol. 2002;33:642–645.

Chapter 4 Special Stains

1. Klatt EC. Special Stains in Histology, http://library.med.utah.edu/WebPath/HISTHTML/STAINS/STAINS.html.
2. Bancroft JD, Gamble M. Theory and Practice of Histological Techniques. 6th ed. Philadelphia: Churchill Livingstone; 2008.
3. Lodish H, Berk A, Kaiser CA, Krieger M, Scott MP, Bretscher A, et al. Molecular Cell Biology. 6th ed. San Francisco: W. H. Freeman; 2007.

Chapter 5 Grading (and Classification) Systems

1. Fan F, Thomas PA. Tumors of the Breast. In: Damjanov I, Fan F, editors. Cancer Grading Manual. New York: Springer; 2007, p.75–81.
2. Guzman G, Cheifec G. Tumors of the Digestive System. In: Damjanov I, Fan F, editors. Cancer Grading Manual. New York: Springer; 2007, p.35–46.
3. Westra WH. The changing face of head and neck cancer in the 21st century: the impact of HPV on the epidemiology and pathology of oral cancer. Head. Neck. Pathol. 2009;3:78–81.
4. Bishop JA, Sciubba J, Westra WH. Squamous cell carcinoma of the oral cavity and oropharynx. Surg. Pathol. Clin.; In Press.
5. Barnes L, Eveson JW, Relchart P, Sidransky D. Tumours of the Oral Cavity and Oropharynx. World Health Organization Classification of Tumours: Pathology and Genetics of Head and Neck TumoursLyon, France: IARC Press; 2005, p.163–208.
6. Lester SC, Bose S, Chen YY, Connolly JL, de Baca ME, Fitzgibbons PL, et al. Protocol for the examination of specimens from patients with ductal carcinoma in situ of the breast. Arch. Pathol. Lab. Med. 2009;133:15–25.
7. Elston CW, Ellis IO. Pathological prognostic factors in breast cancer. I. The value of histological grade in breast cancer: experience from a large study with long-term follow-up. Histopathology 1991;19:403–410.
8. Giri D. Recurrent challenges in the evaluation of fibroepithelial lesions. Arch. Pathol. Lab. Med. 2009;133:713–721.
9. Epstein JI. An update of the Gleason grading system. J. Urol. 2010;183:433–440.
10. Epstein JI, Netto GJ. Biopsy Interpretation of the Prostate. 4th ed. Philadelphia: Lippincott Williams & Wilkins; 2008.
11. Eble JN, Sauter G, Epstein JI, Sesterhenn IA. World Health Organization Classification of Tumours of the Urinary System and Male Genital Organs. Lyon, France: IARC Press; 2004.

12. Miyamoto H, Miller JS, Fajardo DA, Lee TK, Netto GJ, Epstein JI. Non-invasive papillary urothelial neoplasms: the 2004 WHO/ISUP classification system. Pathol. Int. 2010;60:1–8.

13. Ghossein R. Update to the College of American Pathologists reporting on thyroid carcinomas. Head. Neck. Pathol. 2009;3:86–93.

14. Kakudo K, Bai Y, Katayama S, Hirokawa M, Ito Y, Miyauchi A, et al. Classification of follicular cell tumors of the thyroid gland: analysis involving Japanese patients from one institute. Pathol. Int. 2009;59:359–367.

15. Volante M, Collini P, Nikiforov YE, Sakamoto A, Kakudo K, Katoh R, et al. Poorly differentiated thyroid carcinoma: the Turin proposal for the use of uniform diagnostic criteria and an algorithmic diagnostic approach. Am. J. Surg. Pathol. 2007;31:1256–1264.

16. Hiltzik D, Carlson DL, Tuttle RM, Chuai S, Ishill N, Shaha A, et al. Poorly differentiated thyroid carcinomas defined on the basis of mitosis and necrosis: a clinicopathologic study of 58 patients. Cancer 2006;106:1286–1295.

17. Ellis GL, Auclair PL. Tumors of the Salivary Glands. Washington, D.C.: ARP Press; 2008.

18. Goode RK, El-Naggar AK. Mucoepidermoid carcinoma. In: Barnes L, Eveson JW, Reichart P, Sidranksy D, editors. World Health Organization Classification of Tumours. Pathology and Genetics of Head and Neck Tumors.Lyon, France.: IARC Press.; 2005, p.219–220.

19. Cleary KR, Batsakis JG. Biopsy of the lip and Sjogren's syndrome. Ann. Otol. Rhinol. Laryngol. 1990;99:323–325.

20. Greenspan JS, Daniels TE, Talal N, Sylvester RA. The histopathology of Sjogren's syndrome in labial salivary gland biopsies. Oral Surg. Oral Med. Oral Pathol. 1974;37:217–229.

21. Hruban RH, Takaori K, Klimstra DS, Adsay NV, Albores-Saavedra J, Biankin AV, et al. An illustrated consensus on the classification of pancreatic intraepithelial neoplasia and intraductal papillary mucinous neoplasms. Am. J. Surg. Pathol. 2004;28:977–987.

22. Bosman FT, Carneiro F, Hruban RH, Theise ND. WHO Classification of Tumours of the Digestive System. 4th ed. Lyon, France: IARC Press; 2010.

23. Hruban RH, Bishop Pitman M, Klimstra DS. Tumors of the Pancreas. Washington, D.C.: ARP Press; 2007.

24. Maitra A, Fukushima N, Takaori K, Hruban RH. Precursors to invasive pancreatic cancer. Adv. Anat. Pathol. 2005;12:81–91.

25. Montgomery E, Bronner MP, Goldblum JR, Greenson JK, Haber MM, Hart J, et al. Reproducibility of the diagnosis of dysplasia in Barrett esophagus: a reaffirmation. Hum. Pathol. 2001;32:368–378.

26. Theise ND. Liver biopsy assessment in chronic viral hepatitis: a personal, practical approach. Mod. Pathol. 2007;20 Suppl 1:S3–14.

27. Banff schema for grading liver allograft rejection: an international consensus document. Hepatology 1997;25:658–663.

28. Guillou L, Coindre JM, Bonichon F, Nguyen BB, Terrier P, Collin F, et al. Comparative study of the National Cancer Institute and French Federation of Cancer Centers Sarcoma Group grading systems in a population of 410 adult patients with soft tissue sarcoma. J. Clin. Oncol. 1997;15:350–362.

29. Deyrup AT, Weiss SW. Grading of soft tissue sarcomas: the challenge of providing precise information in an imprecise world. Histopathology 2006;48:42–50.

30. Coindre JM. Grading of soft tissue sarcomas: review and update. Arch. Pathol. Lab. Med. 2006;130:1448–1453.

31. Oliveira AM, Nascimento AG. Grading in soft tissue tumors: principles and problems. Skeletal Radiol. 2001;30:543–559.

32. Fisher C. Standards and datasets for reporting cancers: Dataset for cancer histopathology reports on soft tissue sarcomas. Royal College of Pathologists. http://www.rcpath.org/resources/pdf/g094datasetsofttissue.pdf . November 2009.

33. Recommendations for the reporting of soft tissue sarcoma. Association of Directors of Anatomic and Surgical Pathology. Virchows Arch. 1999;434:187–191.

34. Travis WD, Brambilla E, Muller-Hermelink HK, Harris CC(). World Health Organization Classification of Tumours. Pathology and Genetics of Tumours of the Lung, Pleura, Thymus and Heart. Lyon, France: IARC Press; 2004.

35. Rekhtman N. Neuroendocrine tumors of the lung: an update. Arch. Pathol. Lab. Med. 2010;134:1628–1638.

36. Klimstra DS, Modlin IR, Coppola D, Lloyd RV, Suster S. The pathologic classification of neuroendocrine tumors: a review of nomenclature, grading, and staging systems. Pancreas 2010;39:707–712.

37. Shimada H, Ambros IM, Dehner LP, Hata J, Joshi VV, Roald B, et al. The International Neuroblastoma Pathology Classification (the Shimada system). Cancer 1999;86:364–372.

38. Wenig BM, Dulguerov P, Kapadia SB, Prasad ML, Fanburg-Smith JC, Thompson LDR. Neuroectodermal tumours. In: Barnes L, Eveson JW, Reichart P, Sidranksy D, editors. World Health Organization Classification of Tumours. Pathology and Genetics of Head and Neck Tumors.Lyon, France: IARC Press; 2005, p.65–75.

39. Louis DN, Ohgaki H, Wiestler OD, Cavenee WK. WHO Classification of Tumours of the Central Nervous System. 4th ed. Lyon, France: IARC Press; 2007.

40. Burger PC, Scheithauer BW. Tumors of the Central Nervous System. Washington, D.C.: ARP Press; 2007.

41. Fan F, Damjanov I. Tumors of the Female Genital Organs. In: Damjanov I, Fan F, editors. Cancer Grading ManualNew York: Springer; 2007, p.64–74.

42. Tavassoli FA, Devilee P. WHO Classification of Tumours of the Breast and Female Genital Organs. Lyon, France: IARC Press; 2003.

43. Bell SW, Kempson RL, Hendrickson MR. Problematic uterine smooth muscle neoplasms. A clinicopathologic study of 213 cases. Am. J. Surg. Pathol. 1994;18:535–558.

44. Mills AM, Longacre TA. Smooth muscle tumors of the female genital tract. Surg. Pathol. Clin. 2009;2:625–677.

45. Redline RW, Heller D, Keating S, Kingdom J. Placental diagnostic criteria and clinical correlation – a workshop report. Placenta 2005;26 Suppl A:S114–7.

46. Redline RW, Faye-Petersen O, Heller D, Qureshi F, Savell V, Vogler C, et al. Amniotic infection syndrome: nosology and reproducibility of placental reaction patterns. Pediatr. Dev. Pathol. 2003;6:435–448.

47. Swerdlow SH, Campo E, Harris NL, Jaffe ES, Pileri SA, Stein H, et al. WHO Classification of Tumours of Haematopoietic and Lymphoid Tissues. 4th ed. Lyon, France: IARC Press; 2008.

48. Kyle RA, Rajkumar SV. Criteria for diagnosis, staging, risk stratification and response assessment of multiple myeloma. Leukemia 2009;23:3–9.

49. Stewart S, Fishbein MC, Snell GI, Berry GJ, Boehler A, Burke MM, et al. Revision of the 1996 working formulation for the standardization of nomenclature in the diagnosis of lung rejection. J. Heart Lung Transplant. 2007;26:1229–1242.

50. Sale GE, Shulman HM, McDonald GB, Thomas ED. Gastrointestinal graft-versus-host disease in man. A clinicopathologic study of the rectal biopsy. Am. J. Surg. Pathol. 1979;3:291–299.

51. Snover DC. Graft-versus-host disease of the gastrointestinal tract. Am. J. Surg. Pathol. 1990;14 Suppl 1:101–108.

52. Rapini RP. Practical Dermatopathology. Philadelphia: Elsevier Mosby; 2005.

53. Hough AJ, Hollifield JW, Page DL, Hartmann WH. Prognostic factors in adrenal cortical tumors. A mathematical analysis of clinical and morphologic data. Am. J. Clin. Pathol. 1979;72:390–399.

54. van Slooten H, Schaberg A, Smeenk D, Moolenaar AJ. Morphologic characteristics of benign and malignant adrenocortical tumors. Cancer 1985;55:766–773.

55. Weiss LM. Comparative histologic study of 43 metastasizing and nonmetastasizing adrenocortical tumors. Am. J. Surg. Pathol. 1984;8:163–169.

56. Aubert S, Wacrenier A, Leroy X, Devos P, Carnaille B, Proye C, et al. Weiss system revisited: a clinicopathologic and immunohistochemical study of 49 adrenocortical tumors. Am. J. Surg. Pathol. 2002;26:1612–1619.

57. Rosai J. Rosai and Ackerman's Surgical Pathology. 9th ed. St. Louis: Mosby; 2004.

58. DeLellis RA, Lloyd RV, Heitz PU, Eng C. WHO Classification of Tumours of Endocrine Organs. Lyon, France: IARC Press; 2004.

59. Thompson LD. Pheochromocytoma of the Adrenal gland Scaled Score (PASS) to separate benign from malignant neoplasms: a clinicopathologic and immunophenotypic study of 100 cases. Am. J. Surg. Pathol. 2002;26:551–566.

60. Linnoila RI, Keiser HR, Steinberg SM, Lack EE. Histopathology of benign versus malignant sympathoadrenal paragangliomas: clinicopathologic study of 120 cases including unusual histologic features. Hum. Pathol. 1990;21:1168–1180.

61. England DM, Hochholzer L, McCarthy MJ. Localized benign and malignant fibrous tumors of the pleura. A clinicopathologic review of 223 cases. Am. J. Surg. Pathol. 1989;13:640–658.

62. Fine SW, McCarthy DM, Chan TY, Epstein JI, Argani P. Malignant solitary fibrous tumor of the kidney: report of a case and comprehensive review of the literature. Arch. Pathol. Lab. Med. 2006;130:857–861.

63. Gold JS, Antonescu CR, Hajdu C, Ferrone CR, Hussain M, Lewis JJ, et al. Clinicopathologic correlates of solitary fibrous tumors. Cancer 2002;94:1057–1068.

64. Demetri GD, von Mehren M, Antonescu CR, DeMatteo RP, Ganjoo KN, Maki RG, et al. NCCN Task Force report: update on the management of patients with gastrointestinal stromal tumors. J. Natl. Compr. Canc. Netw. 2010;8 Suppl 2:S1-41; quiz S42-4.

65. Miettinen M, Lasota J. Gastrointestinal stromal tumors: pathology and prognosis at different sites. Semin. Diagn. Pathol. 2006;23:70–83.

66. Gill AJ, Clarkson A, Gimm O, Keil J, Dralle H, Howell VM, et al. Loss of nuclear expression of parafibromin distinguishes parathyroid carcinomas and hyperparathyroidism-jaw tumor (HPT-JT) syndrome-related adenomas from sporadic parathyroid adenomas and hyperplasias. Am. J. Surg. Pathol. 2006;30:1140–1149.

67. Delellis RA. Challenging lesions in the differential diagnosis of endocrine tumors: parathyroid carcinoma. Endocr. Pathol. 2008;19:221–225.

68. Borczuk AC, Qian F, Kazeros A, Eleazar J, Assaad A, Sonett JR, et al. Invasive size is an independent predictor of survival in pulmonary adenocarcinoma. Am. J. Surg. Pathol. 2009;33:462–469.

Chapter 6 Potpourri of Quick Morphologic References

1. Coleman H, Altini M. Intravascular tumour in intra-oral pleomorphic adenomas: a diagnostic and therapeutic dilemma. Histopathology 1999;35:439–444.

2. Altini M, Coleman H, Kienle F. Intra-vascular tumour in pleomorphic adenomas – a report of four cases. Histopathology 1997;31:55–59.

3. Cserni G, Bori R, Sejben I. Vascular invasion demonstrated by elastic stain – a common phenomenon in benign granular cell tumors. Virchows Arch. 2009;454:211–215.

4. Miyagawa-Hayashino A, Tazelaar HD, Langel DJ, Colby TV. Pulmonary sclerosing hemangioma with lymph node metastases: report of 4 cases. Arch. Pathol. Lab. Med. 2003;127:321–325.

5. Fanburg-Smith JC, Auerbach A, Marwaha JS, Wang Z, Santi M, Judkins AR, et al. Immunoprofile of mesenchymal chondrosarcoma: aberrant desmin and EMA expression, retention of INI1, and negative estrogen receptor in 22 female-predominant central nervous system and musculoskeletal cases. Ann. Diagn. Pathol. 2010;14:8–14.

6. Fanburg-Smith JC, Auerbach A, Marwaha JS, Wang Z, Rushing EJ. Reappraisal of mesenchymal chondrosarcoma: novel morphologic observations of the hyaline cartilage and endochondral ossification and beta-catenin, Sox9, and osteocalcin immunostaining of 22 cases. Hum. Pathol. 2010;41:653–662.

7. Wehrli BM, Huang W, De Crombrugghe B, Ayala AG, Czerniak B. Sox9, a master regulator of chondrogenesis, distinguishes mesenchymal chondrosarcoma from other small blue round cell tumors. Hum. Pathol. 2003;34:263–269.

8. Argani P, Beckwith JB. Renal Neoplasms of Childhood. In: Mills SE, editor. Sternberg's Diagnostic Surgical Pathology. 5th ed. Philadelphia: Lippincott Williams & Wilkins; 2010, p.1799–1829.

9. Larone DH. Medically Important Fungi. 4th ed. Washington, D.C.: ASM Press; 2002.

10. Merz WG, Roberts GD. Algorithms for detection and identification of fungi. Manual of clinical microbiology Washington, D.C.: American Society for Microbiology Press; 2003, p.1668–1685.

11. Chandler FW, Watts JC. Pathologic Diagnosis of Fungal Infections. Chiacgo: ASCP Press; 1987.

Chapter 7 Tumor Syndromes

1. Genetics Home Reference, http://ghr.nlm.nih.gov/.

2. Hansel DE. Genetic alterations and histopathologic findings in familial renal cell carcinoma. Histol.Histopathol. 2006;21:437–444.

3. Orphanet: an Online Database of Rare Diseases and Orphan Drugs, http://www.orpha.net.

4. Jass JR. Role of the pathologist in the diagnosis of hereditary non-polyposis colorectal cancer. Dis.Markers 2004;20:215–224.

5. Giardiello FM, Welsh SB, Hamilton SR, Offerhaus GJ, Gittelsohn AM, Booker SV, et al. Increased risk of cancer in the Peutz-Jeghers syndrome. N. Engl. J. Med. 1987;316:1511–1514.

6. Jasperson KW, Tuohy TM, Neklason DW, Burt RW. Hereditary and familial colon cancer. Gastroenterology 2010;138:2044–2058.

7. Rustgi AK. The genetics of hereditary colon cancer. Genes Dev. 2007;21:2525–2538.

8. Kimonis VE, Goldstein AM, Pastakia B, Yang ML, Kase R, DiGiovanna JJ, et al. Clinical manifestations in 105 persons with nevoid basal cell carcinoma syndrome. Am. J. Med. Genet. 1997;69:299–308.

9. Gokden N, Gokden M, Phan DC, McKenney JK. The utility of PAX-2 in distinguishing metastatic clear cell renal cell carcinoma from its morphologic mimics: an immunohistochemical study with comparison to renal cell carcinoma marker. Am. J. Surg. Pathol. 2008;32:1462–1467.

10. Merino MJ, Torres-Cabala C, Pinto P, Linehan WM. The morphologic spectrum of kidney tumors in hereditary leiomyomatosis and renal cell carcinoma (HLRCC) syndrome. Am. J. Surg. Pathol. 2007;31:1578–1585.

11. Burkart AL, Sheridan T, Lewin M, Fenton H, Ali NJ, Montgomery E. Do sporadic Peutz-Jeghers polyps exist? Experience of a large teaching hospital. Am. J. Surg. Pathol. 2007;31:1209–1214.

12. Perigny M, Hammel P, Corcos O, Larochelle O, Giraud S, Richard S, et al. Pancreatic endocrine microadenomatosis in patients with von Hippel-Lindau disease: characterization by VHL/HIF pathway proteins expression. Am.J.Surg.Pathol. 2009;33:739–748.

13. Anlauf M, Schlenger R, Perren A, Bauersfeld J, Koch CA, Dralle H, et al. Microadenomatosis of the endocrine pancreas in patients with and without the multiple endocrine neoplasia type 1 syndrome. Am. J. Surg. Pathol. 2006;30:560–574.

14. Umar A, Risinger JI, Hawk ET, Barrett JC. Testing guidelines for hereditary non-polyposis colorectal cancer. Nat. Rev. Cancer. 2004;4:153–158.

15. Lynch HT, Boland CR, Rodriguez-Bigas MA, Amos C, Lynch JF, Lynch PM. Who should be sent for genetic testing in hereditary colorectal cancer syndromes? J. Clin. Oncol. 2007;25:3534–3542.

16. Vasen HF, Watson P, Mecklin JP, Lynch HT. New clinical criteria for hereditary nonpolyposis colorectal cancer (HNPCC, Lynch syndrome) proposed by the International Collaborative group on HNPCC. Gastroenterology 1999;116:1453–1456.

17. Vasen HF, Mecklin JP, Khan PM, Lynch HT. The International Collaborative Group on Hereditary Non-Polyposis Colorectal Cancer (ICG-HNPCC). Dis. Colon Rectum 1991;34:424–425.

18. Greenson JK, Huang SC, Herron C, Moreno V, Bonner JD, Tomsho LP, et al. Pathologic predictors of microsatellite instability in colorectal cancer. Am. J. Surg. Pathol. 2009;33:126–133.

19. Garg K, Soslow RA. Lynch syndrome (hereditary non-polyposis colorectal cancer) and endometrial carcinoma. J. Clin. Pathol. 2009;62:679–684.

20. Hampel H, Frankel WL, Martin E, Arnold M, Khanduja K, Kuebler P, et al. Feasibility of screening for Lynch syndrome among patients with colorectal cancer. J. Clin. Oncol. 2008;26:5783–5788.

21. Hampel H. Point: justification for Lynch syndrome screening among all patients with newly diagnosed colorectal cancer. J. Natl. Compr. Canc. Netw. 2010;8:597–601.

22. Jenkins MA, Hayashi S, O'Shea AM, Burgart LJ, Smyrk TC, Shimizu D, et al. Pathology features in Bethesda guidelines predict colorectal cancer microsatellite instability: a population-based study. Gastroenterology 2007;133:48–56.

23. Shia J, Ellis NA, Paty PB, Nash GM, Qin J, Offit K, et al. Value of histopathology in predicting microsatellite instability in hereditary nonpolyposis colorectal cancer and sporadic colorectal cancer. Am. J. Surg. Pathol. 2003;27:1407–1417.

Chapter 8 Tumor Genetics and Cytogenetics

1. Skalova A, Vanecek T, Sima R, Laco J, Weinreb I, Perez-Ordonez B, et al. Mammary analogue secretory carcinoma of salivary glands, containing the ETV6-NTRK3 fusion gene: a hitherto undescribed salivary gland tumor entity. Am. J. Surg. Pathol. 2010;34:599–608.

2. Mertens F, Fletcher CD, Antonescu CR, Coindre JM, Colecchia M, Domanski HA, et al. Clinicopathologic and molecular genetic characterization of low-grade fibromyxoid sarcoma, and cloning of a novel FUS/CREB3L1 fusion gene. Lab. Invest. 2005;85:408–415.

3. Argani P, Aulmann S, Illei PB, Netto GJ, Ro J, Cho HY, et al. A distinctive subset of PEComas harbors TFE3 gene fusions. Am. J. Surg. Pathol. 2010;34:1395–1406.

4. Williamson D, Missiaglia E, de Reynies A, Pierron G, Thuille B, Palenzuela G, et al. Fusion gene-negative alveolar rhabdomyosarcoma is clinically and molecularly indistinguishable from embryonal rhabdomyosarcoma. J. Clin. Oncol. 2010;28:2151–2158.

5. Jacob K, Albrecht S, Sollier C, Faury D, Sader E, Montpetit A, et al. Duplication of 7q34 is specific to juvenile pilocytic astrocytomas and a hallmark of cerebellar and optic pathway tumours. Br. J. Cancer 2009;101:722–733.

6. Argani P, Lae M, Hutchinson B, Reuter VE, Collins MH, Perentesis J, et al. Renal carcinomas with the t(6;11)(p21;q12): clinicopathologic features and demonstration of the specific alpha-TFEB gene fusion by immunohistochemistry, RT-PCR, and DNA PCR. Am. J. Surg. Pathol. 2005;29:230–240.

7. Woodman SE, Davies MA. Targeting KIT in melanoma: a paradigm of molecular medicine and targeted therapeutics. Biochem. Pharmacol. 2010;80:568–574.

8. Antonescu CR, Zhang L, Chang NE, Pawel BR, Travis W, Katabi N, et al. EWSR1-POU5F1 fusion in soft tissue myoepithelial tumors. A molecular analysis of sixty-six cases, including soft tissue, bone, and visceral lesions, showing common involvement of the EWSR1 gene. Genes Chromosomes Cancer 2010;49:1114–1124.

9. Gleason BC, Fletcher CD. Myoepithelial carcinoma of soft tissue in children: an aggressive neoplasm analyzed in a series of 29 cases. Am. J. Surg. Pathol. 2007;31:1813–1824.

10. Brandal P, Panagopoulos I, Bjerkehagen B, Heim S. t(19;22)(q13;q12) Translocation leading to the novel fusion gene EWSR1-ZNF444 in soft tissue myoepithelial carcinoma. Genes Chromosomes Cancer 2009;48:1051–1056.

11. Haack H, Johnson LA, Fry CJ, Crosby K, Polakiewicz RD, Stelow EB, et al. Diagnosis of NUT midline carcinoma using a NUT-specific monoclonal antibody. Am. J. Surg. Pathol. 2009;33:984–991.

12. Fine SW, Gopalan A, Leversha MA, Al-Ahmadie HA, Tickoo SK, Zhou Q, et al. TMPRSS2-ERG gene fusion is associated with low Gleason scores and not with high-grade morphological features. Mod. Pathol. 2010;.

13. Park K, Tomlins SA, Mudaliar KM, Chiu YL, Esgueva R, Mehra R, et al. Antibody-based detection of ERG rearrangement-positive prostate cancer. Neoplasia 2010;12:590–598.

14. Okabe M, Miyabe S, Nagatsuka H, Terada A, Hanai N, Yokoi M, et al. MECT1-MAML2 fusion transcript defines a favorable subset of mucoepidermoid carcinoma. Clin. Cancer Res. 2006;12:3902–3907.

15. Seethala RR, Dacic S, Cieply K, Kelly LM, Nikiforova MN. A reappraisal of the MECT1/MAML2 translocation in salivary mucoepidermoid carcinomas. Am. J. Surg. Pathol. 2010;34:1106–1121.

16. Behboudi A, Enlund F, Winnes M, Andren Y, Nordkvist A, Leivo I, et al. Molecular classification of mucoepidermoid carcinomas-prognostic significance of the MECT1-MAML2 fusion oncogene. Genes Chromosomes Cancer 2006;45:470–481.

17. Martins C, Fonseca I, Roque L, Pereira T, Ribeiro C, Bullerdiek J, et al. PLAG1 gene alterations in salivary gland pleomorphic adenoma and carcinoma ex-pleomorphic adenoma: a combined study using chromosome banding, in situ hybridization and immunocytochemistry. Mod. Pathol. 2005;18:1048–1055.

18. Shah SP, Kobel M, Senz J, Morin RD, Clarke BA, Wiegand KC, et al. Mutation of FOXL2 in granulosa-cell tumors of the ovary. N. Engl. J. Med. 2009;360:2719–2729.

Chapter 9 Quick Clinical References for Pathologists

1. Umeki S. Association of miliary lung metastases and bone metastases in bronchogenic carcinoma. Chest 1993;104:948–950.
2. Schueller G, Herold CJ. Lung Metastases. Cancer Imaging 2003;3:126–128.
3. Luna MA, Pfaltz M. Cysts of the Neck, Unknown Primary Tumor, and Neck Dissection. In: Gnepp DR, editor. Diagnostic Surgical Pathology of the Head and Neck. 2nd ed. Philadelphia: Saunders; 2009.
4. Marchevsky AM, Gupta R, Balzer B. Diagnosis of metastatic neoplasms: a clinicopathologic and morphologic approach. Arch. Pathol. Lab. Med. 2010;134:194–206.
5. Edge SB, Byrd DR, Compton CC, Fritz AG, Greene FL, Trotti A. AJCC Cancer Staging Manual. 7th ed.; 2010.
6. Burtis CA, Ashwood ER, Bruns DE. Tietz Textbook of Clinical Chemistry and Molecular Diagnostics. 4th ed. Philadelphia: Saunders; 2005.
7. Mino-Kenudson M, Chirieac LR, Law K, Hornick JL, Lindeman N, Mark EJ, et al. A novel, highly sensitive antibody allows for the routine detection of ALK-rearranged lung adenocarcinomas by standard immunohistochemistry. Clin. Cancer Res. 2010;16:1561–1571.
8. Chirieac LR, Dacic S. Targeted Therapies in Lung Cancer. Surg. Pathol. Clin. 2010;3:71–82.
9. Plesec TP, Hunt JL. KRAS mutation testing in colorectal cancer. Adv. Anat. Pathol. 2009;16:196–203.
10. Amado RG, Wolf M, Peeters M, Van Cutsem E, Siena S, Freeman DJ, et al. Wild-type KRAS is required for panitumumab efficacy in patients with metastatic colorectal cancer. J. Clin. Oncol. 2008;26:1626–1634.
11. Dhomen N, Marais R. BRAF signaling and targeted therapies in melanoma. Hematol. Oncol. Clin. North Am. 2009;23:529–45, ix.
12. Woodman SE, Davies MA. Targeting KIT in melanoma: a paradigm of molecular medicine and targeted therapeutics. Biochem. Pharmacol. 2010;80:568–574.
13. Reynoso D, Trent JC. Neoadjuvant and adjuvant imatinib treatment in gastrointestinal stromal tumor: current status and recent developments. Curr. Opin. Oncol. 2010;22:330–335.
14. Bang YJ, Van Cutsem E, Feyereislova A, Chung HC, Shen L, Sawaki A, et al. Trastuzumab in combination with chemotherapy versus chemotherapy alone for treatment of HER2-positive advanced gastric or gastro-oesophageal junction cancer (ToGA): a phase 3, open-label, randomised controlled trial. Lancet 2010;376:687–697.
15. Puxeddu E, Romagnoli S, Dottorini ME. Targeted therapies for advanced thyroid cancer. Curr. Opin. Oncol. 2010.
16. Pratz KW, Levis MJ. Bench to bedside targeting of FLT3 in acute leukemia. Curr. Drug Targets 2010;11:781–789.

Chapter 10 Pathology Web Resources

1. Gabril MY, Yousef GM. Informatics for practicing anatomical pathologists: marking a new era in pathology practice. Mod. Pathol. 2010;23:349–358.
2. Talmon G, Abrahams NA. The Internet for pathologists: a simple schema for evaluating pathology-related Web sites and a catalog of sites useful for practicing pathologists. Arch. Pathol. Lab. Med. 2005;129:742–746.

Chapter 11 CPT coding

1. American Medical Association. CPT 2010 Professional Edition. Chicago: AMA Press; 2009.

Chapter 12 It looks like what? An Illustrated Glossary of Histopathologic Descriptors

1. Indian file definition, http://www.yourdictionary.com/indian-file.
2. Storiform, http://www.biology-online.org/dictionary/Storiform.
3. Trabecular definition, http://www.yourdictionary.com/trabecular.
4. Signet ring definition, http://www.yourdictionary.com/signet-ring.
5. Hyaline definition, http://www.yourdictionary.com/hyaline.
6. Lynch JM, Barrett TL. Collagenolytic (necrobiotic) granulomas: part II – the 'red' granulomas. J. Cutan. Pathol. 2004;31:409–418.
7. Lynch JM, Barrett TL. Collagenolytic (necrobiotic) granulomas: part 1 – the "blue" granulomas. J. Cutan. Pathol. 2004;31:353–361.
8. Amianthoid http://www.biology-online.org/dictionary/Amianthoid.
9. Min KW. Stromal elements for tumor diagnosis: a brief review of diagnostic electron microscopic features. Ultrastruct. Pathol. 2005;29:305–318.

Subject Index

Common conversions:

1in = 2.54cm
1cm = 0.39in
1kg = 2.2lb
1lb = 0.45kg
1g = 0.04oz
1oz = 28g
1gallon = 3.8L
1L = 0.26gallons

CPSIA information can be obtained at www.ICGtesting.com
Printed in the USA
BVOW11s1219300615

406821BV00001B/1/P

9 783642 200854